AF323674

# TUMOR HYPOXIA

# TUMOR HYPOXIA

Editor

## Zhong Yun

*Yale School of Medicine, USA*

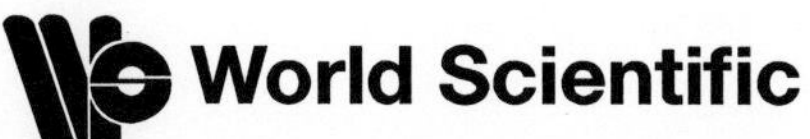


NEW JERSEY • LONDON • SINGAPORE • BEIJING • SHANGHAI • HONG KONG • TAIPEI • CHENNAI • TOKYO

*Published by*

World Scientific Publishing Co. Pte. Ltd.

5 Toh Tuck Link, Singapore 596224

*USA office:* 27 Warren Street, Suite 401-402, Hackensack, NJ 07601

*UK office:* 57 Shelton Street, Covent Garden, London WC2H 9HE

**Library of Congress Cataloging-in-Publication Data**
Names: Zhong, Yun (Associate Professor) author.
Title: Tumor hypoxia / Yun Zhong (Yale School of Medicine, USA).
Description: New Jersey : World Scientific, 2016.
Identifiers: LCCN 2016034582 | ISBN 9789813147317 (hc : alk. paper)
Subjects: LCSH: Tumors--Treatment. | Oxygen therapy.
Classification: LCC RC270.8 .Z48 2016 | DDC 616.99/40636--dc23
LC record available at https://lccn.loc.gov/2016034582

**British Library Cataloguing-in-Publication Data**
A catalogue record for this book is available from the British Library.



Desk Editors: Kalpana Bharanikumar/T. Yugarani

Typeset by Stallion Press
Email: enquiries@stallionpress.com

Printed in Singapore

# **Preface**

Tumors often start out as a benign growth. They gradually progress toward the malignant stage over a relatively long period of time, depending on the nature of the initial transformed cell. Tumor progression likely results from accumulated genetic mutations and inheritable epigenetic modifications that enable clonal evolution and selection of new clonal populations of tumor cells with aggressive characteristics including metastasis and therapy resistance. However, it remains unclear what factors affect or control tumor progression.

Tumor growth results from uncontrolled or autonomous clonal expansion of tumor cells, which inevitably causes disruption of local tissue architecture and leads to the emergence of new tissue structures and cellular hierarchy. Such disruptive and disorganized tissue orders associated with tumor growth are called tumor microenvironment. Tumor microenvironment constantly evolves and changes with tumor progression. Because of the monoclonal origin of individual solid tumor nodules, it is highly possible that tumor microenvironment might play a significant role in directing clonal evolution and determining clonal cell fate, which eventually leads to emergence of malignant tumor cell clones.

One of the most salient features of solid tumors is the presence of hypoxic microenvironment or regions with insufficient oxygen concentrations. If left to run its course, every tumor would become hypoxic. For the most part, tumor hypoxia develops as a result of abnormal vascular formation and function in solid tumors. Hypoxic areas appear randomly throughout the tumor mass. Both the severity and duration of hypoxia are often highly variable and subject to frequent changes with fluctuating blood flow. Most importantly, tumor hypoxia is strongly associated with malignant progression and predicts poor patient outcomes. Increasing amounts of evidence suggest that tumor hypoxia is likely to be a major driving force in tumor microenvironment to elicit cellular adaptation and clonal selection via genetic mutations and epigenetic modifications, to facilitate cancer stem cell maintenance, to enhance metastasis, to augment therapy resistance, and to evade immune surveillance.

From clinical perspectives, Chapter 1 provides a comprehensive discussion on the effects of hypoxia in tumor response to radiation therapy. For X-ray irradiation, oxygen molecules are required to chemically convert initial irradiation-induced DNA free radicals into poorly repairable DNA damages that lead to activation of the cell death pathways. It is commonly observed that tumor cells are two- to three-fold less sensitive to X-ray irradiation in the absence of oxygen than in the presence of physiological levels of oxygen. The half-maximum radiosensitivity is found at approximately 2–3 mmHg of oxygen partial pressure ($pO_2$). Several approaches have been attempted to increase efficiency of radiation therapy including X-ray dose fractionation, radiosensitizers, and irradiation using particles with high linear energy transfer potentials. Despite being a challenge to cancer therapy, tumor hypoxia also offers an opportunity for targeted cancer therapy. Chapter 1 also discusses the potential use of hypoxia-activated cytotoxins that can directly kill hypoxic tumor cells.

In response to hypoxia, specific intracellular signal transduction pathways are activated to cope with the hypoxic stress. The hypoxia-inducible factor (HIF) pathway is arguably the most prominent and ubiquitous signaling pathway that is activated by hypoxia. The HIF transcription factor controls most prominent gene transcription induced by hypoxia. HIF is a heterodimer consisting of an oxygen-sensitive $\alpha$ subunit (HIF-1$\alpha$, HIF-2$\alpha$, or HIF-3$\alpha$) and the stably $\beta$ subunit (HIF-1$\beta$). The HIF-$\alpha$ subunit is subject to extensive post-translational modifications including phosphorylation of serine and threonine, hydroxylation of proline, acetylation of lysine, S-nitrosylation of cysteine, and SUMOylation. These modifications do not only affect protein stability, but also regulate its transcriptional activity. Chapter 2 provides a thorough discourse on post-translational modifications of the HIFs, as well as their impact on the HIF signal transduction pathway.

Metastasis is a hallmark of tumor malignant progression and one of the major causes of death. Chapter 3 provides a detailed discussion of tumor hypoxia and its involvement in the multistage process of metastasis. Hypoxia alters the local matrix microenvironment via differential expression of matrix metalloproteinases (MMPs) and lysyl oxidases (LOX and LOXLs). Hypoxia may promote tumor invasion and extravasation by facilitating epithelial-to-mesenchymal transition (EMT). The ability of hypoxia to promote tumor metastasis illustrates an important role of hypoxia in malignant progression.

Spontaneously arising tumors contain heterogeneous populations of tumor cells at different stages of differentiation. Depending on the tumor stages, there are variable numbers of tumor cells with stem cell-like characteristics and potentials to initiate new tumors. These tumorigenic and stem-like cancer cells are now called cancer stem cells. Similar to normal stem cells, cancer stem cells likely prefer to reside in specific niche microenvironment to remain undifferentiated. Chapter 4 discusses the concept of cancer stem cells, the hypoxic stem cell niche, and the hypoxia-dependent mechanism of cancer stem cell regulation.

On the opposite side of self-renewal and stemness is cellular aging and senescence, a natural progression of cell fate that is also under strong influence by cellular microenvironment. As discussed in Chapter 4, there appears to be a two-sided relationship between hypoxia and senescence. On the one hand, cellular senescence can be suppressed and lifespan of cells, extended under hypoxic conditions. On the other, severe hypoxia appears to have the potential to induce senescence. It is likely that the hypoxia effect on senescence is further determined by other cell intrinsic factors or pathways.

The renewed recognition of the unique energy metabolism in tumor cells has opened up many avenues toward understanding etiology of this deadly disease as well as development of new cancer therapies. One of the most salient metabolic features of hypoxic cells is pronounced glucose uptake and glycolysis, reminiscent of the Warburg Effect. In addition, hypoxia can exert wide-ranging impact on many aspects of energy metabolism including oxidative phosphorylation in mitochondria, glutamine metabolism, and fatty acid synthesis. Chapter 5 discusses several key genes and pathways involved in the hypoxia-dependent regulation of multiple metabolic pathways.

Clonal heterogeneity of solid tumors is well recognized. Genetically distinctive tumor cells are found in different regions of tumor mass. Although it remains to be determined what causes tumor clonal heterogeneity, it is nonetheless possible that hypoxia, especially severe hypoxia, may contribute to clonal evolution. Hypoxia has the potential to suppress DNA repair and to increase mutagenesis. Hypoxia can lead to chromosomal aberrations as well as DNA mutations. The hypoxia-induced genetic instability will likely facilitate emergence of genetically heterogeneous tumor clones. Chapter 6 provides a detailed mechanistic discourse on the impact of hypoxia on genetic instability and epigenetic modifications.

Non-coding RNAs (ncRNAs), such as microRNAs and long ncRNAs (lncRNAs), are important epigenetic regulators in adaptive response to cellular stresses. Hypoxia has been found to modulate the expression of ncRNAs with microRNA-210 (miR-210) being the best characterized hypoxia-induced microRNA. Chapter 7 provides an in-depth discussion of the hypoxia-dependent regulation of ncRNA expression, as well as their biological functions in hypoxic cells.

In addition to gene transcription, hypoxia can affect post-translational protein modifications and assembly. As discussed in Chapter 8, hypoxia is capable of inducing endoplasmic reticulum (ER) stress, which then activates the unfolded protein response (UPR) as an adaptive response to the hypoxia stress. Clinical evidence has shown that UPR is associated with poor patient survival in a variety of human cancers. Chapter 8 will provide a discourse on the current mechanistic studies of hypoxia-induced UPR and its role in tumor cells.

A new exciting direction in the field of tumor microenvironment research is the hypoxia-dependent regulation of anti-tumor immunity. Chapter 10 provides a comprehensive treatise on the role of hypoxia in the regulation of immune cells found in the hypoxic tumor microenvironment. Recognition and understanding of the hypoxic impact on immune surveillance in tumor microenvironment will undoubtedly help the development and clinical application of tumor immunotherapy.

I am sincerely grateful to all the authors for their excellent treatise and expert insights. Their outstanding effort has well represented the exciting advances and new directions, albeit in a few snapshots, of the thriving field of tumor microenvironment research. I am also thankful to the staff members at the World Scientific Publishing: Book Editor Kalpana Bharanikumar, Desk Editor T. Yugarani, and, especially, Executive Editor Christopher B. Davis for their great contributions to bringing this book project to fruition.

Zhong Yun
Department of Therapeutic Radiology
Yale School of Medicine
New Haven, Connecticut, USA

# Contents


*Preface*                                                                    v

Chapter 1    Tumor Hypoxia and Radiotherapy                                  1
             *Olivia J. Kelada and David J. Carlson*

Chapter 2    Post-translational Modifications of the
             Hypoxia Inducible Factors                                       49
             *Ian Cartwright and Chuan-Yuan Li*

Chapter 3    Hypoxia and Metastasis                                          69
             *Elizabeth C. Finger and Amato J. Giaccia*

Chapter 4    Hypoxia and Cancer Stem Cell Regulation                         101
             *Sofie Mohlin, Annika Jögi and Sven Påhlman*

Chapter 5    Hypoxia and Senescence                                          127
             *Yashi Gupta and Scott M. Welford*

Chapter 6    Hypoxic Reprograming of Tumor Metabolism,
             Matching Environmental Supply with
             Biosynthetic Demand                                             147
             *Betina McNeil, Ioanna Papandreou*
             *and Nicholas C. Denko*

Chapter 7    Regulation of DNA Repair by Hypoxia    169
*Yuhong Lu and Peter M. Glazer*

Chapter 8    Regulation of the Hypoxic Response
by Non-coding RNAs    189
*Xin Huang*

Chapter 9    Hypoxia-Induced Endoplasmic Reticulum Stress    225
*Chih-Chien Chou, Rakesh Bam, Zhifen Yang,
Justin L. Bui, Dadi Jiang and Albert C. Koong*

Chapter 10    The Hypoxic Tumor Microenvironment
and the Anti-cancer Immune Response    249
*Joseph Barbi and Fan Pan*

*Index*    293

# Chapter 1

# Tumor Hypoxia and Radiotherapy

Olivia J. Kelada*,†,‡ and David J. Carlson*,§

*Department of Therapeutic Radiology,
Yale University School of Medicine, New Haven, CT, USA
†Department of Medical Physics in Radiation Oncology,
German Cancer Research Center, Heidelberg, Germany
‡okelada@gmail.com
§david.j.carlson@yale.edu

## 1. Tumor Hypoxia and Radiation

Human tumors are not comprised of a homogenous population of cells. The heterogeneity within a tumor consists of two different types: (1) genetic heterogeneity accounting for the genomic differences that generate a diversity of cells with different functions (parenchymal cells) and (2) physiological heterogeneity caused by inconsistency of the supporting structural or connective tissues (stroma) of the tumor. The latter includes hypoxic cells and their presence within a given tumor.[1]

Tumor hypoxia results from several tumor-specific traits as illustrated in Fig. 1. These include: (1) chronic hypoxia caused by the limited-diffusion distance of oxygen from blood vessels to the tumor cells (~150–200 $\mu$m)[2]; (2) acute hypoxia due to the perfusion-limited impairment of the vascular vessels by their structural abnormality and high interstitial pressure caused by the combination of fluid in the tumor matrix and the rapidly

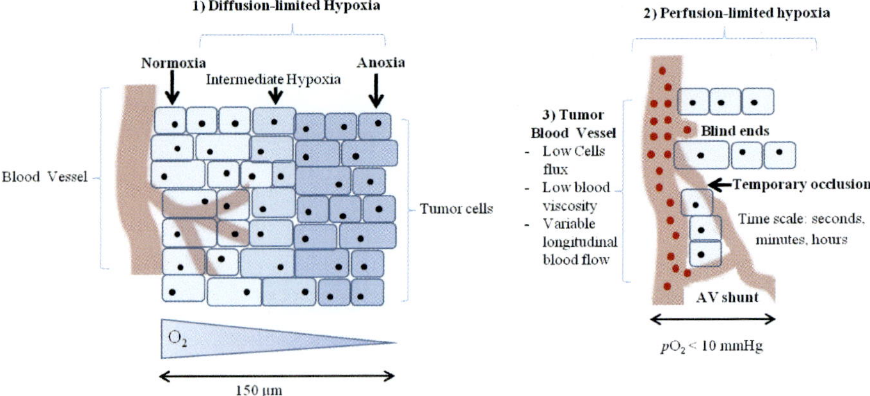


Fig. 1.   Tumor hypoxia is caused by several tumor-specific traits that result in chronic (diffusion-limited), acute (perfusion-limited) hypoxia. In combination with tumor blood vessel abnormalities, tumor hypoxia is a highly complex biological mechanism, making it difficult to counteract with current treatment techniques (with permission from Kelada and Carlson[33]).

proliferating tumor cells leading to constriction of the intra-tumor vasculature[3–8]; and (3) tumor blood vessel traits such as a reduced vascular density and arteriolar supply, poor blood vessels networks, varied red blood cell flux, and high blood viscosity.[9]

## 2. The Oxygen Effect: Timing, Mechanism, and Concentration

Since the 1930's, we have known about the heterogeneity of tumor cell oxygenation and that hypoxic conditions protect cells from the lethal effects of ionizing radiation.[10] Since then, the scientific community believe that the radioresistance of solid neoplasms is due to the presence of hypoxic tumor cells.[11]

Time is a crucial variable that can aid in distinguishing the relative importance of oxygen-dependent biological changes than can influence radiosensitivity. Over 50 years ago, Howard-Flanders and Moore transported cultured cells from a nitrogen environment to an aerobic environment 20 ms after irradiation and saw that the oxygen environment provided no radiosensitizing effect to the cells,[12] as shown in Fig. 2 (top

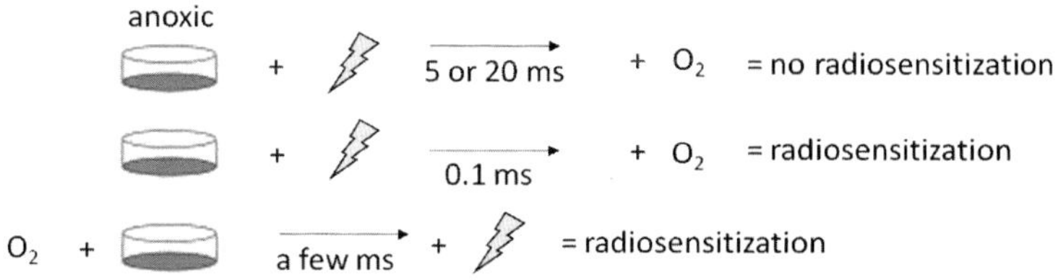

anoxic

+ 5 or 20 ms + $O_2$ = no radiosensitization

+ 0.1 ms + $O_2$ = radiosensitization

$O_2$ + a few ms + = radiosensitization

Fig. 2. The importance of the timing of oxygen administration for anoxic cells to increase radiosensitivity. The top row shows that if oxygen is added to anoxic cells 5 or 20 ms after irradiation, no radiosensitization is observed. The middle row shows that if oxygen is added to anoxic cells 0.1 ms after irradiation, radiosensitization is observed. The last row shows that if oxygen is added a few milliseconds before radiation to anoxic cells, radiosensitization is observed.

row). In addition, Adams and Michael *et al.*[13,14] used a liquid-phase rapid-mix flow technique to reduce the time interval between the irradiation of the anoxic cells by adding an oxygenated buffer solution 5 ms post-irradiation but still found no radiosensitizing effect as illustrated in Fig. 2 (top row). On the contrary, as shown in Fig. 2 (last row), adding oxygen to anoxic cells a few milliseconds preirradiation provided radiosensitization. Further studies use a "gas explosion technique" in bacteria and change the environment from anoxic to normoxic within 0.1 ms of irradiation to determine that radiosensitization was possible post-irradiation, if oxygen was added 0.1 ms later, as illustrated in Fig. 2 (middle row).[14–16] Thus, for oxygen to have an effect on cell radiosensitivity, it must be present at the instance of irradiation or within a fraction of milliseconds after.

Such experiments provided information on the mechanism by which oxygen enhances radiation damage. Due to the short timescale, oxygen effect reactions were likely to involve short-lived free radicals where by reactions involving oxygen lead to DNA strand breaks and causing damage that was different to what occurs under anoxic conditions. This mechanism is referred to as the "oxygen fixation" hypothesis as shown in Fig. 3. When a biological material absorbs radiation, fast charged particles are produced that in turn form ion pairs as they pass through the material. These ion pairs lead to the formation of highly reactive (they contain an unpaired valence electron) free radicals. These radicals break chemical bonds, produce chemical changes and initiate biological damage. DNA damage can be directly caused by the radical as it interacts with the DNA

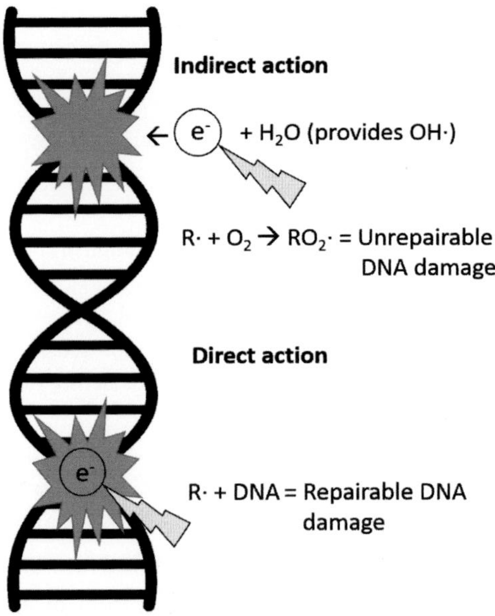


Fig. 3. The oxygen fixation hypothesis: Free radicals are produced either directly when the photon removes a valence electron in the DNA (repairable damage) or indirectly when the radical used oxygen and the subsequent DNA damage is unrepairable.

strand or indirectly via other molecules (e.g. water) found in the cell and diffuse to the DNA to cause damage. As these free radicals are unstable, they can react rapidly with oxygen and change the chemical composition of the DNA strand. In the absence of oxygen, the unstable free radicals can react with hydrogen restoring their original form without causing any DNA damage. Thus the extent of the DNA damage is dependent on the presence or absence of oxygen.

Despite this mechanism being labeled as the "oxygen-fixation" technique, oxygen does not directly "fix" damage but instead modifies the chemical pathways that lead to DNA strand breaks (interaction with free radicals) and releases peroxide by-products during this process. Experiments done over 30 years ago demonstrated that reactions between free-radicals and the DNA sugar backbone led to strand breaks.[17] The routes to these breaks involved base peroxyl radicals via hydrogen abstraction from adjacent sugar complexes and oxygen leads to the migration or

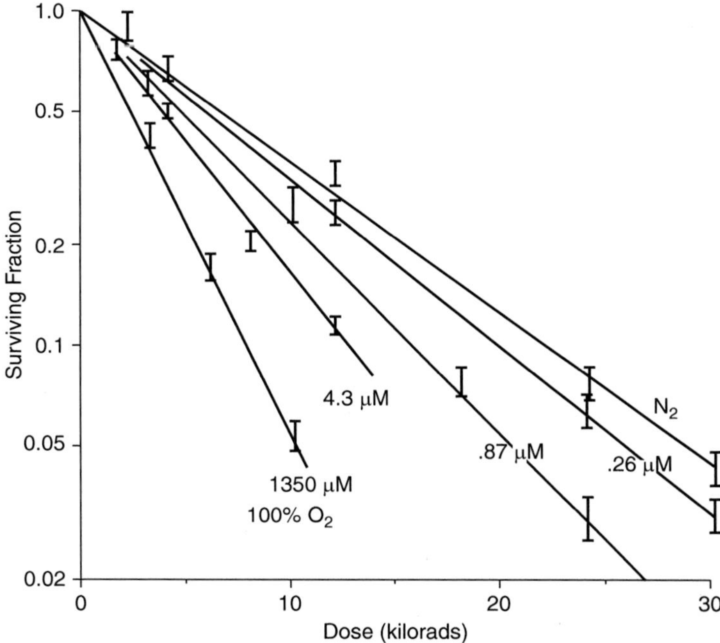



Fig. 4.   Survival curves for *E. coli* held under 100% oxygen to 100% nitrogen and various combinations of oxygen concentration in between. 1 Gy = 0.1 kilorads. (Adapted with permission from Ref. 18.)

change of the DNA damage to a chemically unrepairable form (radical + oxygen = organic peroxide) rather than "fixation" of it.[19]

In keeping with the timing and mechanism of the oxygen effect, what concentration of oxygen is required to potentiate this effect? In Fig. 4, survival curves are shown for *E. coli* held under 100% oxygen, 100% nitrogen and various combinations of oxygen and nitrogen concentrations. It is easy to visualize the effect of oxygen on the slope of the cell survival curves. At 100% $O_2$, the slope is much steeper under oxic conditions than for anoxic conditions shown for cells held under 100% nitrogen. As the oxygen concentration in the cultured cell environment increases, the surviving fraction of cells after irradiation decreases for the same given radiation dose. This introduction of a very small quantity of oxygen, $0.87\,\mu$M (~0.6% $O_2$), results in an increased biological response.

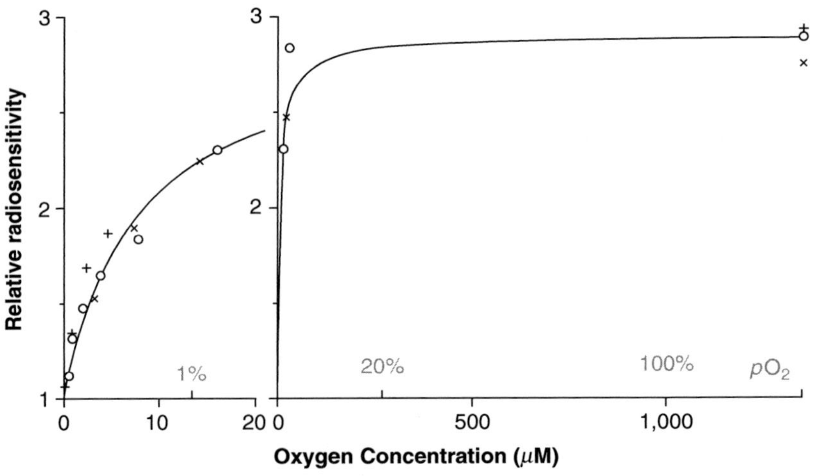



Fig. 5.   The relative radiosensitivity of Ehrlich ascites tumor cells is reduced at lower partial oxygen pressures. (Adapted with permission from Ref. 18.)

Several experiments have shown that at an oxygen concentration of about ~2%, the survival curve of cultured cells after irradiation is very similar to the curve produced under normoxic conditions (21% oxygen). Moreover, increasing the level of oxygen from the level found in air (21%) to 100% does not change the slope of the curve, as shown in Fig. 5. The rapid increase in radiosensitivity occurs between 0% to about 5% oxygen. As the oxygen level increases, the cells become more sensitive to radiation. Anoxic conditions are assigned to be in unity and normoxic conditions a value of 3, i.e. cells in the presence of 100% oxygen are ~3 times more sensitive to radiation than under anoxia. This radiation resistance is attributed to a reduction in DNA damage under reduced oxygen conditions. It is clear that very low concentrations of oxygen are required to dramatically decrease the radiosensitivity of cells to X-rays.

As already mentioned, the response of tumor cells to ionizing radiation is strongly dependent on the presence of oxygen.[2,20] Figure 6 illustrates this effect for mammalian cells *in vitro* irradiated with megavoltage X-rays up to a dose of 30 Gy. The surviving fraction of cell clonogens, is shown as a function of radiation dose in normoxic (fully-oxygenated cells) or hypoxic (oxygen-depleted) cells. The difference in the effectiveness of radiation on cell kill under normoxic versus hypoxic conditions

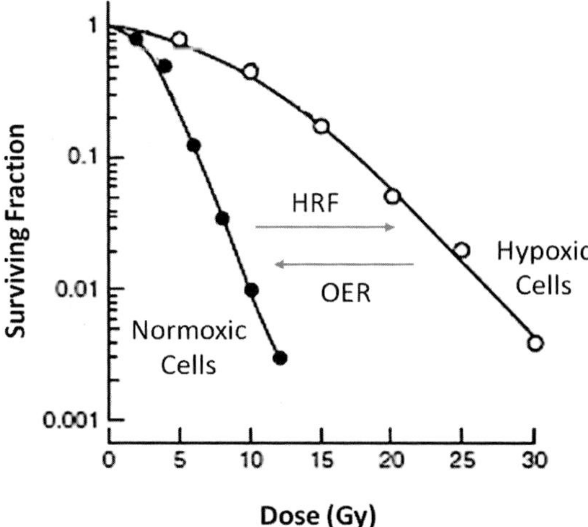


Fig. 6. A clonogenic survival curves for cultured mammalian cells exposed to X-rays under normoxic (solid circles) and hypoxic conditions (open circles), illustrating the dose-modifying effect of oxygen. Adapted from Ref. 3 with permission.

can be defined. This information is used to calculate the enhancement of radiation damage by oxygen and the modification dose needed to provide a particular level of cell survival. That is to say that oxygen has a dose-modifying effect, i.e. it reduces the X-ray dose needed to provide the same level of cell kill under normoxic conditions.

The oxygen enhancement ratio (OER) quantitatively expresses the radioprotective effect of hypoxia and is defined as the radiation dose under hypoxic (or anoxic) conditions divided by the dose under conditions of some partial oxygen pressure $p$ which produces the same biological effect. OER typically increases from unity in anoxic conditions (as $p \to 0$) to 2.5–3.5 for normoxic conditions for most cell types using high dose X-rays.

$$\text{OER}\,(p) = \frac{\text{Radiation dose under anoxic conditions}}{\text{Radiation dose at partial oxygen pressure } p}.$$

Conversely, the hypoxia reduction factor (HRF), another measure of the radiation response-modifying effect of oxygen, is defined as the ratio of the dose at a specific level of hypoxia (at partial oxygen pressure $p$) to the dose under fully aerobic conditions to achieve the same biological effect. The HRF is at its maximum for anoxic conditions and decreases to unity as the cells approach fully aerobic, i.e. normoxic, conditions.

$$\text{HRF}\,(p) = \frac{\text{Radiation dose at partial oxygen pressure } p}{\text{Radiation dose in normoxic conditions}}.$$

Some studies suggest that for lower X-ray doses (<3 Gy), the OER has a smaller value of ~2.5 for cells cultured *in vitro* and this may be due to the variation in OER with phases of the cell cycle i.e. cells in $G_1$ have a lower OER than in S phase as the cells in $G_1$ are more radiosensitive and dominate the low-dose region of the clonogenic survival curve.[21] This is important as conventional radiotherapy is usually delivered in fractions of 2 Gy.

The degree of radiosensitivity of cells to X-rays is dependent on the oxygen partial pressure $p$. Both OER and HRF are a continuous function of oxygen partial pressure. As shown in Fig. 7, as oxygen partial pressure increases, OER increases towards ~3 and HRF decreases towards unity. Figure 7(a) shows OER plotted against a log scale of oxygen partial pressure to show that cells with oxygen tension < 0.15 mmHg are more resistant to ionizing radiation as OER begins to dramatically rise above 1.0 and reaches plateau around 60 mmHg. Most normal tissues (with the exception of cartilage and skin) are well oxygenated and in the range of

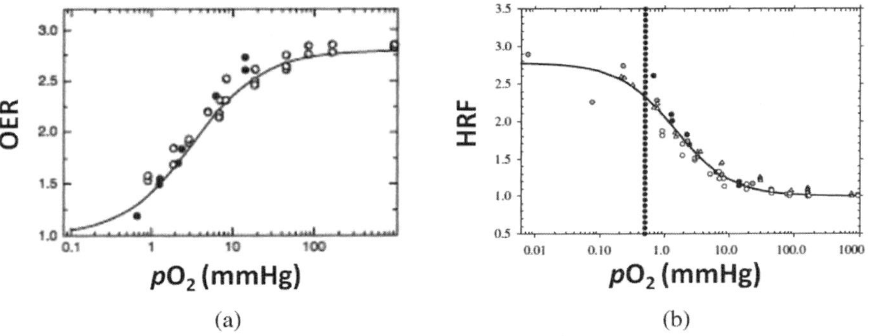



Fig. 7.    (a) Shows the variation OER with oxygen partial pressure ($pO_2$). (b) Shows variation in HRF values with $pO_2$. Both panels used published cell survival data. (Adapted with permission from Ref. 4 (a) and Ref. 5 (b).)

20–60 mmHg with venous to arterial blood in the range as high as 45–100 mmHg.[22] Figure 7(b) shows HRF plotted against a log scale of oxygen partial pressure to show that HRF is dramatically reduced around 1 mmHg reaching almost unity at around 20 mmHg.

## 3. Radioresistance of the Hypoxic Fraction: *in vivo* and Human Tumors

In 1963, it was established that solid rodent tumors contain a subpopulation of clonogenic cells and a radioresistant hypoxic fraction.[23] Powers and Tolmach[23] calculated survival estimates for doses from 2 to 25 Gy using a dilution assay technique to investigate the radiosensitivity of solid subcutaneous lymphosarcoma tumors in mice. The results indicated that the survival curve consisted of two parts, one with slope ~2.5 times shallower than the other suggesting that the tumor consisted of two groups of cells, one oxygenated and the other hypoxic. This was the first study to demonstrate hypoxic cells in solid tumors and show that tumor hypoxia provided a radioprotective effect from cell killing by X-rays that could result in potential tumor re-growth. Hill *et al.*[24] also showed a similar result in KHT mouse sarcomas. Mice were irradiated while breathing air or nitrogen under normal or anemic conditions. Then after irradiation, a lung colony assay was used to estimate tumor cell survival and the resultant survival curves are shown in Fig. 8. Other techniques include the 'clamped tumor growth delay assay' in which the time for tumor growth to a predetermined size is measured after radiation delivery and 'clamped tumor-control assay' in which the percentage of animals with tumor control is recorded at a specific time after treatment.

Using this experimental data, it is possible to calculate the proportion of hypoxic cells in the tumors. At low doses, the dominant cell death is of aerobic tumor cells and the survival curve is similar to that under well-oxygenated conditions. At high doses, the hypoxic fraction influences the dose response curve as the aerobic cells have been killed and the curve becomes parallel to a response curve under hypoxic conditions, as shown in Fig. 8. Thus, the proportion of hypoxic cells (hypoxic fraction) is determined by the distance between the parallel terminal slopes of the hypoxic and air-breathing dose-response curves that are plotted using various

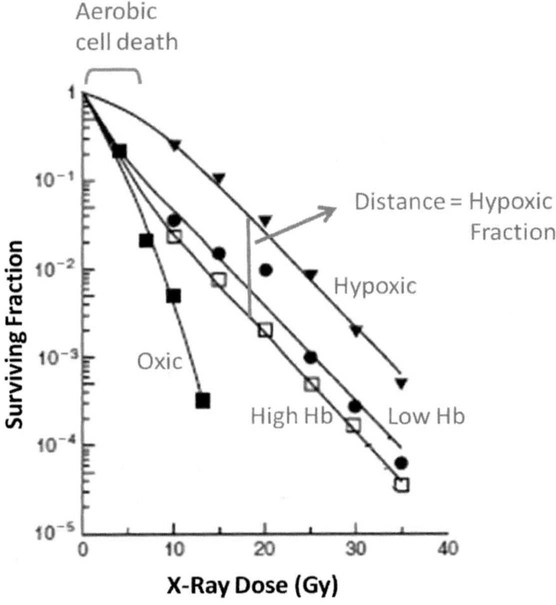



Fig. 8. Dose-response curves for KHT subcutaneous sarcomas irradiated under aerobic and hypoxic conditions. The oxic data was determined using cells irradiated *in vitro*. The two sets of data for tumors in air-breathing mice are shown, with high and low hemoglobin levels. (Adapted with permission from Ref. 6.)

states of animal oxygenation. This distance between the slopes can determine the resistance of the tumor to radiation treatment.

Measuring the level of hypoxia in human tumors has proven more difficult than in animal models as many of the experimental procedures were not translational. Detection techniques will be discussed in the next section. Despite these difficulties, nearly, all solid tumors >1 mm in diameter[25] are positive for some form of hypoxic (severe and intermediate levels) or anoxic (no oxygen present) cells and these areas are often heterogeneously distributed within the tumor.[11,26] The presence of hypoxia does not depend on tumor size, stage, pathology, or nodal status.[3] Moreover, the prevalence of tumor hypoxia and its traits are not cancer-type specific and have been found in a wide range of human malignancies including cancers of the head and neck (H&N), prostate, rectum, breast, uterine cervix as well as brain tumors, soft tissue sarcomas, and malignant melanomas.[27–33]

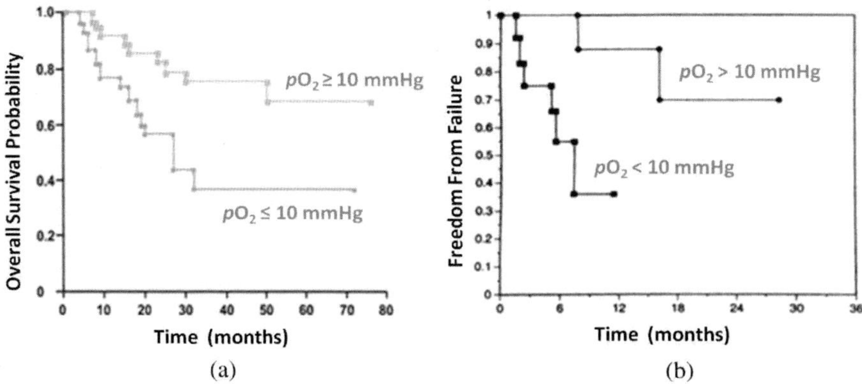



Fig. 9.   (a) The drastic decrease in the overall survival in cervical cancer patients with more hypoxic tumors. (b) An increase in hypoxia-induced invasiveness through metastatic disease in soft tissue sarcoma patients (Adapted with permission from Refs. 7 and 8.)

Using some of the hypoxic measurement techniques described in the next section, many clinical studies have used tumor hypoxia to predict overall survival or treatment failure, emphasizing the radioresistance of the hypoxic fractions in patients. Hockel *et al.*[27] showed a drastic decrease in the overall survival in cervical cancer patients with more hypoxic tumors attributed to hypoxia-induced increased invasiveness and chemoradiation resistance. The corresponding Kaplan–Meier plot is shown in Fig. 9(a). Brizel *et al.*[32] also clinically demonstrated an increase in hypoxia-induced invasiveness through metastatic disease in soft tissue sarcoma patients. The corresponding Kaplan–Meier plot is shown in Fig. 9(b).

Hypoxia-induced radioresistance is a result of a reduction in lethal tumor DNA damage due to lack of oxygen at the site of radiation action. It is well established that the effectiveness of radiation to produce lethal DNA damage is dependent on the presence or absence of oxygen. Thus predicting how a given tumor will be affected by radiation therapy depends upon its state of oxygenation. Reduction in cellular oxygen and nutrients also results in proteomic and genomic changes that create more mutant, adaptive, and aggressive tumor cells.[6,26] However, clinical evidence suggests that hypoxia-induced treatment failure may be more likely attributed to radiation resistance than hypoxia-induced metastasis.[34] Consequently, the hypoxic fraction in tumors has been correlated with a negative treatment outcome[29,31] and a reduction in overall survival.[27,34–38]

## 4. Targeting Hypoxia to Overcome Radioresistance

### 4.1. Methods to quantify tumor hypoxia

It is evident based on the biological complexity, prevalence, and negative prognostic impact of tumor hypoxia in cancer patients that the development of a measurement technique with the capability of easily detecting and accurately quantifying hypoxia would have substantial clinical implications. Over the last 60 years, many techniques have been developed to measure tumor hypoxia and can be divided into two categories, invasive and non-invasive. The invasive group consists of the polarographic needle electrode measurements which are considered to be the 'gold standard' as they provide a direct physical measure of oxygen concentration in tissue. Numerous studies using the Eppendorf $p$O2 electrode[39,40] have found that real-time $p$O$_2$ measurements are correlated with negative survival in patients with various cancer types.[27–32] Although still in use, the Eppendorf electrode is no longer in production or supported by the manufacturer. In 1999, the Oxylite fiber-optic sensor[41] became available to provide $p$O$_2$ measurements, but is not approved to be used on human subjects. Moreover, both methods are user dependent, require expertise and are restricted by sampling error.[42]

Non-invasive methods are proposed as an alternative to invasive hypoxia measurements. These techniques consist of endogenous and exogenous markers. Endogenous markers are cellular proteins whose expression is linked to exposure to hypoxia and are often detected using immunohistochemistry techniques. These include numerous genes that are induced by HIF-1in particular carbonic anhydrase 9 (CA9) and glucose transporter 1 (Glut-1). Exogenous markers are bioreductive drugs that can be systemically administered and include pimonidazole staining and several molecular imaging techniques that have become useful tools to characterize the magnitude and variability of hypoxia within a tumor and to guide clinical treatment decisions.[43,44] These include positron emission

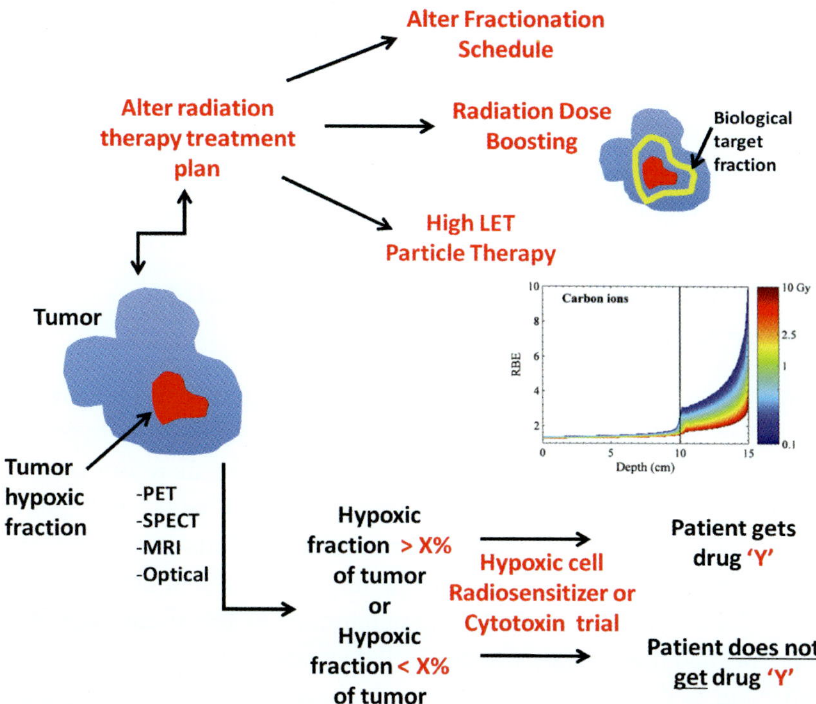



Fig. 10. A schematic illustration of four potential uses of hypoxia PET imaging in a clinical setting in an effort (a) to develop more optimal radiotherapy treatments and (b) to use hypoxia status to stratify patients into a drug trial. (Adapted with permission from Refs. 9 and 32.)

tomography (PET),[33] single-photon emission computed tomography (SPECT), magnetic resonance imaging (MRI),[45–48] and optical imaging.[49] In particular, $^{18}$F-fluoromisonidazole ($^{18}$F-FMISO) PET imaging[50] is the most commonly used non-invasive hypoxia quantification method because the tracer selectively binds in hypoxic cells.[51–54]

Figure 10 shows four potential therapeutic uses of hypoxia imaging and hypoxia-targeted therapies in the clinical setting. It is widely accepted that PET imaging can stratify patients into responding and non-responding groups and provide more targeted treatments for the poor responders.[55–60] Such a process could also prevent some patients from receiving unnecessary treatments and consequential side-effects or indicate the use of hypoxia-selective drugs such as tirapazamine[58] or the hypoxic radiosensitizer nimorazole.[60] Further PET imaging of tumor hypoxia could be used to modify radiation therapy treatment plans via (a) radiation dose boosting,[61,62] (b) the use of high-linear energy transfer (LET) carbon ion therapy, or (c) altered fractionation schedules to allow sufficient time for reoxygenation. Each of these options will be discussed in the following section.

## 4.2. Radiation fractionation: reoxygenation for tumor hypoxia

As previously discussed, at high doses, aerobic tumor cells are preferentially killed as they are the most radiosensitive (relative to hypoxic or anoxic cells). The cells that remain in the tumor are therefore generally more hypoxic relative to the initial distribution of cells, and thus the hypoxic fraction, becomes larger after irradiation. Thus after large single doses, the hypoxic cells can make up the majority of the tumor as the aerobic cells have been eradicated by the radiation.[22] At this point, reoxygenation occurs and the hypoxic fraction will decrease and begin to return to its initial value, as illustrated by the schematic shown in Fig. 11. Reoxygenation is the term that specifically describes the changes in the hypoxic status of the remaining viable cells (i.e. not necrotic) in the tumor after irradiation.

Van Putten and Kallman[63] first demonstrated reoxygenation using a transplanted sarcoma tumor (of spontaneous origin) in mice. The results

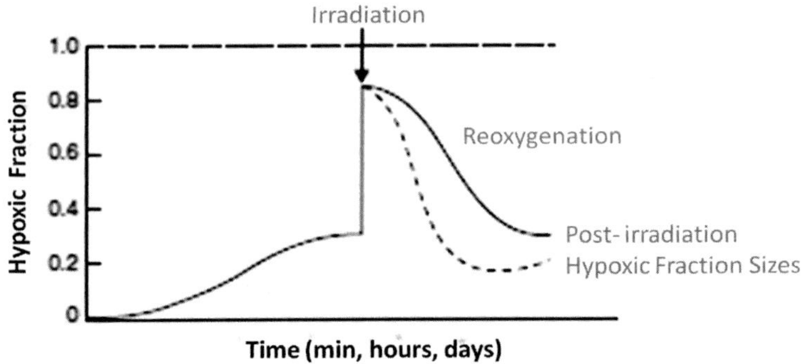


Fig. 11.   A schematic showing the subsequent reoxygenation of the tumor hypoxic fraction after irradiation. (Adapted with permission from Ref. 10.)

showed that the hypoxic fraction was 14% of the total tumor volume preirradiation and after five fractions of 1.9 Gy delivery on five consecutive days the hypoxic fraction was 18%. Thus, the hypoxic fraction was similar to baseline after the delivery of fractionated radiotherapy. This finding demonstrates that hypoxic cells were reoxygenated over the course of treatment, otherwise, the hypoxic fraction would have increased during the fractionated treatment as radiation preferentially kills well-oxygenated cells. This experiment provided the first evidence of the phenomenon of reoxygenation.

The mechanism of reoxygenation is not entirely clear. Each of the possible involved processes occurs over different time scales, as illustrated in Fig. 11. In the first few minutes to hours after radiation, the dominant processes are: (1) recirculation via temporarily closed or shunted blood vessels to decrease the distance oxygen needs to diffuse (minutes); (2) a reduction in the rate of respiration of the irradiated cells (minutes to hours); (3) ischemic cell death (hours); and (4) mitotic death of the aerobic cells (hours). In general, the recirculation mechanism affects the acutely hypoxic (perfusion-limited) cells. For reoxygenation that occurs over days and affects chronically hypoxic (diffusion-limited) cells, this is probably primarily due to cell death and subsequent tumor shrinkage that reduces the distance from the hypoxic cells to the capillary and enables oxygen to reach the cells.

Reoxygenation has been found to occur in a wide variety of tumor systems, but at what time point does reoxygenation begin to occur and at what speed? In general, reoxygenation can occur over a few hours or days but the extent and rapidity is variable and challenging to predict. Van Putten and Kallman[63] showed that the hypoxic fraction of a tumor could return to baseline ~24 hours after irradiation. Kallman and Bleehan[64] demonstrated a similar reoxygenation effect after ~12 hours. Moreover, the hypoxic fraction after reoxygenation maybe larger or smaller than its initial value preirradiation.

The process of reoxygenation plays a crucial role in the clinical delivery of radiotherapy (see Fig. 12). Assuming human tumors reoxygenate as rapidly as animal tumors then a multi-fractionated delivery of radiation should be capable of eradicating all of the hypoxic cells in a tumor. This has been hypothetically illustrated by Wouters and Brown[65] for a

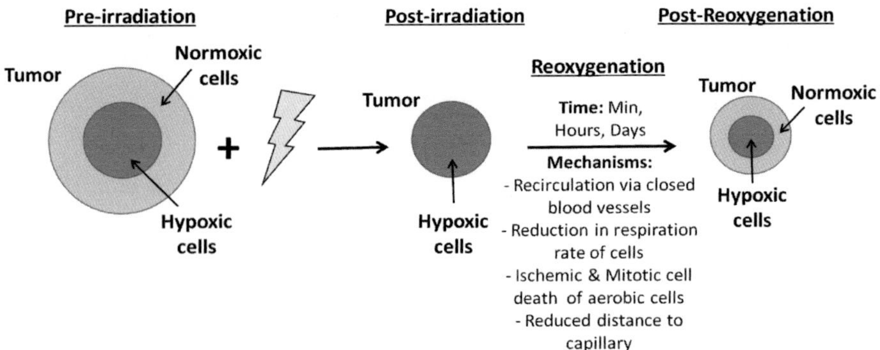


Fig. 12. A simplified schematic illustrating the process of reoxygenation. Before irradiation, the tumor contains a normoxic and hypoxic component, the latter containing cells over a range of low oxygen concentrations. After irradiation, the aerobic cells are preferentially killed and the hypoxic fraction remains. After reoxygenation occurs via various mechanisms and time scales, the tumor contains normoxic cells again, that were hypoxic before reoxygenation.

fractioned radiation schedule of 60 Gy in 2 Gy fractions and a hypothetical tumor comprised of 90% aerobic tumor cells and a 10% hypoxic fraction. Assuming an OER of 2.8, relative to anoxic cells, the tumor surviving fraction after a 60 Gy treatment (in 2 Gy fractions) is a 3$^{rd}$ of the response to radiation that would be obtained in the absence of hypoxic cells. However, assuming reoxygenation occurs between fractions, then the radiation killing of cells that were hypoxic at baseline increases, thus decreasing their impact on tumor radiosensitivity and resulting in a dose-response similar to that of a tumor with only normoxic cells. The process of reoxygenation is therefore crucial to clinical radiotherapy and supports the fact that tumor control is achieved in many tumor types using fractionated radiotherapy of 30–35 Gy in 2 Gy fractions despite the existence of hypoxia. However, the existence of hypoxia, particularly at "intermediate levels" of oxygenation between ~0.5–20 mmHg may be most relevant to the radioresistance of tumors in fractionated radiotherapy. Moreover, classical radiobiological modeling predicts that tumor cell killing is significantly reduced for single doses compared to conventional fractionation for the same biological effective dose in normoxic cells.[68] Stereotactic body radiotherapy (SBRT), also known as stereotactic ablative radiotherapy (SABR), is a hypofractionated regimen that enables the delivery of large radiation doses (8–30 Gy per fraction) to the tumor volume in 5 fractions or fewer.[67] In the SBRT paradigm, hypoxia may have a larger impact on treatment outcome[68] especially if reoxygenation is not allowed to occur between treatment fractions.

## 4.3. Hypoxic cell radiosensitizers and cytotoxins

As the presence of tumor hypoxia results in a reduction in the efficacy of therapy, a variety of experimental and clinical solutions have been designed to combat the radiation resistance to: (1) eliminate hypoxic regions of a tumor, (2) preferentially kill hypoxic cells or (3) mitigate their selective protection.[69] Historically, more direct reoxygenation methods were tried when radiotherapy was combined with hyperbaric oxygen[70,71] or carbogen breathing,[72] oxygenated perfluorochemical emulsions[73] and blood transfusions prior to radiation.[74] Hypoxic cells are considered to be resistant to most anti-cancer drugs due to a number of factors: (1) they are not exposed to adequate doses of the drugs due to their distance from blood vessels[75]; (2) the proliferation of tumor cells decreases as the distance from the blood vessels increases[76]; (3) hypoxic cells may have a reduced sensitivity to p53-mediated apoptosis and therefore the effect of anti-cancer drugs; and (4) the actions of certain anti-cancer drugs is similar to that of radiation and can increase the cytotoxicity of the DNA lesions they induce.[77]

There are essentially two main approaches to drug design that can combat tumor hypoxia. The first is the designing of drugs that radiosensitize the hypoxic cells and these are broadly referred to as 'Radiosensitizers'. The other group, are referred to as 'Cytotoxins' that selectively kill hypoxic cells even in the absence of radiation.

Radiosensitizers are chemical or pharmacological agents that if delivered in conjunction with radiation will increase the lethal effects of radiation on cells. Many kinds of compounds exist that are capable of enhancing the sensitivity of mammalian cells to radiation. However, only a select few have been able to selectively target the tumor instead of increasing the radiosensitivity of the tumor *and* the surrounding normal tissue. Essentially, two types of sensitizers have produced promising clinical results, halogenated pyrimidines and hypoxic-cell radiosensitizers. The aim of both types of drugs is to lower the amount of radiation required to achieve tumor

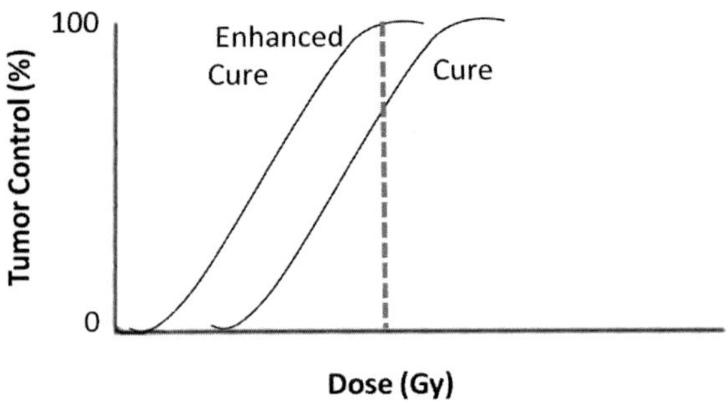


Fig. 13.   Schematic showing the reduction in the amount of radiation required to achieve tumor control with hypoxic specific drugs. (Adapted with permission from Ref. 78.)

control by preferentially increasing the sensitivity of tumor cells to radiation for a given level of normal tissue side effects as shown in Fig. 13.

Halogenated pyrimidines selectively target tumor cells based on the principle that tumor cells have a higher proliferation rate than the surrounding normal tissue and are therefore capable of taking up more of the drug. In short, the halogenated pyrimidine is similar to the thymidine (a DNA precursor) and is incorporated in its place. Unlike thymidine, the halogenated pyrimidine contains a halogen (chlorine, bromine, iodine) in the place of the methyl group, thus weakening the DNA chain. Consequently, the more halogenated the pyrimidine is that is incorporated into the cells (the drug needs to be present for several cell cycles), the more sensitive the DNA becomes to radiation in its already weakened state. Early studies showed that iodine analogue was a better choice than bromine as it did not induce a skin rash caused by exposure to fluorescent light.[79] Clinical studies showed the drug worked better for tumor sites with slowly proliferating normal tissues such as high grade glioblastoma and not H&N tumors.[80]

Hypoxic cell radiosensitizers on the other hand selectively target hypoxic tumor cells and so are not taken up in normal tissues that are not (in general) hypoxic. Thus, radiosensitivity is increased in the low oxygenated regions of a tumor with little to no effect in normal oxygenated cells. Several oxygen substitutes were developed to increase the oxygenation of hypoxic tumor cells, but unlike oxygen, these hypoxic cell radiosensitizers are not rapidly metabolized and thus can penetrate further into the tumor cells with the capability of reaching cells that are far away from the blood supply.[81] Moreover, the efficiency of the sensitization is linked to the

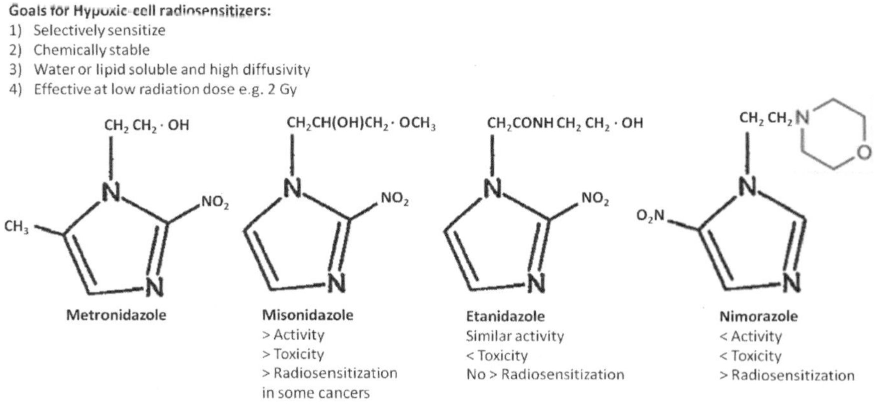

Fig. 14. The chemical structures of hypoxic-cell radiosensitizers and their respective biological differences (relative to metronidazole) to demonstrate the development of these drugs.

electron affinity of the oxygen substitutes and these drugs were found to be specific to hypoxia as they would not be taken up by well oxygenated cells, i.e. therefore not increasing the radiosensitivity of normal tissues.[81]

The nitrobenzenes were the first electron-affinic compounds shown to improve radiosensitization,[81] then nitrofurans and nitroimidazoles lead to the use of both 2-nitroimidazole and misonidazole.[22] Figure 14 shows the chemical structure and biological differences of these compounds.

Adams *et al.*[82] showed survival curves for aerated and hypoxic cells irradiated in the presence or absence of misonidazole and showed that, under hypoxic conditions, the presence of misonidazole increased the radiation sensitivity of the cells and the survival curves were similar to those of cells irradiated under normoxic conditions. Further studies showed an enhancement of radiation damage *in vivo* and the size of this effect is expressed as the sensitizer enhancement ratio (SER) for the same biological effect.

$$\text{SER} = \frac{\text{Radiation dose without sensitizer}}{\text{Radiation dose with sensitizer}}.$$

A number of different animal tumors showed enhancement ratios >2 when the radiosensitizer was delivered prior to irradiation.[83] The enhancement is reduced if the drug is delivered during fractioned radiotherapy most likely due to reoxygenation of the hypoxic fraction between fractions and lower doses.[83] Even if misonidazole is delivered after radiation, cell killing increases (not due to radiosensitization) as the drug alone is toxic to hypoxic cells and increased exposure can increase this effect.[22] In the clinical setting, Overgaard *et al.*[84] tested misonidazole in H&N cancer patients (DAHANCA 2 trial) and found a significant improvement in radiation response in the misonidazole group for pharynx tumors, but the same effect was not seen in cervical tumors.[85–87] The mixed results of many of these trials has often been attributed to the delivery of insufficient doses of misonidazole to achieve a clinically-useful SER because of the associated risk of neurotoxicity.[88]

As a result of the initial mixed clinical results, other radiosensitizers were developed[89,90] such as etanidazole which had a similar sensitizing effect as misonidazole but reduced toxicity due to shorter half-life and lower affinity for neural tissues due to lower lipophilicity.[91] However, the clinical trial data did not show a therapeutic benefit in H&N cancer patients. Pimonidazole was also used clinically due to its increased electron-affinic properties (compared to misonidazole) in cervical cancer patients but the trial was suspended due to decreased tumor response in the radiosensitizer group.[89] Subsequently, nimorazole was tried at higher doses due to lower toxicity despite having a lower radiosensitizing effect compared to misonidazole. The DAHANCA 5 trial showed that patients with supraglottic and pharyngeal carcinomas could benefit from nimorazole with conventional radiation and showed increased tumor control and disease-free survival when compared to receiving radiation alone as shown in Fig. 15.[60] As a result, nimorazole is the standard care in Denmark for H&N cancer patients.[91]

In more recent years, a new hypoxic radiosensitizer called doranidazole (1-[1′,3′,4′-trihydroxy-2′-butoxy]-methyl-2-nitroimidazole), also known as PR-350, another derivative of 2-nitroimidazole was created to reduce neurotoxicity due to its blood–brain barrier impermeability.[92] Doranidazole significantly enhanced radiation-induced tumor cell death *in vitro* in hypoxic but not normoxic conditions and when combined with X-ray radiation treatment, doranidazole significantly inhibited the growth of C6 rat glioblastoma tumors.[93] The compound was successful in a phase Ia trial to evaluate its toxicity and pharmacokinetics in patients undergoing conventional external beam radiotherapy.[94] Although in phase II trial

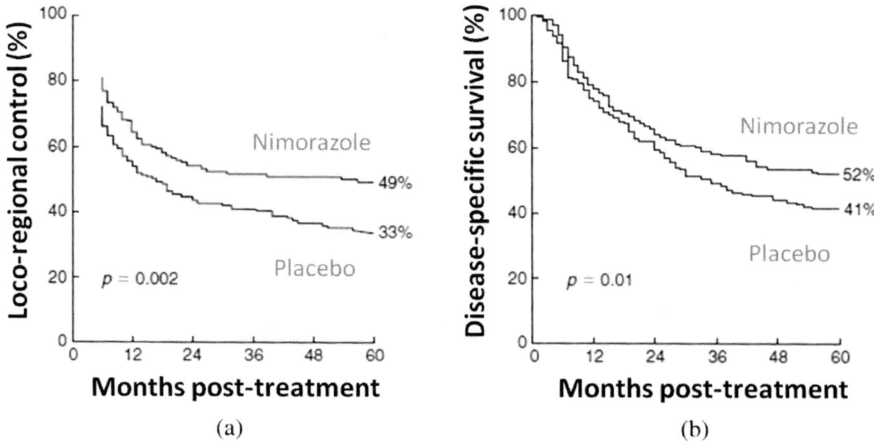


Fig. 15.    (a) Loco-regional control curves showing the effect of nimorazole (219 patients) versus placebo (195 patients) on tumor control. (b) Disease-specific survival curves showing the effect of nimorazole versus placebo on patient survival. (Adapted with permission Ref. 12.)

that evaluated survival at 1-year doranidazole did not demonstrate significantly better survival compared to the control group,[94] at 3-year survival, the sensitizer was shown to be more effective in improving long-term survival for pancreatic cancer patients.[95]

In addition, nitroimidazole compounds have also been historically delivered in combination with conventional radiotherapy using low doses per fraction, e.g. 1.8–2 Gy and these drugs are dependent on oxygen concentration as well as radiation dose. In an effort to improve their efficacy, recent arguments have been made that these same compounds delivered concurrently with hypofractionated radiotherapy, such as SBRT and stereotactic radiosurgery (SRS), should yield a significantly better therapeutic ratio as SER values for hypoxic cell radiosensitizers generally increase with increasing radiation dose per fraction.[66,96]

Hypoxic cell cytotoxins (bio-reductive drugs) are hypoxia-selective drugs that could be administered to counteract the radioprotective effect of tumor hypoxia.[97] They differ from hypoxic cell radiosensitizers as they are designed to selectively kill hypoxic cells and act in the absence of radiation. They are reduced to active cytotoxic species in cells deficient in oxygen.[97] Three groups of hypoxic cell cytotoxins exist: (1) quinone antibiotics, e.g. mitomycin-C, (2) nitroaromatic compounds, e.g. RSU-1069, and (3) benzotriazine di-N-oxides, e.g. tirapazamine. For Mitomycin C, after a long history as a chemotherapeutic drug, it was realized that it had preferential effects in the absence of oxygen as its bioreductive form could produce products to crosslink DNA and kill tumor cells. Clinical trials in H&N patients to combat hypoxia in squamous carcinomas were promising, but despite initial improved local tumor control[98] and no heightened toxicity, subsequent trials showed a small differential killing effect between hypoxic and normoxic cells. This may have been due to infrequent administration of the drug, e.g. 1–2 times per course of radiotherapy.[99]

Clinical trial experience with misonidazole led to the development of other nitro compounds including RSU-1069. This compound exhibited similar radiosensitizing effects to nitroimidazoles with an added azridine ring that provides a cytotoxic effect to hypoxic cells, however, animal studies found that along with killing the tumor cells, the drug caused blindness (the retina is a hypoxic normal tissue).

The benzotriazine di-N-oxides group of hypoxic cytotoxins contains the bioreductive drug tirapazamine. The drug showed very little toxicity to normoxic cells and the bioreductive products are found to be highly toxic in hypoxic environments and increase radiation-induced tumor cell killing. Initially, clinical trials combining tirapazamine with chemotherapy and/or radiation showed little promise. However, once patients were stratified in hypoxic and non-hypoxic groups based on $^{18}$F-FMISO PET imaging, tirapazamine was shown to provide significantly higher levels of local control for H&N squamous cell carcinoma patients in the hypoxic group when combined with cisplatin and 70 Gy radiation versus 70 Gy radiation and fluorouracil as shown in Fig. 16.[58]

In the last three decades, numerous oxygen-breathing and blood transfusion methods, cytotoxins and hypoxic-cell sensitizers have been developed to combat hypoxic radioresistance. Few of these methods have been successful or have yielded inconclusive results. However, a meta-analysis of more than 11,000 patients in 91 clinical trials showed level 1a evidence that overall, when radiation treatment is combined with some form of hypoxic modification treatment (oxygen or carbogen breathing, radiosensitizers, blood transfusions) for patients with solid tumors, local tumor control and overall survival were significantly improved.[11] The improvement

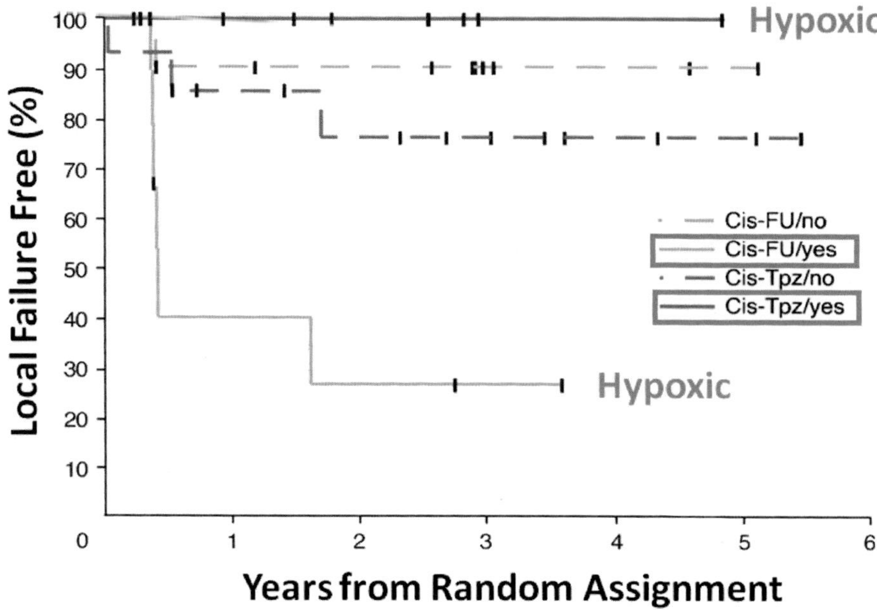


Fig. 16.   A survival curve showing hypoxic H&N squamous cell carcinomas patients and non-hypoxic (based on $^{18}$F-FMISO PET) receiving cisplatin and tirapazamine or cisplatin and 5FU chemotherapy both combined with 70 Gy radiation therapy.

was seen more in squamous cell patients than adenocarcinoma sites, however, overall it seems that there is a need to quantify and combat tumor hypoxia to improve clinical outcomes.

## 4.4.  Radiation dose boosting

Another potential method to combat tumor radioresistance is to increase the radiation dose delivered to a resistant tumor subvolume.[100] The concept of dose-boosting a biological target volume (BTV) requires an imaging biomarker, e.g. a PET radiotracer, that can be used to determine the subvolumes in the treatment plan that are more resistant to radiation, e.g. a hypoxic tumor fraction.[101] Increasing the dose to these regions may increase local control instead of increasing dose to the entire tumor. The latter approach would be limited by normal tissue side-effects and not be necessary as tumors are not heterogeneously resistant. This was first proposed by Ling *et al.*[100,102] who suggested biologically based treatment plans should be implemented in the clinical setting for personalized patient treatment.

Dose escalation can be practically implemented in a clinical setting by either a (1) dose painting by numbers approach, where dose is prescribed to individual voxels,[103] or a (2) dose painting by contours approach, where dose is prescribed to a BTV or tumor subvolumes.[100] The latter method has the advantage of being compatible with current treatment planning techniques to create margins to account for uncertainties in identification of subclinical disease, target motion, and patient setup. Figure 17 shows a PET-positive region for the HX4 radiotracer (indicative of tumor hypoxia) that could be boosted in a radiation treatment plan to combat radioresistance.[104]

Many studies have demonstrated dose painting by numbers *in silico*[105,106]; however, they often yielded clinically implausible boost volumes to achieve the desired tumor-control probability (TCP). In contrast, Zschaeck *et al.*[107] showed in 12 H&N cancer patients that the identification of hypoxic tumor subvolumes is clinically-feasible but requires adaptation during treatment and sufficient target margins.[107] Malinen *et al.*[108] used MRI-derived $pO_2$ measurements in a canine sarcoma model and found a higher TCP could be achieved when the delivered dose was redistributed according to the hypoxic level and an even higher TCP could be obtained if the dose was adapted throughout the treatment. Thorwarth *et al.*[109]

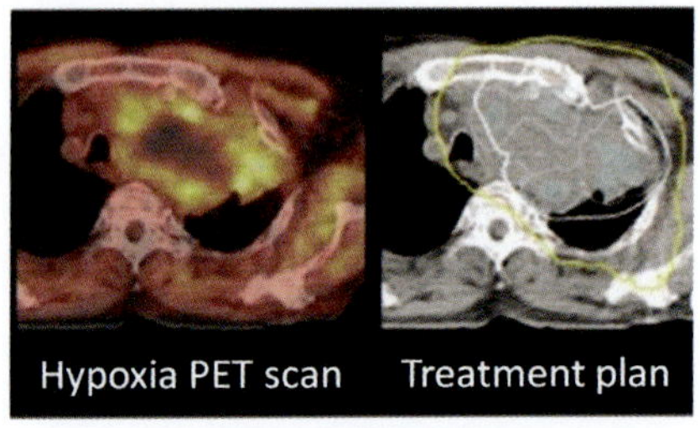


Fig. 17.   Example of pretreatment hypoxia HX4-PET/CT scan and treatment plan dose distributions for the same patient. The cyan region and line represent the $GTV_{HX4}$ and $PTV_{HX4}$ regions, respectively. The isodose line of 90% of the prescribed dose to the lymph nodes is

performed a similar study in patients and showed the potential increase inducted in the clinic.

Much like dose painting, most of the dose escalation studies[62,110–115] are conducted *in silico* i.e. radiation treatment plans are created but are not actually delivered to patients. Such studies have been more successful at achieving clinically-feasible doses. Lee *et al.*[112] showed in a treatment planning feasibility study with 11 patients that boosting the hypoxic volume ($GTV_H$) was feasible based on [18]F-FMISO scans and provided a theoretically improved local tumor control without exceeding the normal tissue tolerance. Henriques de Figueiredo *et al.*[116] also showed dose escalation up to 79.8 Gy guided by [18]F-FMISO-PET with VMAT was feasible in 10 inoperable H&N cancer patients and provided increase TCP without an increase in dose to the parotid glands.[116] Both Eschmann *et al.*[117] and Popple *et al.*[61] simulated escalated doses to [18]F-FMISO-defined hypoxic volumes and predicted a theoretical increase in tumor control. This has also been demonstrated for [64]Cu-ATSM treatment planning studies that showed an IMRT dose boost was feasible with respect to normal tissue constraints.[118] Servagi-Vernat *et al.*[119] showed that [18]F-FAZA PET could be used to identify hypoxic subvolumes for dose escalation protocols and advised that an additional scan be taken during radio-chemotherapy to account for the fluctuation in the hypoxic fraction during treatment.[119] This was further supported by Even *et al.*[104] who found that dose escalation based on metabolic subvolumes, hypoxic subvolumes, and the entire tumor was feasible. In this study, elevated doses were achieved without an increase in dose to normal tissue in 10 non-small cell lung cancer patients imaged with HX4-PET.

Clinical implementation of dose painting or escalation is dependent on accurate quantification of hypoxic regions and the capability of delivering large dose gradients on small spatial scales which may be challenging with current techniques.[120] This challenge in radiation delivery is of particular concern for hypofractionated radiotherapy due to the potential further increase in radioresistance of the hypoxic fraction for higher dose per fraction treatments.[66] In addition, other simulations found that less dose was required for cell kill in a given PET voxel, based on heterogeneous oxygen concentrations and not assuming a homogenous level of hypoxia.[121] The variation of prescribed dose within a GTV has already been clinically-implemented using fluoro-deoxyglucose (FDG) PET imaging data.[122–124] Some propose that for voxels with hypoxia tracer uptake slightly above the background threshold, additional dose could influence the level of tumor cell death, whereas for extremely hypoxic voxels, increasing dose may have little effect.[119] This suggests dose painting by numbers may be useful,[125] but first, a reliable quantitative image of hypoxia must be obtained. Moreover, as the uptake of hypoxia PET radiotracer decreases during treatment (due to a decreasing hypoxic fraction) combined with radiation-induced tumor inflammation and swelling, it becomes more difficult to quantify the hypoxic fraction. In a recent review, Geets *et al.*[126] conclude that, although dose painting is an attractive concept, it is restricted by low contrast, high noise, and poor spatial resolution of the PET image as well as degradation by errors in treatment delivery (set-up error and patient motion). The definition of hypoxia is also limited by the properties of a given PET tracer and its ability to accurately measure hypoxia as well as the method of quantification which is normally based on arbitrary thresholds which vary across studies.[33] Further investigation is needed to confirm the clinical benefit of dose painting or provide evidence for or against uniform target boosting or redistribution of dose to increase local control. Temporal changes in the spatial distribution of hypoxia on $^{18}$F-FMISO may also be problematic and lead to insufficient dose coverage of the tumor hypoxic region if hypoxic volumes change significantly during treatment.[101] Practical dose escalation strategies may therefore require serial imaging and adaptive planning which would be more feasible in a hypofractionation paradigm.[127] In addition, tumor hypoxia is diffusely distributed and thus heterogeneity can restrict the feasibility of defining a hypoxic fraction.[111]

## 4.5. High-LET particle radiotherapy

High-LET radiotherapy has been suggested to be less sensitive to tumor hypoxia when compared to photon radiation.[128] Aside from the increased conformity to the tumor,[129] charged particles can also have an increased relative biological effectiveness (RBE) for the same delivered radiation dose compared to X-rays.[130,131] Charged particles used for radiation therapy differ from X-rays and electrons due to their larger mass[132] and the spatial density of their energy deposition. These include protons as well as the nuclei of heavier ions such as carbon, neon, helium, and silicon.[133] An increase in DSB induction is observed with increasing particle LET, as well as the number of lethal events per unit dose (up to an LET of ~100 keV/$\mu$m).[134] LET is defined as the rate of energy transfer along the track of a charged particle in a medium, while RBE is defined as the ratio of the absorbed dose of a low-LET reference radiation to that of the charged particle of interest to produce the same biological effect or clinical endpoint.

Stewart *et al.*[135] used a Monte Carlo simulation method in combination with the repair–misrepair-fixation (RMF) model[136] (a kinetic reaction-rate model) to predict the RBE of different types of radiation (including high-LET) to account for reductions in DNA damage arising from enhanced chemical repair of DNA radicals under hypoxic conditions; in an effort to exploit the biological potential of protons and carbon ions in radiation therapy.[135] Reductions in the initial DSB yield with decreasing oxygen concentration are consistent with increases in cell survival under hypoxic relative to normoxic conditions.[136] *In vitro* studies showed that OERs decrease monotonously with LET as the OER value was 3 for X-rays but started to decrease at an LET of around 50 keV/$\mu$m. OER values reached < 2 at ~100 keV/$\mu$m and a minimum OER of >1 at an LET of > 300 keV/$\mu$m.[137] Karger *et al.*[138] showed the increased effectiveness of carbon ions (high-LET) relative to photons over the whole dose range for hypoxic and highly radioresistant rat prostate tumors. Further experimental observations provide compelling evidence that the induction of DSBs and other non-DSB clusters is proportional to absorbed dose up to at least several hundred Gy under normoxic and hypoxic conditions. Figure 18 shows the effects of oxygen concentration on the HRF for clonogenic cell survival and DSB induction. It is experimentally observed that initial DSB yield is reduced in cells under reduced oxygen conditions[139–143] and this suggests that average DNA cluster complexity, tends to decrease as oxygen concentration decreases.

In general, as particle LET increases, RBE increases as more ionization events results in a higher probability of causing lethal DNA damage. RBE is dependent on the particle type and energy, as seen in Fig. 19, and is due to variations in particle charge and mass.

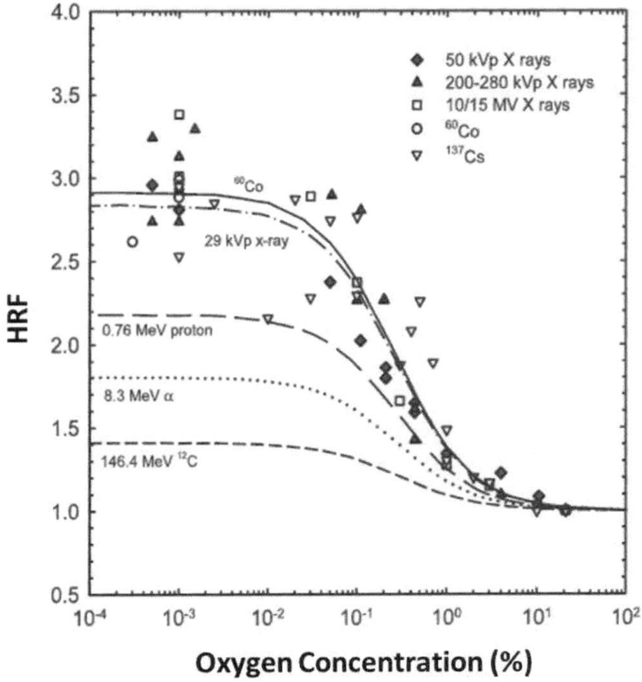



Fig. 18.   Effects of oxygen concentration on the HRF for clonogenic cell survival and DSB induction. Symbols: HRF for clonogenic survival derived from published cell survival experiments for photons. Lines denote the HRF for DSB induction predicted by the Monte Carlo damage simulations for $^{60}$Co (solid line), 29 kVp X rays (dash dot line), 0.76 MeV protons (long dashed line), 8.3 MeV a particles (dotted line) and 146.4 MeV carbon ions (short dashed line). (Adapted with permission from Ref. 13.)

Following unsuccessful experiences with neutrons, protons were chosen for their more favorable dose profile and high dose conformality but like photons lacked a high RBE. Consequently, carbon ions were suggested due to their high RBE, advantageous dose distribution due to a reduction in lateral scattering and range straggling compared to proton ions,[144,145] and superior imaging capabilities of the ion beam fragmentation with PET imaging.[146] Furthermore, due to the high proportion of direct DNA damage, carbon ions are less cell cycle dependent,[147] less influenced by the 5 'R's (radiosensitivity, repair, redistribution, reoxygenation, and repopulation)[148] of radiobiology (relative to photons) and have even been

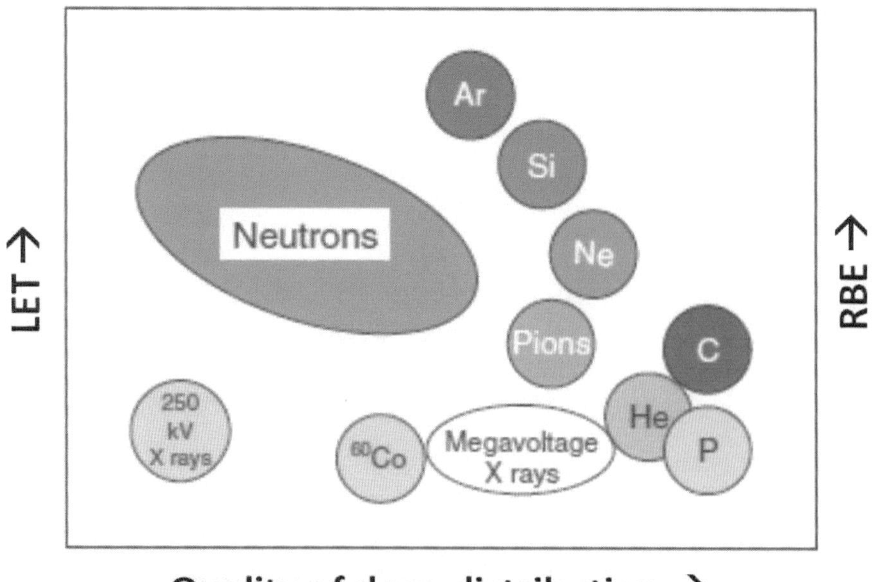



## Quality of dose distribution →

Fig. 19.   The RBE for protons is lower than that of carbon ions or neutrons as it has a lower LET value.[3]

shown to suppress angiogenesis and metastases through the destruction of endothelial cells.[149] Scifoni *et al.*[150] presented a method for adapting a biologically optimized treatment planning for particle beams to tumors with heterogeneous oxygen concentrations using PET imaging.

However, despite these efforts, there is an uncertainty in the value of RBE for carbon ions[151] as the values can range from >1 (at the plateau) up to 4.9 (at the Bragg peak)[131,152] and can even be higher depending on the tissue proliferation rate.[153,154] If carbon ions are to be used clinically, it is necessary to accurately predict: (1) the spatial variation of particle RBE and (2) the clinical RBE values in actual patients. This is of particular clinical consequence when the Bragg peak extends beyond the tumor into normal tissue as carbon ions are known to produce a small tail of dose beyond the Bragg peak due to nuclear fragmentation.[155] In essence, it is vital to know the RBE value of the beam and its position to ensure the tumor or normal tissues are not over or under-dosed. Consequently, some believe that protons may be more favorable than carbon ions (despite lower RBE) due to superior dose distributions and small spatial variation. Despite these potential disadvantages, the use of carbon ions in Japan[156] and Germany[157,158] for over 20 years has shown to produce good results in bone and soft-tissue sarcomas, H&N and pelvis cancers as well as locally recurrent rectal cancer and pancreatic cancer.

## 5. Predicting Radioresistance and Radiation Treatment Outcomes

## 5.1. Predicting treatment response with imaging

As previously discussed, in this and other chapters, there are numerous methods that can be used to measure hypoxia in tumors to develop a treatment strategy to combat its radioresistant effect. These methods can be used to identify a treatment-resistant phenotype and predict patient response. This predictive information is vital to combat the resistant hypoxic phenotype and additional hypoxia specific treatments could be included for more personalized patient care. Predicted treatment response, is usually measured by surrogate markers such as a PET radiotracer because the imaging technique is non-invasive and measurements can be performed serially over several time points. Predicting ineffective treatments means these could be withheld or altered to a more effective option such as with tirapazamine.[58]

Many studies have attempted to derive predictive markers and one of the most widely used is $^{18}$F-FDG, a surrogate for tumor metabolism. PET imaging can also be used to identify tumor hypoxia in cancer patients to predict prognosis to treatment.[109,159–167] Ali *et al.*[168] showed $^{18}$F-[2-(2-nitro-1-H-imidazol-1-yl)-N-(2,2,3,3,3-pentafluoropropyl) acetamide] ($^{18}$F-EF5) PET could predict tumor response to single fraction radiation treatment in a preclinical model. In glioma and rhabdomyosarcoma rat models, a significant correlation was found between $^{18}$F-FAZA uptake and tumor growth delay.[169]

Lee *et al.*[170] reviewed the clinical data of over 300 patients and concluded 18F-FMISO is a predictor of treatment response and provides prognostic information for cancer patients. Direct comparisons between $^{18}$F-FDG and $^{18}$F-FMISO show the latter to be a similar or stronger predictor of outcome.[171,172] Eschmann *et al.*[165] and other groups,[65,159–163,167] reported that 18F-FMISO could predict local recurrence in H&N cancer and NSCLC patients. Zips *et al.*[159] also confirmed that 18F-FMISO PET could predict local recurrence in 25 patients. Additional studies in various cancer types have confirmed that 18F-FMISO is a prognostic factor in glioma[164] and breast[55] cancer patients.

## 5.2. Modeling the effect of hypoxia

In the case that predictive imaging surrogate markers are not available, biophysical models are designed to relate the effect of ionizing radiation to the physical properties of the radiation field. Predicting this effect can be difficult as the radiation interacts with complex and highly structured biological targets, i.e. DNA strands within the cell nucleus. DNA damage models and early chemistry describe the initial events produced by radiation.[173] Biological model parameters are usually derived from the results of *in vitro* clonogenic assays because models are based on the description of the dose-response curve caused and interaction between DNA damage and repair.[174,175] Modeling the effect of oxygen on intrinsic radiation sensitivity is another way to design more biologically-relevant treatments. However, in the past, prescription doses were derived from clinical data through trial and error. A distinct lack of accurate models and response prediction parameters for both tumor and normal tissues was a major factor in the slow development of biologically-relevant treatment in the clinical setting.

Many groups have proposed using the OER concept to incorporate the effects of hypoxia into modeling of *in vitro* and *in vivo* radiation responses. Although the concept of an OER has been applied to end points such as DSB induction[176–178] and chromosomal aberrations,[179] the OER is usually defined as the dose under conditions of extreme hypoxia divided by the dose under conditions of partial oxygen pressure to achieve the same level of cell killing, as previously described. A disadvantage of defining OER in terms of cell killing (or survival) is that the OER becomes a function of dose[21,180] and dose rate.[138] In addition to defining the OER in terms of the cell killing, several groups[65,181–183] have modeled the effects of hypoxia by introducing OER factors that modify radiosensitivity parameters. That is, radiosensitivity parameters for hypoxic cells are determined by reducing $\alpha A$ and $\beta A$ by factors of $OER_\alpha$ and $(OER_\beta)^2$, respectively. A potential advantage of this approach is that the $OER_\alpha$ and $OER_\beta$ factors are presumably independent of dose and dose rate. The $OER_\alpha$ factor is interpreted as the limiting OER for small doses per fraction, and $OER_\beta$ is the OER in the limit of large doses per fraction.[136]

In the literature, the $OER_\alpha$ and $OER_\beta$ are usually treated as statistically independent factors. Wouters and Brown[65] modeled $\alpha$ and $\beta$ for aerobic cells by fixed factors of 2.5 and 9, respectively ($OER_\alpha = 2.5$, $OER_\beta = 3$). Nahum *et al.*[183] estimated hypoxic radiosensitivity parameters for prostate cancer by reducing the aerobic $\alpha$ and $\beta$ parameters by factors of 1.75 and 10.6, respectively ($OER_\alpha = 1.75$, $OER_\beta = 3.26$). In a study by Dasu and Denekamp,[181] the impact of hypoxia on cell killing and on surrogates for treatment effectiveness (hypoxic protection factor) were examined for scenarios in which $OER_\alpha = OER_\beta = 3$ as well as scenarios in which $OER_\alpha$ varies from 1.5 to 3 while keeping $OER_\beta = 3$. Although Carlson *et al.*[136] has suggested, that $OER_\alpha = OER_\beta$ and used several large *in vitro* data sets to explicitly test the hypothesis that $OER_\alpha = OER_\beta$. The study suggested that radiosensitivity parameters $\alpha$ and $\alpha/\beta$ for hypoxic cells can be estimated from parameters for aerobic cells (or vice versa) by introducing a single dimensionless parameter, OER, that is nearly independent of the intrinsic radiosensitivity parameters, $\alpha$ and $\alpha/\beta$. The result of their analysis indicated that OER $pO_2$ of 5 mmHg (clinical relevant) is approximately 1.5 and their formulas can be used for the analysis of clinical data.

Some modeling studies[136,181] have assumed a binary hypoxia distribution in which cells are either anoxic or normoxic. The effect of hypoxia is then modeled using one or two constant factors that effectively decrease intrinsic radiosensitivity. As previously mentioned, Wouters and Brown[65] first quantified differences in cell survival based on a radial oxygen diffusion model and a conventional binary model. They concluded that it is essential to characterize the oxygenation status of tumors in a realistic way (i.e. a dose-response model for hypoxic tumors must include cells at intermediate oxygen levels). Thus a binary model produces estimates of cell killing that would change by more than two orders of magnitude for conventionally fractionated treatments. As illustrated in Fig. 19, a conventional prostate treatment of 39 fractions results in a surviving fraction of

$2.8 \times 10^{-5}$ using a model based on radial oxygen diffusion ($f_{\mathrm{hyp}} = 0.2$). The study[66] notes that if a conventional binary model (distribution of cells that are either anoxic or normoxic) were used, estimates of cell killing would change by more than two orders of magnitude for conventionally fractionated treatments.[66] However, a conventional binary hypoxia model could overpredict the reduction in tumor cell killing expected in hypofractionated radiotherapy as a result of tumor hypoxia. This is unlike a radial oxygen diffusion model that includes cells at intermediate levels of hypoxia and could aid in the temporal optimization of radiation delivery by establishing when the effects of hypoxia on cell survival are most severe.[66]

As shown in Fig. 20, in hypoxic tumors, cell killing may be reduced for single doses compared to fractionated irradiation for the same biologically effective dose under normoxic conditions as predicted by our classical radiobiological models.[66] Others argue that such high doses may trigger a tumor vasculature response that does not occur at lower doses which in turn could provide a secondary mechanism of tumor control.[184,185]

Biophysical models are often tested using clinical data to verify the assumptions of the given model. Such mechanistically-motivated models are often used to describe clinical outcomes such as the probability of local tumor control and may include tumor oxygen heterogeneity.[186] Shuryak *et al.*[187] found that the LQ model combined with heterogeneous radiosensitivity provided the best description of SBRT clinical TCP data when

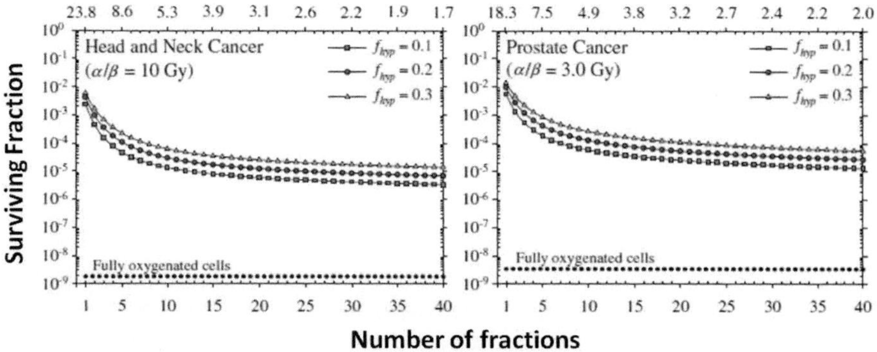


Fig. 20.  Total surviving fraction of tumor clonogens as a function of dose per fraction, assuming daily fractionation and full reoxygenation between fractions for a range of hypoxic tumor fractions. BED = biological effective dose. (Adapted with permission from Ref. 5.)

compared to several models with additional high-dose terms. The study explains that it may be possible that unique tumor cell death mechanisms exist at high doses but their influence could be masked and there is little evidence that single-fraction SBRT produces better tumor control than multi-fraction regimens. Instead, multi-fraction brain SBRT was predicted to produce slightly better TCPs than single-fraction treatments for brain metastases. These conclusions are consistent with expected effects on hypoxic tumors, where fractionation allows tumor reoxygenation between fractions.[66,188,189] Further, it may be expected that such alternate high dose mechanisms would enhance the TCP at high doses per fraction, predicting a steep dose response. However, the conclusions of others[68,187,190,191] support a shallow dose response which may be explained by heterogeneity in radiosensitivity (and perhaps heterogeneity in other factors, such as spatial dose distribution.[192–194] The effects of heterogeneous radiosensitivity dominate the comparatively subtle differences between the dose-response shapes produced by different radiobiological models.[188]

# References


1. Moulder, J. E., and Rockwell, S., Tumor hypoxia: its impact on cancer therapy. *Cancer Metastasis Rev.*, **5**(4), pp. 313–341, 1987.
2. Gray, L. H. *et al.*, The concentration of oxygen dissolved in tissues at the time of irradiation as a factor in radiotherapy. *Br. J. Radiol.*, **26**(312), pp. 638–648, 1953.
3. Vaupel, P., Tumor microenvironmental physiology and its implications for radiation oncology. *Semin. Radiat. Oncol.*, **14**(3), pp. 198–206, 2004.
4. Padera, T. P. *et al.*, Pathology: cancer cells compress intratumour vessels. *Nature*, **427**(6976), p. 695, 2004.
5. Brown, J. M., Tumor hypoxia, drug resistance, and metastases. *J. Natl. Cancer I.*, **82**(5), pp. 338–339, 1990.
6. Vaupel, P., and Harrison, L., Tumor hypoxia: causative factors, compensatory mechanisms, and cellular response. *Oncologist*, **9**(5), pp. 4–9, 2004.
7. Hockel, M., and Vaupel, P., Tumor hypoxia: definitions and current clinical, biologic, and molecular aspects. *J. Natl. Cancer. Inst.*, **93**(4), pp. 266–276, 2001.
8. Brown, J. M., Evidence for acutely hypoxic cells in mouse tumours, and a possible mechanism of reoxygenation. *Br. J. Radiol.*, **52**(620), pp. 650–656, 1979.
9. Dewhirst, M. W., Cao, Y., and Moeller, B., Cycling hypoxia and free radicals regulate angiogenesis and radiotherapy response. *Nat. Rev. Cancer*, **8**(6), pp. 425–437, 2008.

10. Mottram, J. C., A factor of importance in the radio sensitivity of tumours. *Br. J. Radiol.*, **9**(105), pp. 606–614, 1936.

11. Overgaard, J., Hypoxic modification of radiotherapy in squamous cell carcinoma of the head and neck — a systematic review and meta-analysis. *Radiother. Oncol.*, **100**(1), pp. 22–32, 2011.

12. Howard-Flanders, P., and Moore, D., The time interval after pulsed irradiation within which injury to bacteria can be modified by dissolved oxygen. I. A search for an effect of oxygen 0.02 second after pulsed irradiation. *Radiat. Res.*, **9**(4), pp. 422–437, 1958.

13. Adams, G. E., Cooke, M. S., and Michael, B. D., Rapid mixing in radiobiology. *Nature*, **219**(5161), pp. 1368–1369, 1968.

14. Michael, B. D. *et al.*, A posteffect of oxygen in irradiated bacteria: a submillisecond fast mixing study. *Radiat. Res.*, **54**(2), pp. 239–251, 1973.

15. Epp, E. R. *et al.*, Oxygen diffusion times in bacterial cells irradiated with high-intensity pulsed electrons: new upper limit to the lifetime of oxygen-sensitive species suspected to be induced at critical sites in bacterial cells. *Radiat. Res.*, **54**(2), pp. 171–180, 1973.

16. Epp, E. R., Weiss., H., and Ling, C. C., Irradiation of cells by single and double pulses of high intensity radiation: oxygen sensitization and diffusion kinetics. *Curr. Top. Radiat. Res. Q*, **11**(3), pp. 201–250, 1976.

17. von Sonntag, C., Carbohydrate radicals: from ethylene glycol to DNA strand breakage. *Int. J. Radiat. Biol. Relat. Stud. Phys. Chem. Med.*, **46**(5), pp. 507–519, 1984.

18. Alper, T., and Howard-Flanders, P., Role of oxygen in modifying the radiosensitivity of E. coli B. *Nature*, **178**(4540), pp. 978–979, 1956.

19. Schulte-Frohlinde, D., and Bothe, E., Identification of a major pathway of strand break formation in poly U induced by OH radicals in presence of oxygen. *Z. Naturforsch. C.*, **39**(3–4), pp. 315–319, 1984.

20. Wright, E. A., and Howard-Flanders, P., The influence of oxygen on the radiosensitivity of mammalian tissues. *Acta. Radiol.*, **48**(1), pp. 26–32, 1957.

21. Palcic, B., and Skarsgard, L. D., Reduced oxygen enhancement ratio at low doses of ionizing radiation. *Radiat. Res.*, **100**(2), pp. 328–339, 1984.

22. Kogel, A. V. D., and Joiner, M., *Basic Clinical Radiobiology*. 4th edn. Hodder Arnold, 2009.

23. Powers, W. E., and Tolmach, L. J., A multicomponent X-ray survival curve for mouse lymphosarcoma cells irradiated in vivo. *Nature*, **197**, pp. 710–711, 1963.

24. Hill, R. P., Bush, R. S., and Yeung, P., The effect of anaemia on the fraction of hypoxic cells in an experimental tumour. *Br. J. Radiol.*, **44**(520), pp. 299–304, 1971.

25. Stanley, J. A., Shipley, W. U., and Steel, G. G., Influence of tumour size on hypoxic fraction and therapeutic sensitivity of Lewis lung tumour. *Br. J. Cancer.*, **36**(1), pp. 105–113, 1977.

26. Vaupel, P., and Mayer, A., Hypoxia in cancer: significance and impact on clinical outcome. *Cancer Metast. Rev.*, **26**(2), pp. 225–239, 2007.

27. Hockel, M. *et al.*, Association between tumor hypoxia and malignant progression in advanced cancer of the uterine cervix. *Cancer Res.*, **56**(19), pp. 4509–4515, 1996.

28. Fyles, A. W. *et al.*, Oxygenation predicts radiation response and survival in patients with cervix cancer. *Radiother. Oncol.*, **48**(2), pp. 149–156, 1998.

29. Nordsmark, M., Overgaard, M. and Overgaard, J., Pretreatment oxygenation predicts radiation response in advanced squamous cell carcinoma of the head and neck. *Radiother. Oncol.*, **41**(1), pp. 31–39, 1996.

30. Nordsmark, M. *et al.*, Prognostic value of tumor oxygenation in 397 head and neck tumors after primary radiation therapy. An international multicenter study. *Radiother. Oncol.*, **77**(1), pp. 18–24, 2005.

31. Brizel, D. M. *et al.*, Tumor hypoxia adversely affects the prognosis of carcinoma of the head and neck. *Int. J. Radiat. Oncol. Biol. Phys.*, **38**(2), pp. 285–289, 1997.

32. Brizel, D. M. *et al.*, Tumor oxygenation predicts for the likelihood of distant metastases in human soft tissue sarcoma. *Cancer Res.*, **56**(5), pp. 941–943, 1996.

33. Kelada, O. J., and Carlson, D. J., Molecular imaging of tumor hypoxia with positron emission tomography. *Radiat. Res.*, **181**(4), pp. 335–349, 2014.

34. Rofstad, E. K. *et al.*, Hypoxia-induced treatment failure in advanced squamous cell carcinoma of the uterine cervix is primarily due to hypoxia-induced radiation resistance rather than hypoxia-induced metastasis. *Br. J. Cancer*, **83**(3), pp. 354–359, 2000.

35. Vaupel, P., Hockel, M., and Mayer, A., Detection and characterization of tumor hypoxia using pO2 histography. *Antioxid. Redox. Signal.*, **9**(8), pp. 1221–1235, 2007.

36. Graeber, T. G. *et al.*, Hypoxia-mediated selection of cells with diminished apoptotic potential in solid tumours. *Nature*, **379**(6560), pp. 88–91, 1996.

37. Hickman, J. A. *et al.*, Apoptosis and cancer chemotherapy. *Philos. Roy. Soc. B.*, **345**(1313), pp. 319–325, 1994.

38. Nordsmark, M., and Overgaard, J., A confirmatory prognostic study on oxygenation status and loco-regional control in advanced head and neck squamous cell carcinoma treated by radiation therapy. *Radiother. Oncol.*, **57**(1), pp. 39–43, 2000.

39. Vaupel, P. *et al.*, Oxygenation of human tumors: evaluation of tissue oxygen distribution in breast cancers by computerized O2 tension measurements. *Cancer Res.*, **51**(12), pp. 3316–3322, 1991.

40. Donnelly, E. T. *et al.*, Effects of texaphyrins on the oxygenation of EMT6 mouse mammary tumors. *Int. J. Radiat. Oncol. Biol. Phys.*, **58**(5), pp. 1570–1576, 2004.

41. Griffiths, J. R., and Robinson, S. P., The OxyLite: a fibre-optic oxygen sensor. *Br. J. Radiol.*, **72**(859), pp. 627–630, 1999.

42. Adam, M. F., Dorie, M. J., and Brown, J. M., Oxygen tension measurements of tumors growing in mice. *Int. J. Radiat. Oncol. Biol. Phys.*, **45**(1), pp. 171–180, 1999.

43. Tatum, J. L. *et al.*, Hypoxia: importance in tumor biology, noninvasive measurement by imaging, and value of its measurement in the management of cancer therapy. *Int. J. Radiat. Oncol. Biol. Phys.*, **82**(10), pp. 699–757, 2006.

44. Ballinger, J. R., Imaging hypoxia in tumors. *Semin. Nucl. Med.*, **31**(4), pp. 321–329, 2001.

45. Gallez, B., Baudelet, C., and Jordan, B. F., Assessment of tumor oxygenation by electron paramagnetic resonance: principles and applications. *NMR Biomed.*, **17**(5), pp. 240–262, 2004.

46. Pan, X., Xia, D., and Halpern, H., Targeted-ROI imaging in electron paramagnetic resonance imaging. *J. Magn. Reson.*, **187**(1), pp. 66–77, 2007.

47. Landuyt, W. *et al.*, BOLD contrast fMRI of whole rodent tumour during air or carbogen breathing using echo-planar imaging at 1.5 T. *Eur Radiol*, **11**(11), pp. 2332–2340, 2001.

48. Dunn, J. F. *et al.*, Changes in oxygenation of intracranial tumors with carbogen: a BOLD MRI and EPR oximetry study. *J. Magn. Reson. Im.*, **16**(5), pp. 511–521, 2002.

49. Skala, M. C. *et al.*, Longitudinal optical imaging of tumor metabolism and hemodynamics. *J. Biomed. Opt.*, **15**(1), p. 011112, 2010.

50. Rasey, J. S. *et al.*, Radiolabelled fluoromisonidazole as an imaging agent for tumor hypoxia. *Int. J. Radiat. Oncol. Biol. Phys.*, **17**(5), pp. 985–991, 1989.

51. Koh, W. J. *et al.*, Imaging of hypoxia in human tumors with [F-18]fluoromisonidazole. *Int. J. Radiat. Oncol. Biol. Phys.*, **22**(1), pp. 199–212, 1992.

52. Valk, P. E. *et al.*, Hypoxia in human gliomas: demonstration by PET with fluorine-18-fluoromisonidazole. *J. Nucl. Med*, **33**(12), pp. 2133–2137, 1992.

53. Rasey, J. S. *et al.*, Quantifying regional hypoxia in human tumors with positron emission tomography of [18F]fluoromisonidazole: a pretherapy study of 37 patients. *Int. J. Radiat. Oncol. Biol. Phys.*, **36**(2), pp. 417–428, 1996.

54. Rasey, J. S. *et al.*, Determining hypoxic fraction in a rat glioma by uptake of radiolabeled fluoromisonidazole. *Radiat. Res.*, **153**(1), pp. 84–92, 2000.

55. Cheng, J. *et al.*, 18F-fluoromisonidazole PET/CT: a potential tool for predicting primary endocrine therapy resistance in breast cancer. *J. Nucl. Med.*, **54**(3), pp. 333–340, 2013.

56. Hirata, K. *et al.*, (1)(8)F-Fluoromisonidazole positron emission tomography may differentiate glioblastoma multiforme from less malignant gliomas. *Eur. J. Nucl. Med. Mol. Imaging*, **39**(5), pp. 760–770, 2012.

57. McKeage, M. J. *et al.*, PR-104 a bioreductive preprodrug combined with gemcitabine or docetaxel in a phase Ib study of patients with advanced solid tumours. *BMC Cancer*, **12**, p. 496, 2012.

58. Rischin, D. *et al.*, Prognostic significance of [18F]-misonidazole positron emission tomography-detected tumor hypoxia in patients with advanced head and neck cancer randomly assigned to chemoradiation with or without tirapazamine: a substudy of Trans-Tasman Radiation Oncology Group Study 98.02. *J. Clin. Oncol.*, **24**(13), pp. 2098–2104, 2006.

59. Loi, S. *et al.*, Oxaliplatin combined with infusional 5-fluorouracil and concomitant radiotherapy in inoperable and metastatic rectal cancer: a phase I trial. *Br. J. Cancer*, **92**(4), pp. 655–661, 2005.

60. Overgaard, J. *et al.*, A randomized double-blind phase III study of nimorazole as a hypoxic radiosensitizer of primary radiotherapy in supraglottic larynx and pharynx carcinoma. Results of the Danish Head and Neck Cancer Study (DAHANCA) Protocol 5–85. *Radiother. Oncol.*, **46**(2), pp. 135–146, 1998.

61. Popple, R. A., Ove, R., and Shen, S., Tumor control probability for selective boosting of hypoxic subvolumes, including the effect of reoxygenation. *Int. J. Radiat. Oncol. Biol. Phys.*, **54**(3), pp. 921–927, 2002.

62. Alber, M. *et al.*, On biologically conformal boost dose optimization. *Phys. Med. Biol.*, **48**(2), pp. 31–35, 2003.

63. Van Putten, L. M., and Kallman, R. F., Oxygenation status of a transplantable tumor during fractionated radiation therapy. *J. Natl. Cancer*, **40**(3), pp. 441–451, 1968.

64. Kallman, R. F., and Bleehen. N. M., Post-irradiation cyclic radiosensitivity changes in tumors and normal tissues in USAEC Conf. 6801410, 1968.

65. Wouters, B. G., and Brown, J. M., Cells at intermediate oxygen levels can be more important than the "hypoxic fraction" in determining tumor response to fractionated radiotherapy. *Radiat. Res.*, **147**(5), pp. 541–550, 1997.

66. Carlson, D. J. *et al.*, Hypofractionation results in reduced tumor cell kill compared to conventional fractionation for tumors with regions of hypoxia. *Int. J. Radiat. Oncol. Biol. Phys.*, **79**(4), pp. 1188–1195, 2011.

67. Lo, S. S. *et al.*, Stereotactic body radiation therapy: a novel treatment modality. *Nat. Rev. Clin. Oncol.*, **7**(1), pp. 44–54, 2010.

68. Brown, J. M., Carlson, D. J. and Brenner, D. J., The tumor radiobiology of SRS and SBRT: are more than the 5 Rs involved? *Int. J. Radiat. Oncol. Biol. Phys.*, **88**(2), pp. 254–262, 2014.

69. Brown, J. M., Exploiting the hypoxic cancer cell: mechanisms and therapeutic strategies. *Mol. Med. Today*, **6**(4), pp. 157–162, 2000.

70. Churchill-Davidson, I., Sanger, C., and Thomlinson, R. H., Oxygenation in radiotherapy. II. Clinical application. *Br. J. Radiol.*, **30**(356), pp. 406–422, 1957.

71. Dische, S., Hyperbaric oxygen. *Br. J. Radiol.*, **52**(618), p. 508, 1979.

72. Dusault, L. A., The effect of oxygen on the response of spontaneous tumours in mice to radiotherapy. *Br. J. Radiol.*, **36**, pp. 749–754, 1963.

73. Rockwell, S., Use of a perfluorochemical emulsion to improve oxygenation in a solid tumor. *Int. J. Radiat. Oncol. Biol. Phys.*, **11**(1), pp. 97–103, 1985.

74. Overgaard, J. *et al.*, Primary radiotherapy of larynx and pharynx carcinoma — an analysis of some factors influencing local control and survival. *Int. J. Radiat. Oncol. Biol. Phys.*, **12**(4), pp. 515–521, 1986.

75. Tannock, I. F., Conventional cancer therapy: promise broken or promise delayed? *Lancet*, **351** (**2**), pp. 9–16, 1998.

76. Tannock, I. F., The relation between cell proliferation and the vascular system in a transplanted mouse mammary tumour. *Br. J. Cancer*, **22**(2), pp. 258–273, 1968.

77. Teicher, B. A., Lazo, J. S., and Sartorelli, A. C., Classification of antineoplastic agents by their selective toxicities toward oxygenated and hypoxic tumor cells. *Cancer Res.*, **41**(1), pp. 73–81, 1981.

78. Hall, E., *Radiobiology for the Radiologist*. Lippincott Williams & Wilkins, Philadelphia, PA, 2006.

79. Mitchell, J. B. *et al.*, Differing sensitivity to fluorescent light in Chinese hamster cells containing equally incorporated quantities of BUdR versus IUdR. *Int. J. Radiat. Oncol. Biol. Phys.*, **10**(8), pp. 1447–1451, 1984.

80. Kinsella, T. J. *et al.*, A phase I study of intravenous iododeoxyuridine as a clinical radiosensitizer. *Int. J. Radiat. Oncol. Biol. Phys.*, **11**(11), pp. 1941–1946, 1985.

81. Adams, G. E., and Cooke, M. S., Electron-affinic sensitization. I. A structural basis for chemical radiosensitizers in bacteria. *Int. J. Radiat. Biol. Relat. Stud. Phys. Chem. Med.*, **15**(5), pp. 457–471, 1969.

82. Adams, G. E. *et al.*, Electron-affinic sensitization. VII. A correlation between structures, one-electron reduction potentials, and efficiencies of nitroimidazoles as hypoxic cell radiosensitizers. *Radiat. Res.*, **67**(1), pp. 9–20, 1976.

83. Adams, G., *Hypoxic Cell Sensitizers for Radiotherapy. Cancer: A Comprehensive Treatise.* Vol. 6. Plenum Press: New York, pp. 181–223, 1977.

84. Overgaard, J. *et al.*, Misonidazole combined with split-course radiotherapy in the treatment of invasive carcinoma of larynx and pharynx: report from the DAHANCA 2 study. *Int. J. Radiat. Oncol. Biol. Phys.*, **16**(4), pp. 1065–1068, 1989.

85. Dische, S. *et al.*, Clinical experience with nitroimidazoles as radiosensitizers. *Int. J. Radiat. Oncol. Biol. Phys.*, **8**(3–4), pp. 335–338, 1982.

86. Dische, S., Chemical sensitizers for hypoxic cells: a decade of experience in clinical radiotherapy. *Radiother. Oncol.*, **3**(2), pp. 97–115, 1985.

87. Overgaard, J. *et al.*, Misonidazole combined with radiotherapy in the treatment of carcinoma of the uterine cervix. *Int. J. Radiat. Oncol. Biol. Phys.*, **16**(4), pp. 1069–1072, 1989.

88. Brown, J. M., Keynote address: hypoxic cell radiosensitizers: where next? *Int. J. Radiat. Oncol. Biol. Phys.*, **16**(4), pp. 987–993, 1989.

89. Overgaard, J., Clinical evaluation of nitroimidazoles as modifiers of hypoxia in solid tumors. *Oncol. Res.*, **6**(10–11), pp. 509–518, 1994.

90. Coleman, C. N., Hypoxia in tumors: a paradigm for the approach to biochemical and physiologic heterogeneity. *J. Natl. Cancer I*, **80**(5), pp. 310–317, 1988.

91. Overgaard, J. *et al.*, Five compared with six fractions per week of conventional radiotherapy of squamous-cell carcinoma of head and neck: DAHANCA 6 and 7 randomised controlled trial. *Lancet.*, **362**(9388), pp. 933–940, 2003.

92. Hirokawa, K. *et al.*, Pharmacokinetics and radiosensitizing effect of PR-350. *Radiat. Med.*, **15**(1), pp. 45–49, 1997.

93. Yasui, H. *et al.*, The prospective application of a hypoxic radiosensitizer, doranidazole to rat intracranial glioblastoma with blood brain barrier disruption. *BMC Cancer*, **13**, p. 106, 2013.

94. Nemoto, K. *et al.*, Phase Ia study of a hypoxic cell sensitizer doranidazole (PR-350) in combination with conventional radiotherapy. *Anticancer Drugs*, **12**(1), pp. 1–6, 2001.

95. Karasawa, K. *et al.*, Efficacy of novel hypoxic cell sensitiser doranidazole in the treatment of locally advanced pancreatic cancer: long-term results of a placebo-controlled randomised study. *Radiother. Oncol.*, **87**(3), pp. 326–330, 2008.

96. Murata, R., Tsujitani, M., and Horsman, M. R., Enhanced local tumour control after single or fractionated radiation treatment using the hypoxic cell radiosensitizer doranidazole. *Radiother. Oncol.*, **87**(3), pp. 331–338, 2008.

97. McKeown, S. R., Cowen, R. L. and Williams, K. J., Bioreductive drugs: from concept to clinic. *Clin. Oncol. (R Coll Radiol)*, **19**(6), pp. 427–442, 2007.

98. Rewari, A. N. *et al.*, Postoperative concurrent chemoradiotherapy with mitomycin in advanced squamous cell carcinoma of the head and neck: results from three prospective randomized trials. *Cancer J.*, **12**(2), pp. 123–129, 2006.

99. Horsman, M. R, Lindegaard, J. C, Grau, C., Nordsmark, M., and Overgaard, J., Dose-response modifiers in radiation therapy. 2nd edn. *Clinical Radiation Oncology*. Churchill Livingstone, Philadelphia, 2007.

100. Ling, C. C. *et al.*, Towards multidimensional radiotherapy (MD-CRT): biological imaging and biological conformality. *Int. J. Radiat. Oncol. biol. phys.*, **47**(3), pp. 551–560, 2000.

101. Lin, Z. *et al.*, The influence of changes in tumor hypoxia on dose-painting treatment plans based on 18F-FMISO positron emission tomography. *Int. J. Radiat. Oncol. Biol. Phys.*, **70**(4), pp. 1219–1228, 2008.

102. Ling, C. C., and Li, X. A., Over the next decade the success of radiation treatment planning will be judged by the immediate biological response of tumor cells rather than by surrogate measures such as dose maximization and uniformity. *Med. Phys.*, **32**(7), pp. 2189–2192, 2005.

103. Bentzen, S. M., Theragnostic imaging for radiation oncology: dose-painting by numbers. *Lancet Oncol.*, **6**(2), pp. 112–127, 2005.

104. Even, A. J. *et al.*, PET-based dose painting in non-small cell lung cancer: Comparing uniform dose escalation with boosting hypoxic and metabolically active subvolumes. *Radiother. Oncol.*, **116**(2), pp. 281–286, 2015.

105. Thorwarth, D. *et al.*, Hypoxia dose painting by numbers: a planning study. *Int. J. Radiat. Oncol. Biol. Phys.*, **68**(1), pp. 291–300, 2007.

106. Toma-Dasu, I. *et al.*, Dose prescription and treatment planning based on FMISO-PET hypoxia. *Acta. Oncol.*, **51**(2), pp. 222–230, 2012.

107. Zschaeck, S. *et al.*, Spatial distribution of FMISO in head and neck squamous cell carcinomas during radio-chemotherapy and its correlation to pattern of failure. *Acta. Oncol.*, **54**(9), pp. 1355–1363, 2015.

108. Malinen, E. *et al.*, Adapting radiotherapy to hypoxic tumours. *Phys. Med.*, **51**(19), pp. 4903–4921, 2006.

109. Thorwarth, D. *et al.*, Kinetic analysis of dynamic 18F-fluoromisonidazole PET correlates with radiation treatment outcome in head-and-neck cancer. *BMC Cancer*, **5**. p. 152, 2005.

110. Rajendran, J. G. *et al.*, Hypoxia imaging-directed radiation treatment planning. *Eur. J. Nucl. Med. Mol. Im.*, **33**(1), pp. 44–53, 2006.

111. Grosu, A. L. *et al.*, Hypoxia imaging with FAZA-PET and theoretical considerations with regard to dose painting for individualization of radiotherapy in patients with head and neck cancer. *Int. J. Radiat. Oncol. Biol. Phys.*, **69**(2), pp. 541–551, 2007.

112. Lee, N. Y. *et al.*, Fluorine-18-labeled fluoromisonidazole positron emission and computed tomography-guided intensity-modulated radiotherapy for head and neck cancer: a feasibility study. *Int. J. Radiat. Oncol. Biol. Phys.*, **70**(1), pp. 2–13, 2008.

113. Choi, W. *et al.*, Planning study for available dose of hypoxic tumor volume using fluorine-18-labeled fluoromisonidazole positron emission tomography for treatment of the head and neck cancer. *Radiother. Oncol.*, **97**(2), pp. 176–182, 2010.

114. Chang, J. H. *et al.*, Hypoxia-targeted radiotherapy dose painting for head and neck cancer using (18)F-FMISO PET: A biological modeling study. *Acta. Oncol.*, 2013.

115. Hendrickson, K. *et al.*, Hypoxia imaging with [F-18] FMISO-PET in head and neck cancer: potential for guiding intensity modulated radiation therapy in overcoming hypoxia-induced treatment resistance. *Radiother. Oncol.*, **101**(3), pp. 369–375, 2011.

116. Henriques de Figueiredo, B. *et al.*, Hypoxia imaging with [18F]-FMISO-PET for guided dose escalation with intensity-modulated radiotherapy in head-and-neck cancers. *Strahlenther. Onkol.*, **191**(3), pp. 217–224, 2015.

117. Eschmann, S. M. *et al.*, Hypoxia-imaging with (18)F-Misonidazole and PET: changes of kinetics during radiotherapy of head-and-neck cancer. *Radiother. Oncol.*, **83**(3), pp. 406–410, 2007.

118. Chao, K. S. *et al.*, A novel approach to overcome hypoxic tumor resistance: Cu-ATSM-guided intensity-modulated radiation therapy. *Int. J. Radiat. Oncol. Biol. Phys.*, **49**(4), pp. 1171–1182, 2001.

119. Servagi-Vernat, S. *et al.*, A prospective clinical study of (1)(8)F-FAZA PET-CT hypoxia imaging in head and neck squamous cell carcinoma before and during radiation therapy. *Eur. J. Nucl. Med. Mol. Im.*, **41**(8), pp. 1544–1552, 2014.

120. Bowen, S. R. *et al.*, On the sensitivity of IMRT dose optimization to the mathematical form of a biological imaging-based prescription function. *Phys. Med. Biol.*, **54**(6), pp. 1483–1501, 2009.

121. Petit, S. F. *et al.*, Intra-voxel heterogeneity influences the dose prescription for dose-painting with radiotherapy: a modelling study. *Phys. Med. Biol.*, **54**(7), pp. 2179–2196, 2009.

122. Madani, I. *et al.*, Positron emission tomography-guided, focal-dose escalation using intensity-modulated radiotherapy for head and neck cancer. *Int. J. Radiat. Oncol. Biol. Phys.*, **68**(1), pp. 126–135, 2007.

123. Madani, I. *et al.*, Maximum tolerated dose in a phase I trial on adaptive dose painting by numbers for head and neck cancer. *Radiother. Oncol.*, **101**(3), pp. 351–355, 2011.

124. Duprez, F. *et al.*, Adaptive dose painting by numbers for head-and-neck cancer. *Int. J. Radiat. Oncol. Biol. Phys.*, **80**(4), pp. 1045–1055, 2011.

125. Thorwarth, D., and Alber, M., Implementation of hypoxia imaging into treatment planning and delivery. *Radiother. Oncol.*, **97**(2), pp. 172–175, 2010.

126. Geets, X., Gregoire, V., and Lee, J. A., Implementation of hypoxia PET imaging in radiation therapy planning. *Q. J. Nucl. Med. Mol. Imaging.*, **57**(3), pp. 271–282, 2013.

127. Carlson, D. J., Yenice, K. M., and Orton, C. G., Tumor hypoxia is an important mechanism of radioresistance in hypofractionated radiotherapy and must be considered in the treatment planning process. *Med. Phys.*, **38**(12), pp. 6347–6350, 2011.

128. Barendsen, G. W., and Broerse, J. J., Experimental radiotherapy of a rat rhabdomyosarcoma with 15 MeV neutrons and 300 kV X-rays. I. Effects of single exposures. *Eur. J. Cancer*, **5**(4), pp. 373–391, 1969.

129. Wilson, R. R., Radiological use of fast protons. *Radiology*, **47**(5), pp. 487–491, 1946.

130. Wambersie, A., Is there any future for high-LET radiation? *Strahlenther. Onkol.*, **165**(4), pp. 348–356, 1989.

131. Frese, M. C. *et al.*, A mechanism–based approach to predict the relative biological effectiveness of protons and carbon ions in radiation therapy. *Int. J. Radiat. Oncol. Biol. Phys.*, **83**(1), pp. 442–450, 2012.

132. Halperin, E., Perez, C., and Brady, L., *Perez and Brady's principles and practice of radiation oncology.* Lippincott Williams & Wilkins, 2008.

133. Terasawa, T. *et al.*, Systematic review: charged-particle radiation therapy for cancer. *Ann. Intern. Med.*, **151**(8), pp. 556–565, 2009.

134. Carlson, D. J. *et al.*, Combined use of Monte Carlo DNA damage simulations and deterministic repair models to examine putative mechanisms of cell killing. *Radiat. Res.*, **169**(4), pp. 447–459, 2008.

135. Stewart, R. D. *et al.*, Effects of radiation quality and oxygen on clustered DNA lesions and cell death. *Radiat. Res.*, **176**(5), pp. 587–602, 2011.

136. Carlson, D. J., Stewart, R. D., and Semenenko, V. A., Effects of oxygen on intrinsic radiation sensitivity: A test of the relationship between aerobic and hypoxic linear-quadratic (LQ) model parameters. *Med. Phys.*, **33**(9), pp. 3105–3015, 2006.

137. Furusawa, Y. *et al.*, Inactivation of aerobic and hypoxic cells from three different cell lines by accelerated (3)He-, (12)C- and (20)Ne-ion beams. *Radiat. Res.*, **154**(5), pp. 485–496, 2000.

138. Karger, C. P. *et al.*, Relative biological effectiveness of carbon ions in a rat prostate carcinoma in vivo: comparison of 1, 2, and 6 fractions. *Int. J. Radiat. Oncol. Biol. Phys.*, **86**(3), pp. 450–455, 2013.

139. Goodhead, D. T., Initial events in the cellular effects of ionizing radiations: clustered damage in DNA. *Int. J. Radiat. Biol.*, **65**(1), pp. 7–17, 1994.

140. Hirayama, R., *et al.*, Repair kinetics of DNA-DSB induced by X-rays or carbon ions under oxic and hypoxic conditions. *J. Radiat. Res.*, **46**(3), pp. 325–332, 2005.

141. Ward, J. F., The complexity of DNA damage: relevance to biological consequences. *Int. J. Radiat. Biol.*, **66**(5), pp. 427–432, 1994.

142. Pinto, M., Prise, K. M., and Michael, B. D., Evidence for complexity at the nanometer scale of radiation-induced DNA DSBs as a determinant of rejoining kinetics. *Radiat. Res.*, **164**(1), pp. 73–85, 2005.

143. Radford, I. R., DNA lesion complexity and induction of apoptosis by ionizing radiation. *Int. J. Radiat. Biol.*, **78**(6), pp. 457–466, 2002.

144. Blakely, E. A., *Current issues in low and high LET medical radiobiology hadrontherapy in oncology, Excerpta Medica, Int. Congr. Series 1077,* pp. 693–701, 1994.

145. Tobias, C. A. *et al.*, *Radiobiological Basis for Heavy-Ion Therapy in: Treatment of Radioresistant Cancers,* eds. Abe, M., Sakamoto, K., and Phillips., T. J. 1979: Elsevier, North Holland. p. 159.

146. Weber, U., and Kraft, G., Comparison of carbon ions versus protons. *Cancer J.* **15**(4), pp. 325–332, 2009.

147. Tobias, C. A. *et al.*, Molecular and cellular radiobiology of heavy ions. *Int. J. Radiat. Oncol. Phys.*, **8**(12), pp. 2109–2120, 1982.

148. Steel, G. G., McMillan, T. J., and Peacock, J. H., The 5Rs of radiobiology. *Int. J. Radiat. Biol.*, **56**(6), pp. 1045–1048, 1989.

149. Takahashi, Y. *et al.*, Heavy ion irradiation inhibits in vitro angiogenesis even at sublethal dose. *Cancer. Res.*, **63**(14), pp. 4253–4257, 2003.

150. Scifoni, E. *et al.*, Including oxygen enhancement ratio in ion beam treatment planning: model implementation and experimental verification. *Phys. Med. Biol.*, **58**(11), pp. 3871–3895, 2013.

151. Tobias, C. A. *et al.*, Radiological physics characteristics of the extracted heavy ion beams of the bevatron. *Science*, **174**(14), pp. 1131–1134, 1971.

152. Kamp, F. *et al.*, Fast Biological Modeling for Voxel-based Heavy Ion Treatment Planning Using the Mechanistic Repair-Misrepair-Fixation Model and Nuclear Fragment Spectra. *Int. J. Radiat. Oncol. Biol. Phys.,* **93**(3), pp. 557–568, 2015.

153. Kraft, G., The radiobiological and physical basis for radiotherapy with protons and heavier ions. *Strahlenther. Onkol.*, **166**(1), pp. 10–13, 1990.

154. Dale, R. G., Jones, B., and Carabe-Fernandez, A., Why more needs to be known about RBE effects in modern radiotherapy. *Appl. Radiat. Isotopes.*, **67**(3), pp. 387–392, 2009.

155. Kraft, G., Tumor therapy with heavy charged particles. *Progress in Particle and Nuclear Physics* (45), pp. S473–S544, 2000.

156. Kamada, T. *et al.*, Carbon ion radiotherapy in Japan: an assessment of 20 years of clinical experience. *Lancet Oncol.*, **16**(2), pp. e93–e100, 2015.

157. Rieken, S. *et al.*, Proton and carbon ion radiotherapy for primary brain tumors delivered with active raster scanning at the Heidelberg Ion Therapy Center (HIT): early treatment results and study concepts. *Radiat. Oncol.*, **7**, p. 41, 2012.

158. Jensen, A. D. *et al.*, COSMIC: A Regimen of Intensity Modulated Radiation Therapy Plus Dose-Escalated, Raster-Scanned Carbon Ion Boost for Malignant Salivary Gland Tumors: Results of the Prospective Phase 2 Trial. *Int. J. Radiat. Oncol. Biol. Phys.,* **93**(1), pp. 37–46, 2015.

159. Zips, D. *et al.*, Exploratory prospective trial of hypoxia-specific PET imaging during radiochemotherapy in patients with locally advanced head-and-neck cancer. *Radiother. Oncol.*, **105**(1), pp. 21–28, 2012.

160. Askoxylakis, V. *et al.*, Multimodal hypoxia imaging and intensity modulated radiation therapy for unresectable non-small-cell lung cancer: the HIL trial. *Radiat. Oncol.*, **7**, p. 157, 2012.

161. Kikuchi, M. *et al.*, 18F-fluoromisonidazole positron emission tomography before treatment is a predictor of radiotherapy outcome and survival prognosis in patients with head and neck squamous cell carcinoma. *Ann. Nucl. Med.*, **25**(9), pp. 625–33, 2011.

162. Yamane, T. *et al.*, Reduction of [(18)F]fluoromisonidazole uptake after neoadjuvant chemotherapy for head and neck squamous cell carcinoma. *Mol. Imaging. Biol.*, **13**(2), pp. 227–231, 2011.

163. Gagel, B. *et al.*, [18F] fluoromisonidazole and [18F] fluorodeoxyglucose positron emission tomography in response evaluation after chemo-/radiotherapy of non-small-cell lung cancer: a feasibility study. *BMC Cancer*, **6**, p. 51, 2006.

164. Zimny, M. *et al.*, FDG — a marker of tumour hypoxia? A comparison with [18F]fluoromisonidazole and pO2-polarography in metastatic head and neck cancer. *Eur. J. Nucl. Med. Mol. Im.*, **33**(12), pp. 1426–1431, 2006.

165. Eschmann, S. M. *et al.*, Prognostic impact of hypoxia imaging with 18F-misonidazole PET in non-small cell lung cancer and head and neck cancer before radiotherapy. *J. Nucl. Med.*, **46**(2), pp. 253–260, 2005.

166. Hicks, R. J. *et al.*, Utility of FMISO PET in advanced head and neck cancer treated with chemoradiation incorporating a hypoxia-targeting chemotherapy agent. *Eur. J. Nucl. Med. Mol. Im.*, **32**(12), pp. 1384–1391, 2005.

167. Thorwarth, D. *et al.*, Combined uptake of [18F]FDG and [18F]FMISO correlates with radiation therapy outcome in head-and-neck cancer patients. *Radiother. Oncol.*, **80**(2), pp. 151–156, 2006.

168. Ali, R. *et al.*, 18F-EF5 PET Is Predictive of Response to Fractionated Radiotherapy in Preclinical Tumor Models. *PLoS One*, **10**(10), pp. e0139425, 2015.

169. Tran, L. B. *et al.*, Potential role of hypoxia imaging using (18)F-FAZA PET to guide hypoxia-driven interventions (carbogen breathing or dose escalation) in radiation therapy. *Radiother. Oncol.*, **113**(2), pp. 204–209, 2014.

170. Lee, S. T., and Scott, A. M., Hypoxia positron emission tomography imaging with 18f-fluoromisonidazole. *Semin. Nucl. Med.*, **37**(6), pp. 451–461, 2007.

171. Rajendran, J. G. *et al.*, Tumor hypoxia imaging with [F-18] fluoromisonidazole positron emission tomography in head and neck cancer. *Clin. Cancer Res.*, **12**(18), pp. 5435–5441, 2006.

172. Gagel, B. *et al.*, pO(2) Polarography versus positron emission tomography ([[(18)F] fluoromisonidazole, [(18)F]-2-fluoro-2'-deoxyglucose). An

appraisal of radiotherapeutically relevant hypoxia. *Strahlenther. Onkol.*, **180**(10), pp. 616–622, 2004.

173. Goodhead, D. T., The initial physical damage produced by ionizing radiations. *Int. J. Radiat. Biol.*, **56**(5), pp. 623–634, 1989.

174. Braby, L. A., Phenomenological models. *Basic Life Sci.*, **58**, pp. 339–361; discussion 361–365, 1991.

175. Curtis, S. B., Mechanistic models. *Basic Life Sci.*, **58**, pp. 367–382; discussion 382–386, 1991.

176. Whitaker, S. J., and McMillan, T. J., Oxygen effect for DNA double-strand break induction determined by pulsed-field gel electrophoresis. *Int. J. Radiat. Biol.*, **61**(1), pp. 29–41, 1992.

177. Prise, K. M. *et al.*, The irradiation of V79 mammalian cells by protons with energies below 2 MeV. Part II. Measurement of oxygen enhancement ratios and DNA damage. *Int. J. Radiat. Biol.*, **58**(2), pp. 261–277, 1990.

178. Nygren, J., and Ahnstrom, G., The oxygen effect in permeabilized and histone-depleted cells: an enhanced OER for DNA double-strand breaks, compared to single-strand breaks, is abolished by soluble scavengers. *Int. J. Radiat. Biol.*, **72**(2), pp. 163–170, 1997.

179. Darroudi, F, *et al.*, Biochemical and cytogenetical characterization of Chinese hamster ovary X-ray-sensitive mutant cells xrs 5 and xrs 6. V. The correlation of DNA strand breaks and base damage to chromosomal aberrations and sister-chromatid exchanges induced by X-irradiation. *Mutat. Res.*, **235**(2), pp. 119–127, 1990.

180. Skarsgard, L. D., and Harrison, I., Dose dependence of the oxygen enhancement ratio (OER) in radiation inactivation of Chinese hamster V79–171 cells. *Radiat. Res.*, **127**(3), pp. 243–247, 1991.

181. Dasu, A. and Denekamp, J., New insights into factors influencing the clinically relevant oxygen enhancement ratio. *Radiother. Oncol.*, **46**(3), pp. 269–77, 1998.

182. Jones, B., and Dale, R. G., Mathematical models of tumour and normal tissue response. *Acta. Oncol.*, **38**(7), pp. 883–893, 1999.

183. Nahum, A. E. *et al.*, Incorporating clinical measurements of hypoxia into tumor local control modeling of prostate cancer: implications for the alpha/beta ratio. *Int. J. Radiat. Oncol. Biol. Phys.*, **57**(2), pp. 391–401, 2003.

184. Garcia-Barros, M. *et al.*, Tumor response to radiotherapy regulated by endothelial cell apoptosis. *Science*, **300**(5622), pp. 1155–1159, 2003.

185. Park, H. J. *et al.*, Radiation-induced vascular damage in tumors: implications of vascular damage in ablative hypofractionated radiotherapy (SBRT and SRS). *Radiat. Res.*, **177**(3), pp. 311–327, 2012.

186. Harting, C., Peschke, P., and Karger, C. P., Computer simulation of tumour control probabilities after irradiation for varying intrinsic radio-sensitivity using a single cell based model. *Acta. Oncol.*, **49**(8), pp. 1354–1362, 2010.

187. Shuryak, I. *et al.*, High-dose and fractionation effects in stereotactic radiation therapy: Analysis of tumor control data from 2965 patients. *Radiother. Oncol.*, **115**(3), pp. 327–334, 2015.

188. Lindblom, E. *et al.*, Survival and tumour control probability in tumours with heterogeneous oxygenation: a comparison between the linear-quadratic and the universal survival curve models for high doses. *Acta. Oncol.*, **53**(8), pp. 1035–1040, 2014.

189. Lindblom, E. *et al.*, Treatment fractionation for stereotactic radiotherapy of lung tumours: a modelling study of the influence of chronic and acute hypoxia on tumour control probability. *Radiat. Oncol.*, **9**, p. 149, 2014.

190. Brown, J. M., Brenner, D. J., and Carlson, D. J., Dose escalation, not "new biology," can account for the efficacy of stereotactic body radiation therapy with non-small cell lung cancer. *Int. J. Radiat. Oncol. Biol. Phys.*, **85**(5), pp. 1159–1160, 2013.

191. Guckenberger, M. *et al.*, Applicability of the linear-quadratic formalism for modeling local tumor control probability in high dose per fraction stereotactic body radiotherapy for early stage non-small cell lung cancer. *Radiother. Oncol.*, **109**(1), pp. 13–20, 2013.

192. Suit, H. *et al.*, Clinical implications of heterogeneity of tumor response to radiation therapy. *Radiother. Oncol.*, **25**(4), pp. 251–260, 1992.

193. Roberts, S. A., and Hendry, J. H., A realistic closed-form radiobiological model of clinical tumor-control data incorporating intertumor heterogeneity. *Int. J. Radiat. Oncol. Biol. Phys.*, **41**(3), pp. 689–699, 1998.

194. Agren Cronqvist, A. K., *et al.*, Volume and heterogeneity dependence of the dose-response relationship for head and neck tumours. *Acta. Oncol.*, **34**(6), pp. 851–860, 1995.

# Chapter 2

# Post-translational Modifications of the Hypoxia Inducible Factors

Ian Cartwright and Chuan-Yuan Li*

*Departments of Pharmacology and Cancer Biology,*
*Duke University Medical Center,*
*Durham, NC, USA*
**Chuan.Li@duke.edu*

## 1. Introduction

Oxygen is a key ingredient for life and metazoan organisms face constant changes in oxygen levels at both the macro- and microenvironmental levels. Multicellular organisms have evolved complex pathways to respond to these changes in oxygen levels. The hypoxia inducible factors (HIFs) play a key part in this process.

HIF-1 was first discovered by the identification of a hypoxia response element (HRE) in the 3′ enhancer region of the gene encoding erythropoietin (EPO). EPO is a hormone that stimulates erythrocyte proliferation and undergoes hypoxia-induced transcription.[1,2] Further study of HRE revealed a protein that is bound to HRE under hypoxic conditions; this protein was identified as HIF-1. HIF-1 is a heterodimeric complex consisting of a hypoxia inducible subunit, HIF-1$\alpha$, and a constitutively active subunit HIF-1$\beta$.[3] HIF-1 is the primary regulator of oxygen homeostasis,

49

but is also implicated in angiogenesis, energy metabolism, erythropoiesis, cell proliferation and viability, vascular remodeling, and vasomotor responses.[4] HIF-1 has been shown to activate roughly 60 direct target genes, including genes encoding angiogenic factors, glucose transporters and glycolytic enzymes, survival factors and invasion factors.[5–7] Vascular endothelial growth factor (VEGF) is one of the HIF-1 target genes that is expressed under hypoxic conditions in nearly all cell types, the vast majority of HIF-1 target genes are expressed in a cell-type-specific manner under hypoxic conditions.[8] Despite only directly targeting 60 genes, it is believed that 1–5% of all human genes are expressed in response to hypoxia in a HIF-1 dependent manner.[9]

Since HIF-1's discovery, 2 additional HIF variants, HIF-2 and 3, have been discovered. HIFs 2 and 3 are also composed of two subunits, a constitutively present subunit HIF-2/3$\beta$ and the oxygen-regulated subunit HIF-2/3$\alpha$. HIF-1 is ubiquitously and constitutively expressed in nearly all tissues, whereas, HIF-2 and HIF-3 are more tissue specific.

The activities of HIF factors are mainly regulated through the stabilities of the HIF-$\alpha$ subunits, which are in turn regulated by various post-translational modifications. In this chapter, we will review these modifications and how they influence HIF activities, and efforts to manipulate the modifications for therapeutics development.

## 1.1. HIF-$\alpha$s: A brief introduction

### 1.1.1. *HIF-1$\alpha$*

HIF-1 $\alpha$ is the hypoxic inducible subunit of the HIF-1 heterodimer complex.[3] This protein contains four distinct domains, two transactivation domains (N-terminal and C-terminal), an oxygen-dependent degradation domain (ODD), and a basic helix-loop-helix-Per-ARNT-Sim (bHLH-PAS) domain) In addition, HIF-1$\alpha$, as well as the HIF-2/3$\alpha$, contains two nuclear localization signals (N-NLS and C-NLS) which direct the $\alpha$ subunit to the nucleus.[12] The bHLH-PAS domain is required for the formation of the heterodimer between HIF-1$\alpha$ and HIF-1$\beta$.[13] There are currently five splicing isoforms of HIF-1$\alpha$, HIF-1$\alpha^{FL,736,\ 557,\ 516,\ 785}$.[14] The ODD domain and the COOH-terminal activation domain (CAD) are involved with hypoxia signaling. They are both subject to post-translational modification in an oxygen-dependent manor.[15] In addition to oxygen-dependent post-translational modifications, HIF-1$\alpha$ also undergoes several oxygen-independent modifications, including SUMOylation, S-nitrosylation, and phosphorylation. These post-translational modifications will be covered in more detail later in the chapter. HIF-1$\alpha$ is rapidly degraded, half-life of HIF-1$\alpha$ is <1–5 min, under normoxic conditions and will rapidly accumulate under hypoxic conditions, $O_2$ concentrations of less than 6% trigger accumulation of HIF-1$\alpha$.[3,16,17] When combined, HIF-1$\alpha$'s ability to be regulated in both an oxygen dependent and independent fashion and extremely short half-life allow the cell to exert precise control over HIF-1$\alpha$ levels and its transcriptional activities.

## 1.1.2. *HIF-2$\alpha$*

HIF-2$\alpha$ shares 48% of its amino acid sequence with HIF-1$\alpha$ and accordingly shares several structural and biochemical similarities. HIF-2$\alpha$ differs from HIF-1$\alpha$ the most in the N-TAD region, this region is primarily responsible for target gene specificity.[18] The HIF-2$\alpha$ subunit heterodimerizes with HIF-2$\beta$. This forms the complex HIF-2 and ultimately allows for binding to HRE.[19,20] Unlike HIF-1$\alpha$, HIF-2$\alpha$ is not expressed in all cell types and can be sequestered in the cytoplasm after activation.[21] The N-TAD region of HIF-2$\alpha$ facilitates binding of target genes primarily associated with tumor growth, cell cycle progression, and maintaining stem cell pluripotency.[22] As with HIF-1$\alpha$, HIF-2$\alpha$ contains an ODD containing several proline residues that under normoxic conditions undergo hydroxylation via PHDs resulting in the ultimate degradation of the protein.

## 1.1.3. *HIF-3$\alpha$*

HIF-3$\alpha$ was the third protein in the HIF-1 family to be identified. HIF-3$\alpha$ has not been well studied, but it has been shown that a splice variant of HIF-3$\alpha$ has the ability to bind to and inhibit HIF-1$\alpha$.[23,24] Additionally, HIF-3$\alpha$ lacks the oxygen sensing domain found in HIF-1 and HIF-2$\alpha$.

## 2. Post-translational Modifications of HIF-$\alpha$s

Post-translational modifications play a key role in regulating the steady-state levels and transcriptional activities of the HIF-$\alpha$s. There is a multitude of post-translational modifications that participate in regulating HIF-$\alpha$s (Fig. 1). In the ensuing sections, we will review the major known post-translational modifications of HIF-$\alpha$s.

## 2.1. Hydroxylation of proline 402/564

HIF-1 is primarily regulated via a von Hippel–Lindau (pVHL)-mediated ubiquitin-proteasome pathway which relies on the hydroxylation of HIF-$\alpha$.[25] Under normal circumstances, prolines, conserved in both HIF-1/2$\alpha$, are rapidly hydroxylated by a family of 2-oxoglutarate (2-OG)-dependent dioxygenases (proline 402 and 564 for HIF-1$\alpha$ and proline 405/531 for HIF-2$\alpha$) within the ODD.[26–30] In HIF-1$\alpha$, the hydroxylation of Pro402/564 results in the interaction between HIF-1$\alpha$ and pVHL ubiquitin (UB) E3 ligase complex resulting ubiquitination and ultimate degradation. A mutation in both proline residues results in the disruption in interaction of HIF-1$\alpha$ and pVHL UB E3 ligase complex resulting in increased HIF-1$\alpha$ stabilization. Additionally, a mutation in either proline

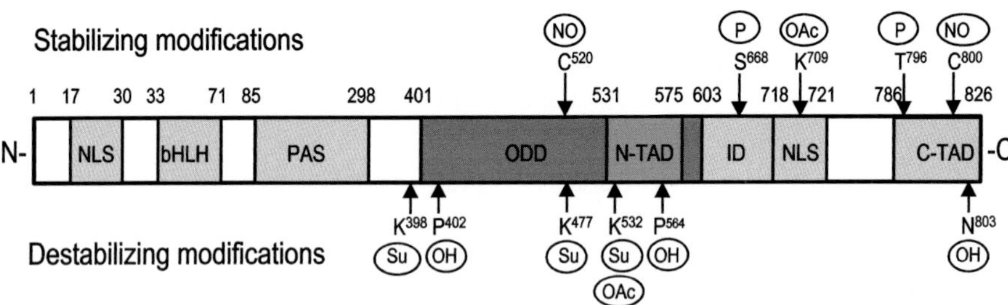


Fig. 1.   Domain structure and post-translational modifications sites. Numbers indicate amino acid bordering the domains. The amino acid with arrows indicate sites of amino acid modifications. NLS, nuclear localization signal; bHLH, basic helix-loop-helix domain; PAS, Per-ARNT-Sim homology domain; N-,C-TAD, N- and C- terminal transactivation domains; ID, inhibitory domain. Labels in circles indicate post-translational modifications. OH, hydroxilation; Su, sumoylation; OAc, acetylation; NO, nitrosylation; P, phosphorylation.

alone only partially stabilizes HIF-1$\alpha$ under normoxia conditions.[27] The human HIF-1$\alpha$ dioxygenase are known as either prolyl hydroxylase domain (PHD), HIF-prolyl hydroxylase (HPH), or Egg-laying Nine (EGLN). There have been three isoforms of PHD identified, PHD1/2/3.[29-31] PHD2 has the highest specificity for the hydroxylation of HIF-1$\alpha$.[32] PHDs require the presence of oxygen, $Fe^{2+}$ and ascorbate as cofactors in order to hydroxylate the proline residues in HIF-1$\alpha$. The requirement of oxygen allows for hydroxylation of proline 402/564 to regulate HIF-1$\alpha$ stability in an oxygen dependent manor, in the presence of oxygen HIF-1$\alpha$ is rendered instable whereas the lack of oxygen prevents hydroxylation and stabilization of HIF-1$\alpha$.[29-31] In addition to mutations to proline 402/564, inhibition of PHDs by 2-OG analogs can significantly increase the half-life of HIF-1$\alpha$ under normoxia conditions.[33] These PHDs are the primary regulatory aspect of HIF-1$\alpha$ due to the absolute requirement of oxygen for their function.[30] In the presence of oxygen, PHDs are highly active and quickly hydroxylate the prolines within HIF-1$\alpha$ creating a recognition signal for the binding of pVHL and the subsequent ubiquitination, followed by degradation of HIF-1$\alpha$.[34,35]

## 2.1.1. *Hydroxylation of asparagine by FIH-1*

In contrast to hydroxylation of proline 402/564 in HIF-1$\alpha$, hydroxylation of asparaginyl residue (Asn803 in HIF-1$\alpha$ and Asn851 in HIF-2$\alpha$) does not affect the stabilization of HIF-1$\alpha$, but instead effects its' transcriptional activation.[36-38] Under normoxic conditions, the Asn803 residue in the C-TAD region of HIF-1$\alpha$ is hydroxylated by factor inhibiting HIF-1 (FIH-1). This hydroxylation prevents the interaction of HIF-1$\alpha$ with a transcriptional coactivator, CBP/p300.[15,39,40] Like PHD's, FIH-1, a 2-OG-dependent dioxygenase, requires oxygen, $Fe^{2+}$, and ascorbate as cofactors allowing FIH-1 to serve as a second oxygen sensor.[41] It should be noted that FIH has a Michaelis constant ($K_M$) roughly three times lower then PHD, this allows FIH to remain active in $O_2$ concentrations which would inactivate PHD. This differential inactivation allows HIF-1$\alpha$ to stabilize and localize to the nucleus without being activated.[42] It appears that FIH-1 hydroxylation of HIF-1$\alpha$ at Asn803 acts as an inhibitor of HIF-1$\alpha$ activity and is not necessarily involved in HIF-1$\alpha$

stability. Not only does hydroxylation of Asn803 inhibit transactivation of HIF-1, but it has been shown that FIH-1 and HIF-1 can form a tertiary structure with pVHL; this can lead to the eventual degradation of HIF-1$\alpha$.

It is interesting to note that HIF-2$\alpha$ has the ability to be hydroxylated by FIH-1; however, FIH-1 has been shown to preferentially hydroxylate HIF-1$\alpha$ over HIF-2$\alpha$. HIF-1$\alpha$ contains a valine near Asn803 whereas HIF-2$\alpha$ contains an alanine near Asn851 and it is believed that FIH-1 binding is enhanced by the valine residue.[43]

## 2.1.2. *Polyubiquitination of HIF-$\alpha$ by pVHL*

A key step in the degradation of HIF-1$\alpha$ under normoxia conditions is the polyubiquitination of hydroxylated HIF-1$\alpha$. The hydroxyprolines are recognized and bound by pVHL, once bound the HIF-1$\alpha$/pVHL complex associates with proteins elongin C, elongin B, cullin-2 and Rbx1 to form the VCB-Cul2 E3 ligase complex which causes polyubiquitination of HIF-1$\alpha$.[34,44,45] Interestingly, pVHL was first identified in VHL disease, an inherited human cancer syndrome characterized by multiple tumors at multiple sites.[46] When pVHL is lacking, both HIF-1$\alpha$ and HIF-2$\alpha$ are stable and active under normoxia, resulting in the expression of hypoxia-inducible genes under normal oxygen concentrations.[47]

Recent studies have also shown that deubiquitinases oppose the function of E3 ligases by hydrolyzing UB chains. More specifically, UB-specific protease 20 binds pVHL resulting in deubiquitination and stabilization of HIF-1$\alpha$.[48,49] More interesting is the deubiquitinase Cezanne, a Lys11 linkage-specific ovarian tumor deubiquitinase, essential for HIF-1$\alpha$ protein stability independent of hydroxylase and proteasome activity. Loss of Cezanne resulted in an overall decrease in HIF-1$\alpha$ stability and transcriptional activity under hypoxic conditions. Additionally, it was shown that HIF-1$\alpha$ transcriptional activity in Cezanne null cells in the absence of proteasome activity or hydroxylases was decreased.[50]

## 2.1.3. *Acetylation of HIF-$\alpha$s*

The ODD domain of HIF-1$\alpha$ contains a lysine residue (Lys532) which can be acetylated by an acetyltransferase known as arrest-defective-1 (ARD1).

ARD1 acetylates HIF-1$\alpha$ by transferring an acetyl group from Ac-CoA to Lys532. The acetylation of Lys532 increases HIF-1$\alpha$ interaction with pVHL, and thus destabilizing HIF-1$\alpha$. It has been shown that a K532R mutant stabilizes HIF-1$\alpha$ and decreases its interaction with pVHL.[51] Unlike PHD and FIH, ARD1 operates in an oxygen independent fashion.

An additional route by which HIF-1$\alpha$ is modulated via acetylation is by sirtuins, a family of redoxsensitive, NAD$^+$-dependent deacetylases and/or ADP-ribosyltransferases, the mammalian homolog being SIRT1-7.[52] SIRT1-7 binds to HIF-2$\alpha$ where it deacetylates the lysine residues in the N-TAD domain, enhancing HIF-2$\alpha$ transcriptional activity both *in vitro* and *in vivo*.[53]

A recent study has shown that HIF-1$\alpha$ can also be acetylated at Lys709. Lys709 is acetylated in a p300 dependent manor. Acetylation of HIF-1$\alpha$ is facilitated by p300 results in the stabilization and an increase in HIF-1$\alpha$ transcriptional activity. K709A mutants have been shown to stabilize HIF-1$\alpha$, resulting in decreased polyubiquitination and less dependency on p300.[54] Additionally, it has been shown that cancer cells expressing a K709A mutation are more transcriptionally active and less sensitive to hypoxia-induced growth arrest than cells containing a wild-type Hif-1$\alpha$.[54]

## 2.1.4. *Phosphorylation of HIF-1$\alpha$ by MAPK*

It has been shown that HIF-1$\alpha$ is phosphorylated by the mitogen-activated protein kinase (MAPK) at threonine 796.[55-57] HIF-1$\alpha$/HIF-2$\alpha$ are both phosphorylated by p42/44 and p38 kinases. Inhibition of either of these kinases leads to a loss in HIF-1$\alpha$/2$\alpha$-mediated reporter gene expression.[58,59] One proposed mechanism by which threonine 796 phosphorylation increases HIF-1 activity is that Hif-1$\beta$ preferentially binds to phosphorylated Hif-1$\alpha$.[60] In addition to increasing binding of HIF-1$\alpha$ and HIF-1$\beta$, it has also been shown that phosphorylation increases interaction between HIF-1$\alpha$ and p300, resulting in increased transcriptional activity. Recent studies have also shown that in addition to threonine 796, HIF-1$\alpha$ can also be phosphorylated at serine 668 by cyclin dependent kinase 1 (CDK1). Phosphorylation of serine 668 results in stabilization of HIF-1$\alpha$ under normoxic conditions. HIF-1$\alpha$ containing a phosphor-mimetic at Ser668 is significantly more stable under normoxic and hypoxic conditions and the mutants also display increased tumor angiogenesis, proliferation, and tumor growth *in vivo*.[61]

Interestingly, phosphorylation of HIF-1$\alpha$ and HIF-2$\alpha$ result in activation of two cohorts of overlapping but non-redundant genes. Additionally, it has been shown that phosphorylation of HIF-1$\alpha$ represses that MYC-dependent expression of nibrin, a DNA damage response protein, by displacing the SP1 transcription factor from MYC. Whereas, HIF-2$\alpha$ is inhibited from interacting with SP1 when Thr324 is phosphorylated by protein kinase D1.[62]

## 2.1.5. *SUMOylation*

It has been shown that small UB-like modifier (SUMO)-1 expression is increased during hypoxia, this increase in SUMO-1 leads to the SUMOylation and stabilization of HIF-1$\alpha$.[63,64] HIF-1$\alpha$ is SUMOylated at Lys398/477 by SUMO-1. These Lys residues are located in the ODD domain of HIF-1$\alpha$ and SUMOylation of these lysines results in stabilization of HIF-1$\alpha$ under normoxic conditions.[64,65] It has been shown that HIF-1$\beta$ can be SUMOylated by SUMO-1 at Lys245. Lys245 is located within the PAS domain of HIF-1$\alpha$; unlike HIF-1$\alpha$, SUMOylation of this Lys resulted in decreased transcriptional activity.[66]

However, there has been a recent finding which indicates that SUMOylation of HIF-1$\alpha$ can also lead to HIF-1$\alpha$ degradation. Hypoxia-induced HIF-1$\alpha$ SUMOylation can promote hydroxyproline-independent HIF-1$\alpha$-pVHL E3 ligase complex binding, ultimately leading to HIF-1$\alpha$ ubiquitylation and proteasomal degradation.[65]

## 2.1.6. *S-Nitrosylation*

It has been shown that exposure to various growth factors, insulin-like growth factor, epidermal growth factor, or platelet-derived growth factor, results in the stabilization of HIF-1$\alpha$ under normoxic conditions. HIF-1$\alpha$ can be nitrosylated at Cys800, increasing transactivation of HIF-1 through its interaction with CBP/p300.[67] Under normoxic conditions, cellular exposure to nitric oxide leads to HIF-1$\alpha$ stabilization and transcriptional activation.[68,69] In addition, HIF-1$\alpha$ can be S-nitrosylated at cys520, which is located in the ODD region of HIF-1$\alpha$, this S-nitrosylation disrupts the prolylhydroxylases which leads to the stabilization of HIF-1$\alpha$.[69]

It has also been shown that NO is required for activation of HIF-1 in macrophages during bacterial infection.[70] In the tumor microenvironment, it was shown that NO was a key mediator of tumor associate macrophages (TAM) induced tumor angiogenesis.[69]

## 3. Targeting Post-translational Modifications in Tumor Therapy

Tumors are often associated with both transient and chronic hypoxia and because of this, HIF-1 plays a critical role in tumor progression. HIF-1 has the ability to activate angiogenic growth factors, glucose transporters, and glycolytic enzymes. The loss or dysfunction of HIF-1$\alpha$ has been shown to inhibit tumor growth, whereas overexpression of HIF-1$\alpha$ promotes tumor growth and progression.[71–74] HIF-1$\alpha$ overexpression in tumors can be the result of tumor hypoxia, nitrogen species, loss of function of a tumor suppressor, gain of function of an oncogene, or proteins encoded by transforming viruses.

Therapies targeting post-translational modifications of HIF-1$\alpha$ offer a unique opportunity to treat tumors over expressing HIF-1$\alpha$. One study has shown that bortezomib, a proteasome inhibitor, has the ability to inhibit HIF-1 activity. It was shown that bortezomib was able to reinforce the interaction of FIH-1 with the CAD domain of HIF-1$\alpha$, even at decreased $O_2$ concentrations, ultimately inhibiting recruitment of the p300 coactivator.[75]

Another interesting approach is by targeting HIF-1$\alpha$ stability under both normoxic and hypoxic conditions. There have also been several reports that have shown that treatment with histone deacetylase inhibitors also inhibit HIF-1$\alpha$ activity. Histone deacetylase inhibitors are able to inhibit HIF-1$\alpha$ activity by promoting pVHL binding and UB-independent proteasomal degradation.[76–78] In a recent study, it has also been shown that Hif-1$\alpha$ stability can be altered by targeting CDK1. It was shown that CDK1 inhibitors were able to enhance proteasomal degradation of HIF-1$\alpha$ by inhibiting phosphorylation of Ser668.[61]

In addition, inhibitors of nitric oxide syntheses, which participate in hypoxia-independent stabilization of HIF-1$\alpha$, can potently enhance radiotherapy of cancer by decreasing tumor HIF-1$\alpha$ levels and inhibiting angiogenesis.[69]

Finally, HIF-1$\alpha$ stability can be altered by inhibiting chaperone proteins. One such protein, is heat-shock protein 90 (HSP90), another potential target for inhibiting HIF-1. Two drugs, geldanamycin and KF58333, have both been shown to destabilize HIF-1$\alpha$ by inhibiting HSP90 binding.[79,80]

## 3.1. Stabilization of HIF-$\alpha$ through manipulating its post-translational modifications for vascular and tissue regeneration

There is a significant body of work highlighting the potential pharmacological advantages of activating HIF-1. Being able to selectively activate HIF-1 under nomoxic condition has the potential to greatly improve wound healing and vascular regeneration.[81] Currently, there is no evidence that dysregulation of HIF is sufficient to cause tumorigenesis. Coupling this with the relatively short duration of therapy for wound healing, HIF makes an excellent target for potential therapies when dealing with chronic wounds.[82,83]

Chronic wounds, characterized by persistent inflammation and chronic ischemia, appear to be the best targets for HIF-1$\alpha$ therapies.[84] One type of chronic wound which often heals very slowly are 2$^{nd}$ and 3$^{rd}$ degree burns. A recent study showed that aged mice injected with a stable HIF-1$\alpha$ mutant protein and bone marrow-derived angiogenic cells experienced more rapid wound closure of burns than the controlled aged mice.[85] Diabetic individuals often suffer from chronic wounds which are extremely slow to heal. It has been shown that both stabilization and over expression of HIF-1 through gene therapy improves wound healing in aged diabetic mice.[86,87] Further research has provided evidence that diabetic tissues contain methylglyoxalation events on HIF-1 transcriptional cofactor p300; this modification prevents assembly of the transcriptome and ultimate activation of HIF-1$\alpha$ responsive genes. In aged tissue, it has been shown that several PHD's are upregulated resulting in an overall decrease in HIF-1$\alpha$ stabilization. Both aged and diabetic tissues suffer from a decreased HIF-1 activity and inability to adapt to wound associated hypoxia.[88,89]

There is a fine line between therapeutic over expression of HIF-1$\alpha$ and levels of HIF-1$\alpha$ resulting in adverse outcomes, elevated levels of HIF-1$\alpha$ for an extended period of time can result in detrimental outcomes in wound healing. Consistent over expression of HIF-1$\alpha$ is often observed in keloid and scleroderma tissues, two painful skin conditions arising from faulty wound repair.[90,91] The potential to target post-translational modifications would allow for the rapid accumulation of HIF-1$\alpha$ for a specific amount of time before allowing it to return to basal levels. The most promising therapy is the use of PHD inhibitors to increase the stability of HIF-1 and promote expression of downstream HIF-1 targets.[92] These types of drugs have had success in improving diabetic ischemic wounds in mice and are currently undergoing clinical trials for treatment of human-ischemia-based wounds.[93]

Currently, there are several PHD inhibitors being researched for their effects on wound healing and angiogenesis stimulation. One such PHD inhibitor, simvastatin, was shown to increase angiogenesis after myocardial infarction in diabetic rats. Rats treated with simvastatin were observed having decreases in PHD-3 expression and better prognostic outcomes than control rats.[94] Two other PHD inhibitors, dimethyl–oxalylglycine (DMOG) and desferrioxamine (DFX), have been shown to increase HIF-1$\alpha$ expression by inhibiting PHD's expression in diabetic mice.[92]

## 4.1. Summary

As key mediators of mammalian cellular response to low oxygen tension, HIF factors regulate a wide range of biological processes such as angiogenesis, glucose metabolism, cellular survival, etc. The main mechanism of HIF regulation is through post-translational modifications of HIF-$\alpha$. In this chapter, we reviewed some of the most important post-translational modifications that regulate HIF-1$\alpha$ stability. Many of those modifications regulate HIF-1$\alpha$ activities under hypoxic conditions while others influence its activities in a hypoxia-independent manner. Why does HIF-1$\alpha$ possess so many different post translational modifications (PTMs)? We speculate that it is caused by (1) the necessity for HIF-$\alpha$ to respond to or associate with different upstream factors or environmental conditions; (2) the necessity for HIF-$\alpha$ to be regulated with a great degree of precision under many different conditions.

The existence of different PTMs allow for the development of different therapeutics to regulate cellular HIF-1$\alpha$ levels for treatment, such as inhibiting cancer growth or promoting wound healing.

In summary, PTMs play a crucial role in regulating HIF activities. It is likely that new PTMs or novel functions of the already identified PTMs will be revealed in future studies.

# References


1. Goldberg, M. A., Dunning, S. P., and Bunn, H. F., Regulation of the erythropoietin gene: Evidence that the oxygen sensor is a heme protein. *Science*, **242**(4884), pp. 1412–1415, 1988.
2. Semenza, G. L., Nejfelt, M. K., Chi, S. M., and Antonarakis, S. E., Hypoxia-inducible nuclear factors bind to an enhancer element located 3′ to the human erythropoietin gene in *P. Natl. Acad. Sci.*, **88**(13), pp. 5680–5684, 1991.
3. Wang, G. L., Jiang, B. H., Rue, E. A., and Semenza, G. L., Hypoxia-inducible factor 1 is a basic-helix-loop-helix-PAS heterodimer regulated by cellular O2 tension, in *P. Natl. Acad. Sci.*, **92**(12), pp. 5510–5514, 1995.
4. Semenza, G. L., and HIF-1: Mediator of physiological and pathophysiological responses to hypoxia. *J. Appl. Physiol.*, **88**(4), pp. 1474–1480, 2000.
5. Semenza, G. L., and Wang, G. L., A nuclear factor induced by hypoxia via de novo protein synthesis binds to the human erythropoietin gene enhancer at a site required for transcriptional activation. *Mol. Cell. Biol.*, **12**(12), pp. 5447–5454, 1992.
6. Krishnamachary, B., Berg-Dixon, S., Kelly, B., Agani, F., Feldser, D., Ferreira, G. *et al.*, Regulation of colon carcinoma cell invasion by hypoxia-inducible factor 1. *Cancer Res.*, **63**(5), pp. 1138–1143, 2003.
7. Pennacchietti, S., Michieli, P., Galluzzo, M., Mazzone, M., Giordano, S., and Comoglio, P. M., Hypoxia promotes invasive growth by transcriptional activation of the met protooncogene. *Cancer Cell*, **3**(4), pp. 347–346, 2003.
8. Iyer, N. V., Kotch, L. E., Agani, F., Leung, S. W., Laughner, E., Wenger, R. H. *et al.*, Cellular and developmental control of O2 homeostasis by hypoxia-inducible factor 1 alpha. *Gene. Dev.*, **12**(2), pp. 149–162, 1998.
9. Carmeliet, P., Dor, Y., Herbert, J. M., Fukumura, D., Brusselmans, K., Dewerchin, M. *et al.*, Role of HIF-1alpha in hypoxia-mediated apoptosis, cell

proliferation and tumour angiogenesis. *Nature*, **394**(6692), pp. 485–490, 1998.

10. Ruas, J. L., Poellinger, L., and Pereira, T., Functional analysis of hypoxia-inducible factor-1 alpha-mediated transactivation. Identification of amino acid residues critical for transcriptional activation and/or interaction with CREB-binding protein. *J. Biol. Chem.*, Oct 11; **277**(41), pp. 38723–38730, 2002.

11. Pugh, C. W., O'Rourke, J. F., Nagao, M., Gleadle, J. M., and Ratcliffe, P. J., Activation of hypoxia-inducible factor-1; definition of regulatory domains within the alpha subunit. *J. Biol. Chem.*, **272**(17), pp. 11205–11214, 1997.

12. Zagorska, A., and Dulak, J., HIF-1: the knowns and unknowns of hypoxia sensing. *Acta Biochim. Pol.*, **51**(3), pp. 563–585, 2004.

13. Crews, S. T., Control of cell lineage-specific development and transcription by bHLH-PAS proteins. *Gene. Dev.*, **12**(5), pp. 607–620, 1998.

14. Gothie, E., Richard, D. E., Berra, E., Pages, G., and Pouyssegur, J., Identification of alternative spliced variants of human hypoxia-inducible factor-1alpha. *J. Biol. Chem.*, **275**(10), pp. 6922–6927, 2000.

15. Lando, D., Peet, D. J., Whelan, D. A., Gorman, J. J., and Whitelaw, M. L., Asparagine hydroxylation of the HIF transactivation domain a hypoxic switch. *Science*, 1; **295**(5556), pp. 858–861, 2002.

16. Jewell, U. R., Kvietikova, I., Scheid, A., Bauer, C., Wenger, R. H., and Gassmann, M. Induction of HIF-1alpha in response to hypoxia is instantaneous. *FASEB J.*, **15**(7), pp. 1312–1314, 2001.

17. Yu, A. Y., Frid, M. G., Shimoda, L. A., Wiener, C. M., Stenmark, K., and Semenza, G. L., Temporal, spatial, and oxygen-regulated expression of hypoxia-inducible factor-1 in the lung. *Am. J. Physiol.*, **275**(4.1), pp. L818–826, 1998.

18. Hu, C. J., Sataur, A., Wang, L., Chen, H., and Simon, M. C., The N-terminal transactivation domain confers target gene specificity of hypoxia-inducible factors HIF-1alpha and HIF-2alpha. *Mol. Biol. Cell.*, **18**(11), pp. 4528–4542, 2007.

19. Ema, M., Taya, S., Yokotani, N., Sogawa, K., Matsuda, Y., and Fujii-Kuriyama, Y. A novel bHLH-PAS factor with close sequence similarity to hypoxia-inducible factor 1alpha regulates the VEGF expression and is potentially involved in lung and vascular development. *P. Natl. Acad. Sci. USA.*, **94**(9), pp. 4273–4278, 1997.

20. Tian, H., McKnight, S. L., and Russell, D. W., Endothelial PAS domain protein 1 (EPAS1), a transcription factor selectively expressed in endothelial cells. *Gene. Dev.*, **11**(1), pp. 72–82, 1997.

21. Park, S. K., Dadak, A. M., Haase, V. H., Fontana, L., Giaccia, A. J., and Johnson, R. S., Hypoxia-induced gene expression occurs solely through the

action of hypoxia-inducible factor 1alpha (HIF-1alpha): role of cytoplasmic trapping of HIF-2alpha. *Mol. Cell. Biol.*, **23**(14), pp. 4959–4971, 2003.

22. Gordan, J. D., Bertout, J. A., Hu, C. J., Diehl, J.A. and Simon, M. C., HIF-2alpha promotes hypoxic cell proliferation by enhancing c-myc transcriptional activity. *Cancer Cell*, **11**(4), pp. 335–347, 2007.

23. Gu, Y. Z., Moran, S. M., Hogenesch, J. B., Wartman, L. and Bradfield, C. A., Molecular characterization and chromosomal localization of a third alpha-class hypoxia inducible factor subunit, HIF3alpha. *Gene Expression*, **7**(3), pp. 205–213, 1998.

24. Makino, Y., Kanopka, A., Wilson, W. J., Tanaka, H., and  Poellinger, L., Inhibitory PAS domain protein (IPAS) is a hypoxia-inducible splicing variant of the hypoxia-inducible factor-3alpha locus. *J. Biol. Chem.*, **277**(36), pp. 32405–32408, 2002.

25. Huang, L. E., Arany, Z., Livingston, D. M., and Bunn, H. F., Activation of hypoxia-inducible transcription factor depends primarily upon redox-sensitive stabilization of its alpha subunit. *J. Biol. Chem.*, **271**(50), pp. 32253–32259, 1996.

26. Srinivas, V., Zhang, L. P., Zhu, X. H., and Caro, J., Characterization of an oxygen/redox-dependent degradation domain of hypoxia-inducible factor alpha (HIF-alpha) proteins. *Biochem. Bioph. Res. Co.*, **260**(2), pp. 557–561, 1999.

27. Masson, N., Willam, C., Maxwell, P. H., Pugh, C. W., and Ratcliffe, P. J., Independent function of two destruction domains in hypoxia-inducible factor-alpha chains activated by prolyl hydroxylation. *EMBO J.*, **20**(18), pp. 5197–5206, 2001.

28. Masson, N., and Ratcliffe, P. J., HIF prolyl and asparaginyl hydroxylases in the biological response to intracellular O(2) levels. *J. Cell Sci.*, **116**(15), pp. 3041–3049, 2003.

29. Bruick, R. K., and McKnight, S. L., A conserved family of prolyl-4-hydroxylases that modify HIF. *Science*, **294**(5545), pp. 1337–1340, 2001.

30. Epstein, A. C., Gleadle, J. M., McNeill, L. A., Hewitson, K. S., O'Rourke, J., Mole, D. R. *et al.*, C. elegans EGL-9 and mammalian homologs define a family of dioxygenases that regulate HIF by prolyl hydroxylation. *Cell*, **107**(1), pp. 43–54, 2001.

31. Huang, J., Zhao, Q., Mooney, S. M., and Lee, F. S., Sequence determinants in hypoxia-inducible factor-1alpha for hydroxylation by the prolyl hydroxylases PHD1, PHD2, and PHD3. *J. Biol. Chem.*, **277**(42), pp. 39792–39800, 2002.

32. Hewitson, K. S., McNeill, L. A., and Schofield, C. J., Modulating the hypoxia-inducible factor signaling pathway: applications from cardiovascular disease to cancer. *Curr. Pharm. Design*, **10**(8), pp. 821–833, 2004.

33. Ivan, M., Haberberger, T., Gervasi, D. C., Michelson, K. S., Gunzler, V., Kondo, K. *et al.*, Biochemical purification and pharmacological inhibition of a mammalian prolyl hydroxylase acting on hypoxia-inducible factor. *P. Natl. Acad. Sci. USA.*, **99**(21), pp. 13459–13464, 2002.

34. Ivan, M., Kondo, K., Yang, H., Kim, W., Valiando, J., Ohh, M., *et al.*, HIFalpha targeted for VHL-mediated destruction by proline hydroxylation: implications for O2 sensing. *Science*, **292**(5516), pp. 464–468, 2001.

35. Jaakkola, P., Mole, D. R., Tian, Y. M., Wilson, M. I., Gielbert, J., Gaskell, S.J. *et al.*, Targeting of HIF-alpha to the von Hippel-Lindau ubiquitylation complex by O2-regulated prolyl hydroxylation. *Science*, **292**(5516), pp. 468–472, 2001.

36. Arany, Z., Huang, L. E., Eckner, R., Bhattacharya, S., Jiang, C., Goldberg, M. A. *et al.*, An essential role for p300/CBP in the cellular response to hypoxia. *P. Natl. Acad. Sci. USA*, **93**(23), pp. 12969–12973, 1996.

37. Ebert, B. L. Bunn, H. F. Regulation of transcription by hypoxia requires a multiprotein complex that includes hypoxia-inducible factor 1, an adjacent transcription factor, and p300/CREB binding protein. *Mol. Cell. Biol.*, Jul; **18**(7), pp. 4089–4096, PubMed PMID: 9632793. PMCID: 108993, 1998.

38. Ema, M., Hirota, K., Mimura, J., Abe, H., Yodoi, J., Sogawa, K. *et al.*, Molecular mechanisms of transcription activation by HLF and HIF1alpha in response to hypoxia: their stabilization and redox signal-induced interaction with CBP/p300. *EMBO J.*, **18**(7), pp. 1905–1914, 1999.

39. Hewitson, K. S., McNeill, L. A., Riordan, M. V., Tian, Y. M., Bullock, A. N., Welford, R. W. *et al.*, Hypoxia-inducible factor (HIF) asparagine hydroxylase is identical to factor inhibiting HIF (FIH) and is related to the cupin structural family. *J. Biol. Chem.*, **277**(29), pp. 26351–26355, 2002.

40. Sang, N., Fang, J., Srinivas, V., Leshchinsky, I. and Caro, J., Carboxyl-terminal transactivation activity of hypoxia-inducible factor 1 alpha is governed by a von Hippel-Lindau protein-independent, hydroxylation-regulated association with p300/CBP. *Mol. Cell. Biol.*, **22**(9), pp. 2984–2992, 2002.

41. Lando, D., Peet, D. J., Gorman, J. J., Whelan, D. A., Whitelaw, M. L., and Bruick, R. K., FIH-1 is an asparaginyl hydroxylase enzyme that regulates the transcriptional activity of hypoxia-inducible factor. *Gene. Dev.*, **16**(12), pp. 1466–1471, 2002.

42. Koivunen, P., Hirsila, M., Gunzler, V., Kivirikko, K. I., and Myllyharju, J., Catalytic properties of the asparaginyl hydroxylase (FIH) in the oxygen

sensing pathway are distinct from those of its prolyl 4-hydroxylases. *J. Biol. Chem.*, **279**(11), pp. 9899–9904, 2004.

43. Bracken, C. P., Fedele, A. O., Linke, S., Balrak, W., Lisy, K., Whitelaw, M. L., *et al.*, Cell-specific regulation of hypoxia-inducible factor (HIF)-1alpha and HIF-2alpha stabilization and transactivation in a graded oxygen environment. *J. Biol. Chem.*, **281**(32), pp. 22575–22585, 2006.

44. Min, J. H., Yang, H., Ivan, M., Gertler, F., Kaelin, W. G., Jr., and Pavletich, N.P. Structure of an HIF-1alpha -pVHL complex: hydroxyproline recognition in signaling. *Science*, **296**(5574), pp. 1886–1889, 2002.

45. Hon, W. C., Wilson, M. I., Harlos, K., Claridge, T.D., Schofield, C. J., Pugh, C. W. *et al.*, Structural basis for the recognition of hydroxyproline in HIF-1 alpha by pVHL. *Nature*, **417**(6892), pp. 975–978, 2002.

46. Ivan, M., and Kaelin, W. G., Jr., The von Hippel-Lindau tumor suppressor protein. *Curr. Opin. Genet. Dev.*, **11**(1), pp. 27–34, 2001.

47. Iliopoulos, O., Levy, A. P., Jiang, C., Kaelin, W. G., Jr., and Goldberg, M. A., Negative regulation of hypoxia-inducible genes by the von Hippel-Lindau protein. *P. Natl. Acad. Sci. USA*, **93**(20), pp. 10595–10599, 1996.

48. Komander, D., Clague, M. J., and Urbe, S., Breaking the chains: structure and function of the deubiquitinases. *Nat. Rev. Mol. Cell Biol.*, **10**(8), pp. 550–563, 2009.

49. Li, Z., Wang, D., Na, X., Schoen, S. R., Messing, E. M., and Wu, G., Identification of a deubiquitinating enzyme subfamily as substrates of the von Hippel-Lindau tumor suppressor. *Biochem. Biophys. Res. Comm.*, **294**(3), pp. 700–709, 2002.

50. Bremm, A., Moniz, S., Mader, J., Rocha, S., and Komander, D., Cezanne (OTUD7B) regulates HIF-1alpha homeostasis in a proteasome-independent manner. *EMBO Reports* **15**(12), pp. 1268–1277, 2014.

51. Jeong, J. W., Bae, M. K., Ahn, M. Y., Kim, S. H., Sohn, T. K., Bae, M. H. *et al.*, Regulation and destabilization of HIF-1alpha by ARD1-mediated acetylation. *Cell*, **111**(5), pp. 709–720, 2002.

52. Finkel, T., Deng, C. X., and Mostoslavsky, R., Recent progress in the biology and physiology of sirtuins. *Nature*, **460**(7255), pp. 587–591, 2009.

53. Dioum, E. M., Chen, R., Alexander, M. S., Zhang, Q., Hogg, R. T., Gerard, R. D. *et al.*, Regulation of hypoxia-inducible factor 2alpha signaling by the stress-responsive deacetylase sirtuin 1. *Science*, **324**(5932), pp. 1289–1293.

54. Geng, H., Liu, Q., Xue, C., David, L. L., Beer, T. M., Thomas, G. V. *et al.*, HIF1alpha protein stability is increased by acetylation at lysine 709. *J. Biol. Chem.*, **287**(42), pp. 35496–35505, 2012.

55. Richard, D. E., Berra, E., Gothie, E., Roux, D., and Pouyssegur, J., p42/p44 mitogen-activated protein kinases phosphorylate hypoxia-inducible factor 1alpha (HIF-1alpha) and enhance the transcriptional activity of HIF-1. *J. Biol. Chem.*, **274**(46), pp. 32631–32637.

56. Sodhi, A., Montaner, S., Patel, V., Zohar, M., Bais, C., Mesri, E. A. *et al.,* The Kaposi's sarcoma-associated herpes virus G protein-coupled receptor up-regulates vascular endothelial growth factor expression and secretion through mitogen-activated protein kinase and p38 pathways acting on hypoxia-inducible factor 1alpha. *Cancer Res.*, **60**(17), pp. 4873–4880, 2000.

57. Minet, E., Arnould, T., Michel, G., Roland, I., Mottet, D., Raes, M. *et al.,* ERK activation upon hypoxia: involvement in HIF-1 activation. *FEBS Lett.*, **468**(1), pp. 53–58, 2000.

58. Hur, E., Chang, K. Y., Lee, E., Lee, S. K., and Park, H., Mitogen-activated protein kinase kinase inhibitor PD98059 blocks the trans-activation but not the stabilization or DNA binding ability of hypoxia-inducible factor-1alpha. *Mol. Pharmacol.*, **59**(5), pp. 1216–1224, 2001.

59. Chun, S. Y., Johnson, C., Washburn, J. G., Cruz-Correa, M. R., Dang, D. T., and Dang, L.H., Oncogenic KRAS modulates mitochondrial metabolism in human colon cancer cells by inducing HIF-1alpha and HIF-2alpha target genes. *Mol. Cancer*, **9**: 293, 2010.

60. Suzuki, H., Tomida, A., and Tsuruo, T., Dephosphorylated hypoxia-inducible factor 1alpha as a mediator of p53-dependent apoptosis during hypoxia. *Oncogene.*, **20**(41), pp. 5779–5788, 2001.

61. Warfel, N. A., Dolloff, N. G., Dicker, D. T., Malysz, J., and El-Deiry, W. S., CDK1 stabilizes HIF-1alpha via direct phosphorylation of Ser668 to promote tumor growth. *Cell Cycle*, **12**(23), pp. 3689–3701, 2013.

62. To, K. K., Sedelnikova, O. A., Samons, M., Bonner, W. M., and Huang, L. E., The phosphorylation status of PAS-B distinguishes HIF-1alpha from HIF-2alpha in NBS1 repression. *EMBO J.*, **25**(20), pp. 4784–4794, 2006.

63. Shao, R., Zhang, F. P., Tian, F., Anders Friberg, P., Wang, X., Sjoland, H. *et al.,* Increase of SUMO-1 expression in response to hypoxia: direct interaction with HIF-1alpha in adult mouse brain and heart in vivo. *FEBS Lett.*, 569(1–3), pp. 293–300, 2004.

64. Bae, S. H., Jeong, J. W., Park, J. A., Kim, S. H., Bae, M. K., Choi, S. J. *et al.,* Sumoylation increases HIF-1alpha stability and its transcriptional activity. *Biochem. Biophys. Res. Comm.*, **324**(1), pp. 394–400, 2004.

65. Cheng, J., Kang, X., Zhang, S., and Yeh, E. T., SUMO-specific protease 1 is essential for stabilization of HIF1alpha during hypoxia. *Cell*, **131**(3), pp. 584–595, 2007.

66. Tojo, M., Matsuzaki, K., Minami, T., Honda, Y., Yasuda, H., Chiba, T. *et al.*, The aryl hydrocarbon receptor nuclear transporter is modulated by the SUMO-1 conjugation system. *J. Biol. Chem.*, **277**(48), pp. 46576–46585, 2002.

67. Yasinska, I. M., and Sumbayev, V. V., S-nitrosation of Cys-800 of HIF-1alpha protein activates its interaction with p300 and stimulates its transcriptional activity. *FEBS Lett.*, **549**(1–3), pp. 105–109, 2003.

68. Metzen, E., Zhou, J., Jelkmann, W., Fandrey, J., and Brune, B., Nitric oxide impairs normoxic degradation of HIF-1alpha by inhibition of prolyl hydroxylases. *Mol. Biol. Cell*, **14**(8), pp. 3470–3481, 2003.

69. Li, F., Sonveaux, P., Rabbani, Z. N., Liu, S., Yan, B., Huang, Q. *et al.*, Regulation of HIF-1alpha stability through S-nitrosylation. *Mol. Cell*, **26**(1), pp. 63–74, 2007.

70. Peyssonnaux, C., Datta, V., Cramer, T., Doedens, A., Theodorakis, E. A., Gallo, R. L. *et al.*, HIF-1alpha expression regulates the bactericidal capacity of phagocytes. *J. Clin. Invest.*, **115**(7), pp. 1806–1815, 2005.

71. Semenza, G. L., Hypoxia-inducible factor 1: oxygen homeostasis and disease pathophysiology. *Trends Mol. Med.*, **7**(8), pp. 345–350.

72. Seagroves, T. N., Ryan, H. E., Lu, H., Wouters, B. G., Knapp, M., Thibault, P. *et al.*, Transcription factor HIF-1 is a necessary mediator of the pasteur effect in mammalian cells. *Mol. Cell Biol.*, **21**(10), pp. 3436–3444, 2001.

73. Ravi, R., Mookerjee, B., Bhujwalla, Z. M., Sutter, C. H., Artemov, D., Zeng, Q. *et al.*, Regulation of tumor angiogenesis by p53-induced degradation of hypoxia-inducible factor 1alpha. *Gene. Dev.*, **14**(1), pp. 34–44, 2000.

74. Kung, A. L., Wang, S., Klco, J. M., Kaelin, W. G., and Livingston, D. M., Suppression of tumor growth through disruption of hypoxia-inducible transcription. *Nat. Med.*, **6**(12), pp. 1335–1340, 2000.

75. Shin, D. H., Chun, Y. S., Lee, D. S., Huang, L. E., and Park, J. W., Bortezomib inhibits tumor adaptation to hypoxia by stimulating the FIH-mediated repression of hypoxia-inducible factor-1. *Blood*, **111**(6), pp. 3131–3136, 2008.

76. Fath, D. M., Kong, X., Liang, D., Lin, Z., Chou, A., Jiang, Y. *et al.*, Histone deacetylase inhibitors repress the transactivation potential of hypoxia-inducible factors independently of direct acetylation of HIF-alpha. *J. Biol. Chem.*, **281**(19), pp. 13612–13619, 2006.

77. Kong, X., Lin, Z., Liang, D., Fath, D., Sang, N., and Caro, J., Histone deacetylase inhibitors induce VHL and ubiquitin-independent proteasomal degradation of hypoxia-inducible factor 1alpha. *Mol. Cell. Biol.*, **26**(6), pp. 2019–2028, 2006.

78. Qian, D. Z., Kachhap, S. K., Collis, S. J., Verheul, H. M., Carducci, M. A., Atadja, P. *et al.,* Class II histone deacetylases are associated with VHL-independent regulation of hypoxia-inducible factor 1 alpha. *Cancer Res.,* **66**(17), pp. 8814–8821, 2006.

79. Isaacs, J. S., Jung, Y. J., Mimnaugh, E. G., Martinez, A., Cuttitta, F., and Neckers, L. M. Hsp90 regulates a von Hippel Lindau-independent hypoxia-inducible factor-1 alpha-degradative pathway. *J. Biol. Chem.,* **277**(33), pp. 29936–29944, 2002.

80. Mabjeesh, N. J., Post, D. E., Willard, M. T., Kaur, B., Van Meir, E. G., Simons, J. W. *et al.,* Geldanamycin induces degradation of hypoxia-inducible factor 1alpha protein via the proteosome pathway in prostate cancer cells. *Cancer Res.,* **62**(9), pp. 2478–2482, 2002.

81. Vincent, K. A., Feron, O., and Kelly, R. A., Harnessing the response to tissue hypoxia: HIF-1 alpha and therapeutic angiogenesis. *Trends Cardiovas. Med.,* **12**(8), pp. 362–367, 2002.

82. Vincent, K. A., Shyu, K. G., Luo, Y., Magner, M., Tio, R. A., Jiang, C. *et al.,* Angiogenesis is induced in a rabbit model of hindlimb ischemia by naked DNA encoding an HIF-1alpha/VP16 hybrid transcription factor. *Circulation,* **102**(18), pp. 2255–2261, 2000.

83. Elson, D. A., Thurston, G., Huang, L. E., Ginzinger, D. G., McDonald, D. M., Johnson, R. S. *et al.,* Induction of hypervascularity without leakage or inflammation in transgenic mice overexpressing hypoxia-inducible factor-1alpha. *Gene. Dev.,* **15**(19), pp. 2520–2532, 2001.

84. Palolahti, M., Lauharanta, J., Stephens, R. W., Kuusela, P., and Vaheri, A., Proteolytic activity in leg ulcer exudate. *Exp. Dermatol.,* **2**(1), pp. 29–37, 1993.

85. Du, J., Liu, L., Lay, F., Wang, Q., Dou, C., Zhang, X. *et al.,* Combination of HIF-1alpha gene transfection and HIF-1-activated bone marrow-derived angiogenic cell infusion improves burn wound healing in aged mice. *Gene Ther.,* **20**(11), pp. 1070–1076, 2013.

86. Loh, S. A., Chang, E. I., Galvez, M. G., Thangarajah, H., El-ftesi, S., Vial, I. N. *et al.,* SDF-1 alpha expression during wound healing in the aged is HIF dependent. *Plast. Reconstr. Surg.,* **123**(2), pp. 65S–75S, 2009.

87. Zhang, X., Liu, L., Wei, X., Tan, Y. S., Tong, L., Chang, R. *et al.,* Impaired angiogenesis and mobilization of circulating angiogenic cells in HIF-1alpha heterozygous-null mice after burn wounding. Wound repair and regeneration: official publication of the Wound Healing Society [and] the European Tissue Repair Society, **18**(2), pp.193–201, 2010.

88. Thangarajah, H., Yao, D., Chang, E. I., Shi, Y., Jazayeri, L., Vial, I. N. *et al.*, The molecular basis for impaired hypoxia-induced VEGF expression in diabetic tissues. *P. Natl. Acad. Sci. USA.*, **106**(32), pp. 13505–13510, 2009.

89. Chang, E. I., Loh, S. A., Ceradini, D. J., Chang, E. I., Lin, S. E., Bastidas, N. *et al.*, Age decreases endothelial progenitor cell recruitment through decreases in hypoxia-inducible factor 1alpha stabilization during ischemia. *Circulation*, **116**(24), pp. 2818–2829, 2007.

90. Bayat, A., McGrouther, D. A., and Ferguson, M. W., *Skin Scarring BMJ.*, **326**(7380), pp. 88–92, 2003.

91. Distler, J. H., Jungel, A., Pileckyte, M., Zwerina, J., Michel, B. A., Gay, R. E. *et al.*, Hypoxia-induced increase in the production of extracellular matrix proteins in systemic sclerosis. *Arthritis Rheum.*, **56**(12), pp. 4203–4215, 2007.

92. Botusan, I. R., Sunkari, V. G., Savu, O., Catrina, A. I., Grunler, J., Lindberg, S. *et al.*, Stabilization of HIF-1alpha is critical to improve wound healing in diabetic mice. *P. Natl. Acad. Sci. USA.*, **105**(49), pp. 19426–19431, 2008.

93. Smith, T. G., and Talbot, N. P., Prolyl hydroxylases and therapeutics. *Antioxidants & Redox Signaling*, **12**(4), pp. 431–433, 2010.

94. Thirunavukkarasu, M., Selvaraju, V., Dunna, N. R., Foye, J. L., Joshi, M., Otani, H. *et al.*, Simvastatin treatment inhibits hypoxia inducible factor 1-alpha-(HIF-1alpha)-prolyl-4-hydroxylase 3 (PHD-3) and increases angiogenesis after myocardial infarction in streptozotocin-induced diabetic rat. *Int. J. Cardiol.*, **168**(3), pp. 2474–2480, 2013.

# Chapter 3

# Hypoxia and Metastasis

Elizabeth C. Finger and Amato J. Giaccia*

*Department of Radiation Oncology, Stanford University,
CCSR-S, Rm. 1255,269 Campus Dr. Stanford,
CA 94305-5152, USA
*giaccia@stanford.edu.*

## 1. Introduction — Cancer Metastasis

One of the hallmarks of cancer, metastasis, has long been an area of intense research among cancer biologists worldwide. Metastasis can be broadly defined as the process in which cells spread from a primary tumor site in one organ to a distant site in another organ of the body, creating a new tumor mass that is a derivative of the initial tumor. The intense research interest in this topic is largely due to the fact that metastasis of a primary tumor to distant organs is the main cause of death in most cancer patients, accounting for approximately 90% of all cancer related deaths.[1,2]

Metastasis is a common feature of solid tumors, such as: lung, pancreatic and brain cancers. The major sites where metastatic disease arises include the lungs, liver, and bone; though other organs can be affected, depending on the primary tumor type.[3] Why is metastatic disease so lethal compared to primary tumor growth? A major reason is because distant metastases often grow undetected until they reach a stage at which they are already so advanced, little can be done clinically to eradicate them.

69

Often, patients complain of ailments common to other more prevalent diseases, such as back pain and shortness of breath, and it is only after many lab tests that metastatic cancer is discovered. Once metastasis is detected, common therapies for primary tumors, such as surgery and radiation, are less effective in eradicating the disease and instead serve as palliative treatment options to improve quality of life.

The process of metastasis can be thought of as a series of steps a tumor cell takes on its journey to a distant organ. First, a cancer cell within a primary tumor must obtain signals, both intrinsic and extrinsic, that alter its overall shape and function to allow it to be more invasive.[4] This process is termed epithelial-to-mesenchymal transition (EMT).[4] The tumor cell then invades through the extracellular matrix (ECM) to enter the blood stream.[4] Once in the blood stream, the circulating tumor cell (CTCs) travels to a distant organ, exits the blood stream and colonizes a distant site, forming a new tumor completely separate from its site of origin (Fig. 1).[4]

In this chapter, we will introduce the concept of tumor hypoxia, and how this component of the tumor microenvironment is involved in each step of the metastatic cascade. As discussed in earlier chapters, hypoxia is broadly defined as a region of a tumor that has low levels of oxygen present. Hypoxia induces the transcription of genes involved in biological processes important for tumor growth and metastatic disease such as: cell proliferation, migration, invasion, and ECM remodeling.[5,6] This increase

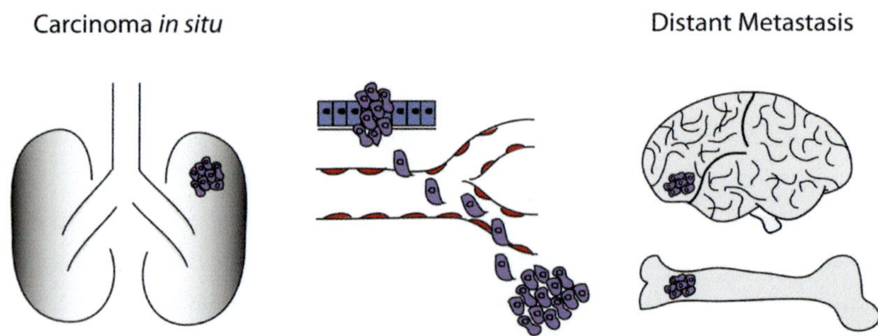



Fig. 1.  The metastatic cascade. The process of metastasis involves tumor cells undergoing EMT in which they become more invasive and invade through the basement membrane and ECM at the primary tumor site. The tumor cells then enter the blood stream, and those that survive can home to distant organs, where they can seed and grow into a distant metastasis.

in gene expression by hypoxia is typically accomplished through the hypoxia-inducible family of transcription factors (HIFs).[7] Importantly, many research groups have shown a link between HIF-1$\alpha$ expression and metastatic disease. Early studies in breast cancer showed that HIF-1$\alpha$ was overexpressed in 69% of breast cancer metastases, 29% of primary breast tumors and not expressed in benign tissue, indicating hypoxia, and HIF specifically, correlates with metastatic disease progression.[8] Many studies have been published since, linking hypoxia and HIF, as well as downstream genes, with metastatic tumor burden and decreased survival. Some of these studies will be discussed in this chapter.

## 2. Hypoxia and the Tumor Microenvironment

A critical component for tumor development and metastasis is the complex makeup of the region surrounding the tumor, called the tumor microenvironment. Specifically, this includes endothelial cells, fibroblasts, infiltrating immune cells, growth factors and the ECM itself (Fig. 2).[9,10] Each of these components plays a role in supporting tumor development by regulating angiogenesis, desmoplasia, lymphangiogenesis, and the immune response.[9] Hypoxia, the consequence of insufficient or inadequate angiogenesis has been shown to be involved in regulation of the other components of the microenvironment, which will each be described in more detail within this section.

## 2.1. The extracellular matrix

The ECM is a dynamic 3D structure that helps regulate cell proliferation, differentiation and migration through interactions with integrins, matrix metalloproteases and soluble growth factors.[11,12] In addition, tumor cells often have to migrate through a specialized ECM called the basement membrane, a barrier which serves to separate endothelial and epithelial cells from stromal components, in order to undergo metastasis.[13] The basement membrane is composed of collagen IV, fibronectin, heparansulfate proteoglycans, entactin, and laminin.[14] Components of and interactors with the ECM which are hypoxia-regulated, such as integrins, MMPs and growth factors, will be discussed in this section.

 *Tumor Hypoxia*

## Tumor Microenvironment

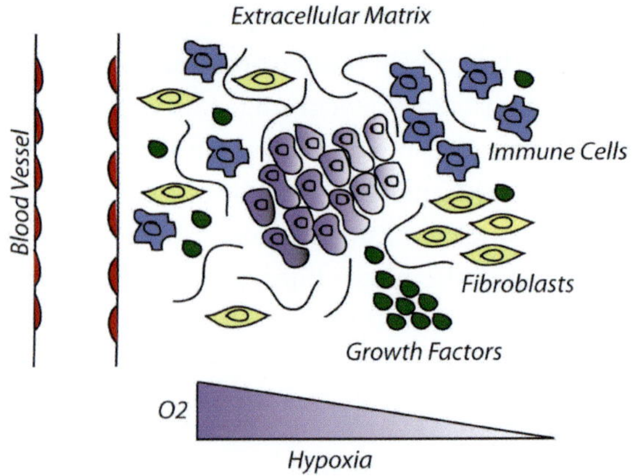



Fig. 2.   The tumor microenvironment is made up of many cell types and factors that influence tumor growth. First there are infiltrating immune cells (including tumor-associate macrophages, dendritic cells, lymphocytes, eosinophils, neutrophils and mast cells), and fibroblasts. Many types of extrinsic factors are located within the tumor microenvironment, including LOX and the CTGF. Additional components of the tumor microenvironment include integrins, matrix metalloproteinases (MMPs), and ECM structural components such as: fibronectin, collagen, and laminin.[139]

## 2.1.1. *Integrins*

Integrins, or adhesion proteins, form heterodimeric transmembrane proteins consisting of an $\alpha$-subunit and a $\beta$-subunit, and commonly interact with the ECM.[9,15] The multitude of possible heterodimer combinations of the 18 known $\alpha$-subunits and 8 $\beta$-subunits allows for specific crosstalk between growth factor receptors and oncogenes, and serve to regulate cell proliferation, survival, and migration.[9] Some of the signaling cascades integrins target include protein kinase B (AKT/PKB), Src-family kinases, and focal adhesion kinase (FAK).[4] In addition, there are often differences in expression of integrin heterodimers combinations in tumor cells versus normal epithelial cells.[9] For example, $\alpha v\beta 3$ integrin expression is strongly linked with growth and metastasis of pancreatic, breast, ovarian, cervical, and prostate cancer as well as gliomas.[16] The connection between hypoxia and integrin expression has also been examined. In the context of human keratinocytes, it was found that exposure to hypoxia (1% oxygen) leads to increased migration through the upregulation of $\alpha v \beta 6$ integrin.[17] In a study of lung cancer patients, it was found that $\alpha v \beta 5$ was highly expressed and associated with HIF-1$\alpha$ expression in tissues derived from brain metastases.[18] A study in pancreatic cancer utilized anti-sense HIF-1$\alpha$ and demonstrated a corresponding decrease in $\beta 1$-integrin, suggesting a link between HIF and $\beta 1$-integrin expression.[19] Another study with gastric cancer cells showed that RNA interference to HIF-1$\alpha$ increased the levels of $\alpha 5$ integrin, which resulted in increased anoikis.[20] Taken together, these studies demonstrate that within the tumor microenvironment, hypoxia and altered integrin expression are coordinated and associated with the metastatic cascade.

## 2.1.2. *Matrix metalloproteinases*

Another component of the tumor microenvironment involved in metastasis are MMPs.[21] There are over 24 metalloproteinases that are members of a larger group of proteases.[21] Some MMPs are secreted in an inactive state and have to be proteolytically cleaved to allow activation.[22] Once activated, MMP enzymatic activity allows them to degrade components of the ECM including, but not limited to, growth factors, fibronectin and numerous types of collagen.[21] MMPs are normally expressed at low levels, and their expression is regulated by tissue inhibitors of metalloproteinases (TIMPs), which are normally found at a 1:1 ratio with MMPs.[23] During the process of tumorigenesis, there is a shift in this balance, with alterations in expression of MMPs and TIMPs seen in many cancer types.[24–26] MMPs act to remodel the tumor microenvironment, such as degrading collagen, and activating cell surface receptors and their downstream signaling cascades.[27] One main alteration that commonly occurs during remodeling of the tumor microenvironment is degradation of the ECM component, Type IV collagen. This is a critical step in metastasis because Type IV collagen is the main component of the basement membrane.[28] The main MMPs that regulate this degradation of Type IV collagen are MMP-2 and MMP-9.[29] These MMPs have been shown to be upregulated in cancers including: lung, breast, prostate, ovarian and colorectal cancers.[24,29–32]

Interestingly, numerous papers have linked hypoxia and HIF with regulation of MMP expression and activity in human cancer cells.[33–36] For example, a study by Jae Young Choi *et al.* demonstrated HIF-1$\alpha$ induction of MMP-9 in NCI-H-1299 lung cancer cells, MDA-MB-231 breast cancer cells, and in breast cancer tissue.[34] In lung adenocarcinoma cells, Kou-Gi Shyu *et al.* demonstrated that cells overexpressing HIF-1$\alpha$ show an increase in MMP-1 expression and active MMP-2.[35] Another study demonstrated that in the absence of the Von Hippel–Lindau (VHL) tumor suppressor gene in renal cell carcinoma cell lines, HIF-2$\alpha$ is stabilized and in coordination with Sp1 leads to an increase in MT1–MMP expression at both the RNA and protein level.[36] Also, shRNA to HIF-1$\alpha$ in a hepatocellular carcinoma cell line caused downregulation of MMP-2 protein expression under hypoxia.[37]

## 2.1.3. *Extrinsic factors*

A notable hypoxia-regulated factor, which regulates extracellular collagen and elastin, is lysyl oxidase (LOX).[38] It is a member of a family of secreted proteins consisting of LOX, LOXL (LOXL1), LOXL2, LOXL3, and LOXL4.[39] LOX is secreted into the ECM as a precursor version of the protein that requires proteolytic cleavage to release a 32 kDa catalytically active protein.[40,41] Once activated, the protein serves as an amine oxidase that is involved in premetastatic niche formation and cross-linking collagen and elastin within the ECM.[42,43]

Numerous studies have linked LOX and its family members with aggressive metastatic disease.[44–46] Early studies demonstrated strong association of LOX, as well as LOXL2, in highly invasive breast cancer cell lines.[45] The first paper to clearly link LOX with metastatic cancer showed that HIF-1 regulated LOX expression in human breast cancer, and head and neck (H&N) tumors, and that patients with high levels of LOX had decreased distant metastasis free and overall survival.[46] The study went on to show that LOX is acting through FAK and cell-to-matrix adhesion to elicit these prometastatic activities in human hypoxic cancer cells.[46] The fact LOX is hypoxia-regulated and clearly involved in metastatic disease makes it a good therapeutic target. Indeed, numerous studies have been performed using *in vivo* mouse models to examine the potential of targeting LOX and its family members to inhibit the spread of tumor cells. Using an orthotopic mouse model of breast cancer, one group found that treatment with $\beta$-aminoproprionitrile (BAPN), an irreversible LOX inhibitor, or treatment with a purified LOX antibody did not affect primary tumor growth but significantly reduced metastatic tumor burden.[46] Another study examined use of an inhibitory monoclonal antibody, AB0023, which targets LOXL2 in an ovarian tumor cell line model that metastasizes *in vivo* and demonstrated decreased metastasis to the lung, pancreas and liver in the mice treated with AB0023.[47] The humanized variant of this antibody, GS-6624 (simtuzumab, formerly AB0024), is being tested in Phase II trials for treatment of idiopathic pulmonary fibrosis (IPF) and also has potential for treatment of solid tumors.

Another hypoxia-regulated growth factor that is involved in metastasis is the connective tissue growth factor (CTGF, CCN2). This secreted protein is a member of the larger CCN family of matricellular proteins.[48] CTGF has been shown to be involved in normal physiological processes, as well as cell proliferation, migration, and adhesion.[48] CTGF is multimodular and is composed of four domains known to bind to (and be induced by) other growth factors and signaling molecules including transforming growth factor beta (TGF-$\beta$) and vascular endothelial growth factor (VEGF).[49–51] Paradoxically, no unique CTGF receptor has been identified, and it is thought to elicit its effects through interaction with other growth factors, including IGF-1/2, TGF-$\beta$, and VEGF, cell surface receptors as well as interactions with cell surface heparin sulfate proteoglycans and integrins.[52]

There is a strong foundation in the literature linking hypoxia and CTGF to metastatic disease. Studies in melanoma have demonstrated a role for HIF-1$\alpha$ (and HIF-2$\alpha$) dependent increases in CTGF expression.[53,54] In addition, HIF-1$\alpha$ directly regulates CTGF expression in primary tubular epithelial cells, and loss of HIF-1$\alpha$ using a HIF-1$\alpha$ knockout mouse model resulted in decreased CTGF expression.[55] *In vitro*, secretion of CTGF from pancreatic tumor cells is elevated under hypoxic conditions with HIF playing a role.[48] This same study showed that clinical specimens from human pancreatic adenocarcinomas demonstrated colocalization between CTGF and a marker of hypoxia.[48] Another *in vitro* study in breast cancer demonstrated that CTGF messenger RNA and protein are both elevated in response to hypoxia.[56] What is the consequence of elevated CTGF? In broad terms, CTGF overexpression makes cells more migratory and thereby leads to increased cell metastasis. The specific mechanism by which this occurs varies between cancer types. For example, one *in vitro* study utilizing a human breast cancer cell line demonstrated that elevated levels of CTGF enhance their metastatic potential through $\alpha v\beta 3$-ERK1/2 upregulation of S100A4.[57] Another study in human osteosarcoma demonstrated that CTGF induces expression of MMP-2 and MMP-3 through downregulation of miR-519d through the MEK/ERK pathway, which in turn promotes tumor metastasis.[58] Overall, these studies show the importance of hypoxia on regulating components of the tumor microenvironment, such as CTGF and LOX, and demonstrate the ways in which they regulate tumor growth.

## 2.2. Epithelial to mesenchymal transition

EMT is a term that was developed to define the process that occurs when non-motile, polarized epithelial cells transition to motile, non-polarized mesenchymal cells.[4] This process is commonly used to refer to the early event in the metastatic process when cancer cells become more motile as they locally invade into surrounding tissue. One of the most critical steps is termed "cadherin switching," when epithelial cells lose their expression of E-cadherin and increase their expression of N-cadherin.[16] E-cadherin is a cell adhesion molecule present in epithelial cells.[4] N-cadherin on the other hand is a mesenchymal marker that facilitates a change in the adhesion properties of a cell, leading to a mesenchymal phenotype.[4] With the loss of E-cadherin and resulting dissolution of adherens junctions, as well as increase in N-cadherin, cells therefore become less adhesive to other surrounding epithelial cells and are able to become more invasive.[4]

Hypoxia is a critical regulator of many of the important transcription factors involved in the process of EMT. One study in renal cancer derived RCC10 cells showed that expression of constitutively active HIF-1$\alpha$ or HIF-2$\alpha$ were each able to reduce the expression of E-cadherin RNA and protein.[59] Mechanistically, Twist-related protein 1 (Twist 1), a basic helix-loop-helix transcription factor that is a transcriptional target of HIF, decreases E-cadherin expression and increases N-cadherin expression in multiple model systems.[60] One study in pancreatic cancer determined that a 48 hour exposure to hypoxia caused elevated levels of Twist in all cell lines tested (MiaPaCa-2, Panc-1, AsPC-1, Capan-1, and HPAF-2).[61] In addition to Twist, another transcription factor that reduces expression of E-cadherin is the Zinc-finger protein SNAIL1 (Snail).[60] It has been shown that the Snail promoter contains a hypoxia-response element (HRE) site within its promoter and is directly bound and regulated by HIF-$1\alpha$.[62] Recent work has linked HIF-$1\alpha$ expression with Snail in ovarian cancer cell lines and ovarian cancer tissues.[63] Expression of HIF-$1\alpha$, E-cadherin and Snail were significantly correlated with clinically pathological features of ovarian cancer.[63] Another zinc-finger transcription factor known to repress E-cadherin is Slug.[60] Hypoxia induces Notch signaling, which in turn elevates the levels of Slug, and inhibits E-cadherin.[64] Other transcription factors that are involved in the process of EMT include Zinc-finger E-box-binding homeobox 1 and 2 (ZEB1 and ZEB2).[60] The regulation of the ZEB transcription factors by HIF-$1\alpha$ is not as well understood. A new investigation of colorectal cancer-derived cell lines has identified a HRE within the proximal promoter of ZEB1, and showed that HIF-$1\alpha$ is able to directly bind and regulate ZEB1.[65] Importantly, HIF regulation of these transcription factors causes a decrease in E-cadherin and increase in N-cadherin that are necessary for the "cadherin switch" as well as EMT itself (Fig. 3).[60] Even though there is plenty of evidence of EMT occurring both *in vitro* as well as *in vivo*, and the evidence of hypoxia being involved in this process is solid, more work needs to be performed to elucidate the significance of EMT within the clinical setting of human metastatic cancer.

## 3. Hypoxia and Circulating Tumor Cells

In the last section, we established factors within the tumor microenvironment that serve to induce the migratory and invasive potential of primary tumor cells. What happens once they leave the primary tumor site and get to the blood stream to begin their journey to colonize distant organs in the body? The cells that migrate to and intravasate into the blood stream are

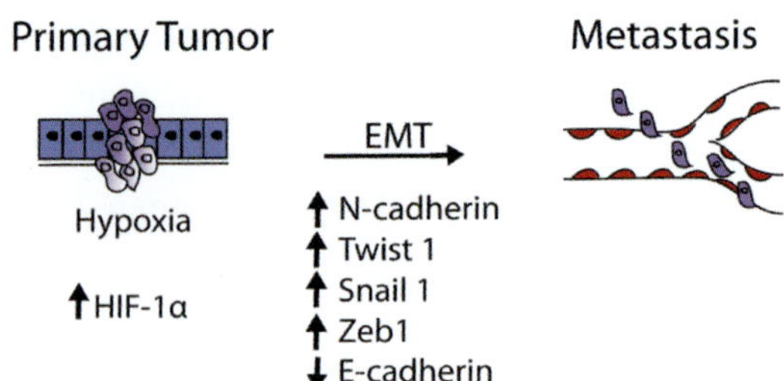



Fig. 3.   EMT. Hypoxia induces expression of HIF-1α, which can lead to changes in expression of various proteins (E-cadherin, N-cadherin) and transcription factors (Twist 1, Snail 1, Zeb 1) involved in the transition of cells from an epithelial (non-motile) phenotype to a mesenchymal (motile) phenotype. EMT is a necessary transition for tumor cells, allowing them to undergo the process of cell invasion and metastasis through the blood stream to a distant site.

termed CTCs.[66] These cells are very rare and represent a challenge to detect in humans, with approximately 1–10 CTCs present in 10 mL of a cancer patient's blood.[67] The ability of these cells to survive in the bloodstream and home to a distant site is a relatively low probability event. This is demonstrated by the estimation that only 0.01% of CTCs will give rise to metastasis.[66] Indeed, CTCs are challenged by physical damage due to hemodynamic shear forces, immune-mediated attack and anoikis (cell death due to loss of adhesion).[13] What role does hypoxia play in this step of the metastatic cascade? One might argue a very small one, since the blood vessels themselves are not hypoxic. But, the time in which CTCs are in the blood stream could be very short, from a few minutes to a few hours, allowing the transcriptional changes induced by hypoxia to still be expressed under aerobic conditions.[39,68] Indeed, one study demonstrated that the half-life of CTCs in breast cancer dormancy patients is between 1 and 2.4 hours.[69] In this section, we will detail the challenges faced by tumor cells in the blood stream and how hypoxia might be contributing to their survival.

## 3.1. Anoikis

A very real threat to CTCs is cell death due to lack of attachment to the ECM or anoikis.[13] The role of hypoxia in anoikis varies depending on the cancer type. One study showed that BNIP3 (a Bcl-2 binding protein) is upregulated through a HIF-1$\alpha$/ERK pathway that leads to anoikis resistance in hepatocellular carcinoma cells.[70] Another study using the breast cancer cell line MCF-10A overexpressing ERBB2 demonstrated that HIF-1$\alpha$ was required for anoikis resistance.[71] This group also showed that suspended MCF10A cells, as well as those grown in 3D culture systems, under hypoxia, had suppression of the Bcl-2-homology domain 3 (BH-3)-only family protein (Bim), a factor required for anoikis.[72] Importantly, this was not unique to breast cancer cells, but Bim suppression in the absence of adhesion under hypoxia also occurred in breast carcinoma cells, primary mammary epithelial cells, and immortalized prostate cells.[72] Resistance to anoikis in Ewing tumor (ET) sarcoma cell spheroids was shown to occur through the upregulation of E-cadherin, activation of the receptor tyrosine kinase ErbB4, which in turn activates the PI3K/Akt pathway.[73] The exact mechanism of how these individual factors work together to lead to resistance in ET sarcomas still remains to be defined. While we can conclude that the mechanism of anoikis suppression varies between cancer types, the significance of anoikis in circulating human cancer cells is still up for debate, since CTCs can attach to a distant vascular wall and begin the process of extravasation from the blood before anoikis becomes activated.[13] Further studies need to be performed to conclusively link anoikis with the metastatic process in human cancer patients.

## 3.2. Shear forces

As discussed above in Section 3.1, the environment in which a tumor cell resides plays a large role in its aggressive nature. There is a difference in environmental influences between a tumor cell growing attached to the ECM at a primary site exposed to hypoxia and a tumor cell circulating within the vasculature. During the process of metastasis, tumor cells enter the bloodstream, and there the CTCs encounter a number of obstacles which regulate their route and survival, including speed of blood flow, diameter of blood vessels, intracellular adhesion and shear flow.[74] It is hypothesized that shear forces are a major factor that impact the ability of a CTC to survive in circulation.[74,75] Fluid stresses develop from the flow of blood in the vessels themselves as well as interstitial pressure that can be found at the primary tumor site, partly due to leaky vasculature. It is estimated that shear stress in venous circulation is ~0.5–4.0 dyn/cm$^2$ and can reach even higher levels in the arteries (~4.0–30.0 dyn/cm$^2$).[75] To put these numbers in perspective, fluid shear stresses are only ~0.007–0.015 dyn/cm$^2$ for interstitial flow rates of $1\mu$m/s.[75] This dramatic increase in shear stress in the vasculature is a significant obstacle for CTCs to overcome. Shear forces also influence the location of tumor seeding at distant sites. Specifically, shear forces can influence the rotation and movement of CTCs, affecting their ability to interact with and adhere to the blood vessel wall, a necessary step a CTC must take before exiting the blood stream.[74]

## 3.3. The immune response

Tumor cells, whether they are at a primary site or growing as a distant metastasis, release cytokines and chemokines that cause a "pro-tumor" inflammatory response at the site of the tumor.[76] This response includes an influx of leukocytes (eosinophils, mast cells, neutrophils, macrophages, dendritic cells and lymphocytes) that then produce factors such as tumor necrosis factor-$\alpha$ (TNF-$\alpha$), interferons and interleukins.[76]

Hypoxic areas of tumors have an increased population of tumor-associated macrophages (TAMs), which stabilize HIF and serve to dampen adaptive immunity ("anti-tumor" response) by suppressing T-cell actions and enhancing the tumor's ability to survive and proliferate.[77,78] More specifically, it has been shown that HIF-2$\alpha$ is increased in M2-polarized macrophages.[77,79] The association between HIF-2$\alpha$ expression and TAMs has been reported in numerous solid tumors, including: brain, breast, colon, prostate, pancreatic, and renal carcinomas.[78]

Once inflammatory cells have infiltrated the tumor, they greatly influence the tumor microenvironment by releasing growth factors, cytokines, interleukins, and interferons.[76] One such proinflammatory cytokine, TNF-$\alpha$, is secreted by macrophages.[80] TNF-$\alpha$ can improve tumor growth through several mechanisms, including enhanced tumor cell survival through NF$\kappa$B signaling to anti-apoptotic downstream factors.[81] In addition, TNF-$\alpha$ has also been shown to promote angiogenesis.[82] In addition to cytokines, interleukins, such as IL-6, IL-10, IL-18, and IL-19 are also upregulated in the tumor microenvironment.[83–86] Interleukins play a variety of roles within different types of cancer, and some of their general functions include: promoting proliferation, inhibiting apoptosis, and increasing metastatic invasiveness.[82,87] One study examined serum from breast cancer patients and found that high levels of IL-6 were correlated to poor clinical outcome.[86] Another study examined gastric cancer cell lines, AGS, Hs-746T, and NCI-N87 that were cocultured with TAMs, and found higher expression of IL-10, IL-11, and IL-18 under hypoxia.[85] Even with this influx of inflammatory cells and cytokines within the tumor microenvironment, the overall host's anti-tumor immune response is blunted.[76]

## 4. Hypoxia and Distant Metastasis

CTC that are able to survive in circulation must then be home to and extravasate into a distant organ and survive at a distant site. There are individual components of each of these processes that are hypoxia-mediated, such as the homing itself, mesenchymal to epithelial transition, cell proliferation and angiogenesis. These processes and the role of hypoxia in mediating them will be discussed in this section.

## 4.1. Homing of circulating tumor cells

The step of homing of the CTCs to distant organs is a complex process that is not well understood. It is known that tumor cells, as well as endothelial cells, demonstrate hypoxia-dependent upregulation of CXCR4 and its ligand is stromal cell-derived factor-1 (SDF-1, CXCL12).[68,88] CXCR4 is a chemokine receptor, which is a member of the large CXC chemokine family.[89] Multiple biological effects that contribute to the metastatic process, including invasion, migration, and angiogenesis are regulated by chemokines and their receptors.[90] Interestingly, it has been shown that CXCL12, the only known ligand for CXCR4, is preferentially expressed in bone marrow, lymph nodes, liver and lung, suggesting that tumor cells expressing CXCR4 will home to these organs when undergoing metastatic spread.[91] Indeed, it was shown that in an *in vivo* breast cancer model, inhibition of CXCL12/CXCR4 decreases metastasis to lung and lymph nodes.[91] More recently, a second receptor of CXCL12 has been identified, CXCR7, which is thought to have some similar roles as CXCR4, but also has novel independent roles in neoplastic growth *in vivo* as well as maintenance of the tumor vasculature.[92] There are other chemokine/receptor interactions, such as CCL19/CCR7, that are thought to be involved in metastatic spread as well as invasion and migration at distant organs.[93] Perhaps not unexpectedly, expression of either CXCR4 or CCR7 is correlated with poor patient prognosis.[93–96] These chemokines, along with their receptors, play a critical role in homing of cancer cells to distant organs (Fig. 4).[97,98]

## 4.2. Mesenchymal to epithelial transition

Once a CTCs successfully reaches a distant organ and exits the blood stream (extravasation), it now has to colonize the distant site, undergoing the final step in the metastatic cascade. In order to seed in the new tissue,

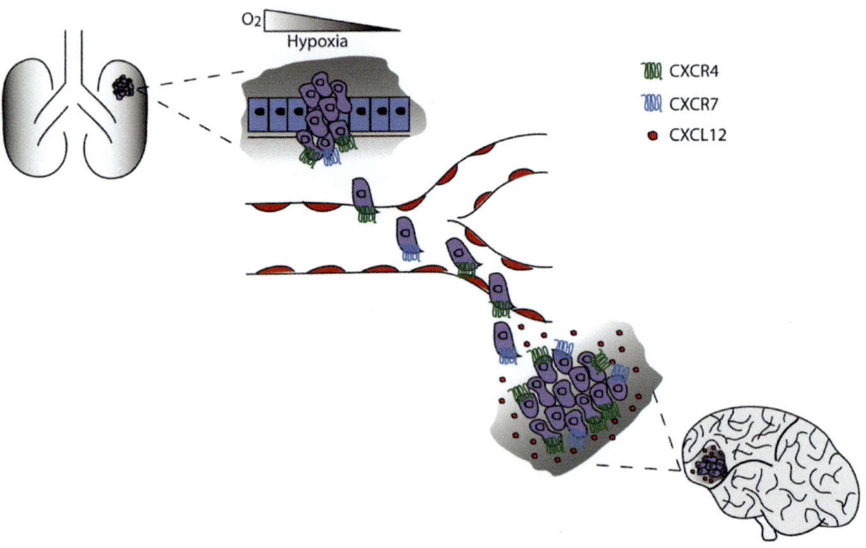


Fig. 4. Homing of CTC. Tumor cells at a primary site are exposed to a hypoxic microenvironment, this leads to upregulation of chemokine receptors, such as CXCR4 and/or CXCR7. This directs the tumor cells to distant organs that express the ligand for these receptors, CXCL12.

it is hypothesized that the invasive mesenchymal cells have to once again undergo a morphological change to a less invasive phenotype.[99] The term "mesenchymal to epithelial transition" has been coined for this process, though whether this actual transition occurs in human cancers is still hotly debated.[99,100] For example, hypoxia, and HIF-1$\alpha$ specifically, could increase levels of E-cadherin and decrease vimentin in osteosarcoma cells.[101] Another group examined the effects of hyperoxia on a DMBA-induced mammary tumor in a rat adenocarcinoma model and found that hyperbaric oxygen (HBO) treatment caused the tumors to be more differentiated and less aggressive.[102] They also found a downregulation in genes associated with EMT, such as *Cdh2*, *Snail*, and *Twist2*.[102] This was one of the first examples utilizing an *in vivo* model of how oxygen could be playing a role in the MET "switch".[102] Another study, in ovarian carcinoma, suggests that once cells reach the peritoneal cavity, they actually reoxygenate, which then leads to the reversal of the hypoxia-regulated EMT phenotype. This MET is hypothesized to allow them to survive and grow in this new normoxic environment.[103] While there is solid evidence of changes in markers of epithelial and mesenchymal phenotypes *in vitro*, more research needs to be done to clarify whether or not MET occurs in patients and to define the mechanisms through which this process happens.

## 4.3. Tumor cell survival and growth

Once established at a metastatic site, tumor cells are thought to be able to either stay as micrometastases for an unknown length of time until they start to grow and give rise to macrometastases.[39,104] One thought is that a small percentage of tumor cells are cancer stem cells, and that hypoxia has the capacity to regulate these cells, which likely play a role in the development and growth of macrometastases.[105] The topic of hypoxia and cancer stem cells will be described in greater detail in Chapter 11. In this section, we will focus on tumor cell survival and growth events that are hypoxia-mediated.

Depending on where metastasis occurs, tumor cells will either be exposed to hypoxia quickly, such as in the hematopoietic stem cell niche in the bone or portions of the liver, or they will be exposed to hypoxia as the tumor grows.[106] It is known that hypoxia influences a tumor cell's ability to survive and grow, both at the metastatic site as well as at the site of the primary tumor.[107] This occurs through a number of routes, such as through the expression of growth factors. For example, hepatocyte growth factor (HGF), which can be regulated by HIF-1$\alpha$, has been shown to increase both proliferation and tube formation of endothelial progenitor cells (EPCs).[108] In addition, HIF-1$\alpha$ also induces VEGF and VEGFR1 expression, which serve to increase blood vessel formation which is necessary for tumor cell growth.[6,109]

## 4.4. Angiogenesis

Once tumor cells have colonized at the metastatic site, they are only able to grow to 1–2mm in diameter without a supply of nutrients and oxygen.[110–112] This problem is resolved with the growth of new blood vessels, termed angiogenesis, to supply these necessary components to the growing tumor.[39] Why would the tumor become hypoxic if there is angiogenesis occurring? The disconnect between angiogenesis and tumor hypoxia is in large part due to the fast rate of growth of the tumor, which causes the tumor to outgrow the blood vessel supply.[113] In addition, many of the blood vessels associated with hypoxic tumors are both structurally and functionally "abnormal," with leaky vessels and a lack of strong interconnections.[114,115] Both insufficient and inadequate angiogenesis limits the supply of nutrients and oxygen to the growing tumor.

Hypoxia is known to induce a number of mitogenic factors associated with initiation and progression of angiogenesis, such as: VEGF, Platelet-derived growth factor (PDGF), fibroblat growth factor (FGF) and Angiopoietin-2 (Ang-2).[107,113,116–118] The most well characterized of these proangiogenic factors is VEGF (also known as VEGF-A). VEGF-A has a number of roles in the formation of new blood vessels including: chemotaxis of EPCs detachment of pericytes and increases in overall vascular permeability.[119] Many studies have conclusively demonstrated that hypoxia drives the increased expression of VEGF-A through its hypoxia responsive element.[120–122] Specifically, one study examined hepatic micrometastasis using a murine B16 melanoma cell line and showed with pimonizadole staining that regions of hypoxia can be found even in micrometastasis.[123] Within this same model, they demonstrated that hypoxia induces hepatic stellate cells (HSCs) to produce VEGF.[123] Therefore, hypoxia provides the proangiogenic microenvironment needed for the generation of new vasculature.

In addition to VEGF, another hypoxia-inducible angiogenic factor is angiopoietin 2 (Ang-2, ANGPT2).[113] This factor plays a role in angiogenesis by binding to its receptor, TIE2[124], and is involved in vessel remodeling.[125,126] In fact, HIF-1$\alpha$ directly binds to a HRE within the Ang-2 gene in human microvascular endothelial cells, linking hypoxia to regulation of this gene.[126] In addition to upregulation of proangiogenic factors, hypoxia also downregulates anti-angiogenic factors, such as the secreted glycoprotein thrombospondin-1 (TSP-1).[127] Thus hypoxia can suppress expression of TSP-1 in both rodent fibroblasts and select human cells, while also inducing VEGF and promoting angiogenesis.[127]

## 5.  Targeting Hypoxia and Metastasis in the Clinic

There is a well-established link between hypoxia and clinical disease. In human patients, hypoxia can be classified as either physiological hypoxia (~2% $O_2$), pathological hypoxia (~1% $O_2$) or radiobiological hypoxia (~0.4% $O_2$).[128] Studies have demonstrated that tumor cells under anoxic conditions are approximately three times more resistant to conventional radiotherapy than well-oxygenated tumors.[129,130] Hypoxic tumor cells are also more resistant to chemotherapy, partly due to hypoxia's ability to impair drug delivery through leaky vasculature as well as inducing genetic instability.[39,130] In addition, hypoxia can slow cell proliferation, and since cytotoxic chemotherapies require proliferating cells to be effective, hypoxia can also impede chemotherapies effectiveness in this regard.[131,132]

Retrospective studies have utilized patient samples to determine hypoxia gene signatures and link these signatures with human survival and time to recurrence in patients. For example, one group developed a hypoxia response signature that was successful in predicting poorer overall survival and a higher risk of disease recurrence in breast and ovarian cancer patient samples.[133] Importantly, this group also compared their hypoxia signature to other well-established prognostic and clinical decision-making factors, such as tumor size, grade and ER status in a multivariate COX model. They determined that their signature contributed more significantly than these other factors to predicting patient prognosis.[133] Another group used *in vivo* selected MDA–MB-231 breast cancer cell subpopulations with varying metastatic potential to come up with a metastasis signature that predicts metastatic potential to bone in their model.[134] Interestingly, none of the genes in their highly bone-metastatic gene signature overlapped with the previously identified poor prognosis breast cancer signature.[135] Also, the signature for metastasis to bone was different than the signature identified for metastasis to the adrenal gland.[134] While these studies all demonstrate the vast amount of data available to classify metastatic disease in individual patients, how they will be used clinically remains to be seen. Likely, the use of hypoxia signatures, as well as signatures of metastasis, to predict the aggressiveness of individual cancers will be translated to the clinic as targeted therapies and individualized cancer treatment regimes become more popular.

Since both HIF-$1\alpha$ and HIF-$2\alpha$ have been shown to be upregulated in primary tumors, such as breast, renal, colon, and pancreatic cancers, as well as in metastatic disease, targeting hypoxia and the HIF pathway for therapy should theoretically enhance anti-metastatic therapy.[136] However, due to the reasons outlined above, hypoxia poses problems for the treatment of cancers by traditional radiation and chemotherapy. Initially, treatments to target hypoxia were performed using HBO chambers, which exposed the whole patient to high levels of oxygen and pressure.[137] This allowed increased oxygen in the patient's plasma and delivery to the tumor tissue.[137] There was concern that increased levels of oxygen in the body could lead to long-term deleterious effects, such as actually causing increased recurrence of disease, since oxygen is required for cellular processes including wound healing and angiogenesis.[137] Thorough reviews of the literature show that studies failed to show that HBO leads to increased disease recurrence or tumor growth, with only 10% of studies over the course of 50 years showing a "tumor-stimulatory" effect of HBO.[137,138] However, HBO has not become a standard treatment in the clinic, likely due to safety concerns as well as the emergence of other promising therapies, discussed below.

Table 1 outlines a small subset of the hypoxia-regulated proteins discussed in this chapter that are (or were recently) targeted in clinical trials for cancer treatment. Since hypoxia regulates proteins involved in each step of the metastatic cascade, drugs targeting these various steps

Table 1.   Selection of hypoxia regulated genes and clinical trials.

| Hypoxia-inducible Protein | Acronym | Drug(s) | Drug Type/ Administation | Target | Clinical Trial |
|---|---|---|---|---|---|
| Connective Tissue Growth Factor | CTGF | FG-3019 | I.V. (mAb) | CTGF | Pancreatic cancer, Phase II |
| Lysyl Oxidase | LOX | ATN-224, Tetrathiomolybdate | Small molecule (Copper Binding Agent) | | Non-squamous NSCLC, Phase I Esophageal Carcinoma, Phase II Prostate Cancer, Phase II (completed) Hepatocellular Carcinoma, Phase II (completed) |
| Lysyl Oxidase-like 2 | LOXL2 | Simtuzumab (GS-6624) | I.V. (mAb) | LOXL2 | Metastatic Pancreatic Adnocarcinoma, Phase II (completed) Colorectal Carcinoma, Phase II (completed) |
| Vascular endothelial growth factor | VEGF | hVEGF26-104/ RFASE | I.M. (vaccine) | VEGF | Metastatic Solid Tumors Phase I |

*(Continued)*

Table 1.  (*Continued*)

| Hypoxia-inducible Protein | Acronym | Drug(s) | Drug Type/ Administation | Target | Clinical Trial |
|---|---|---|---|---|---|
| | | Nintedanib | Oral | VEGF, FGF and PDGF (receptors) | Thyroid Cancer Phase II |
| | | Sevacizumab | Injection (mAb) | VEGF | Advanced or Metatatic Solid Tumors, Phase Ia |
| | | Lucitanib | Oral | FGFR 1-3, VEGFR 1-3, and PDGFR $\alpha/\beta$ | Advanced/Metastatic Lung Cancer, Phase II |
| | | Axitinib | Oral | VEGF receptor | Clear-cell Metastatic Renal Cell Carcinoma, Phase II |
| Matrix Metalloproteinases | MMPs | COL-3 | Oral | MMP Inhibitor | Refractory Metastatic Cancer, Phase I (completed) |
| | | PCK3145 | I.V. (peptide) | MMP-9 | Metastatic Prostate Cancer, Phase I (completed) |

| | | | | | |
|---|---|---|---|---|---|
| | | GS-5745 | I.V. (mAb) | MMP-9 | Soild Tumors, Phase I |
| E-cadherin | E-cad | SNDX-275 | Oral | EGFR, E-cadherin and ErbB3 (reactivation) | NSCLC, Phase II (completed) |
| CXC chemokine receptor type 4 | CXCR4 | BKT-140 | S.C. | CXCR4 | Multiple Myeloma , Phase I/IIa (completed) |
| | | BL-8040 | S.C. | CXCR4 | Chronic Myelogenous Leukemia Phase I/II |
| | | Plerixafor (Mozobil) | I.V. | CXCR4 | Advanced Pancreatic, Ovarian and Colorectal cancers, Phase I |
| $\alpha v\beta 3$ integrin | $\alpha v\beta 3$ | 99mTc-3PRGD2 (SPECT/CT) | I.V. | $\alpha v\beta 3$ | Diagnosis and Evaluation of Lung Cancer Patients, Phase 0 |

Hypoxia-inducible proteins are listed in the first column, with drugs targeting them in the "Drugs" column. Target specificity is indicated in the "target" column. The listed drugs are used either as monotherapies or combined therapies in the cancer types listed in the right column. The stage of the clinical trial the drug is currently in (or completed) is listed in the "clinical trial" column on the right. Information obtained from Clinicaltrials.gov – June 2015.

are represented in clinical trials being conducted in the United States as well as at institutions in other countries around the world. Some of these targets include components of the tumor microenvironment involved in the initial steps of cell migration and invasion, such as CTGF, LOX, and MMPs, described in Section 2.1. Other hypoxia-inducible targets in clinical trails include proteins involved in angiogenesis, such as VEGF, and these are also outlined in Table 1. Targeting angiogenesis has proven successful in the past, with Bevacizumab (Avastin) targeting VEGF-A receiving approval by the FDA in 2004, and is currently being used to treat a wide range of cancer types. As more is understood about the role of hypoxia in metastasis, additional hypoxia-regulated targets will likely be identified and added to the growing list of therapeutic targets.

## 6. Conclusions

With such a large number of cancer deaths due to metastasis, it is necessary to characterize the mechanisms of the spread of disease. A lot of work has been done in this regard, breaking down the metastatic process into individual steps that can each be thoroughly examined. In this chapter, we have linked one component of the tumor microenvironment, hypoxia, with individual steps of the metastatic cascade including: EMT, intravasation, survival in the blood stream, extravasation, and growth at a distant site. Clinically, studies are underway to target components of each of these steps of the metastatic process to attempt to decrease metastatic disease in patients and improve overall survival.

## References


1. Hanahan, D., and Weinberg, R. A., The hallmarks of cancer. *Cell*, **100**(1), pp. 57–70, 2000.
2. Chaffer, C. L., and Weinberg, R. A., A perspective on cancer cell metastasis. *Science*, **331**(6024), pp. 1559–1564, 2011.
3. Disibio, G., and French, S. W., Metastatic patterns of cancers: results from a large autopsy study. *Arch. Pathol. Lab. Med.*, **132**(6), pp. 931–939, 2008.

4. Yilmaz, M., and Christofori, G., EMT, the cytoskeleton, and cancer cell invasion. *Cancer Metastasis Rev.*, **28**(1–2), pp. 15–33, 2009.

5. Gilkes, D. M., Semenza, G. L., and Wirtz, D., Hypoxia and the extracellular matrix: drivers of tumour metastasis. *Nat. Rev. Cancer*, **14**(6), pp. 430–439, 2014.

6. Ruan, K., Song, G., and Ouyang, G., Role of hypoxia in the hallmarks of human cancer. *J. Cell. Biochem.*, **107**(6), pp. 1053–1062, 2009.

7. Rankin, E. B., and Giaccia, A. J., The role of hypoxia-inducible factors in tumorigenesis. *Cell Death Differ.*, **15**(4), pp. 678–685, 2008.

8. Zhong, H. *et al.*, Overexpression of hypoxia-inducible factor 1alpha in common human cancers and their metastases. *Cancer Res.*, **59**(22), pp. 5830–5835, 1999.

9. Desgrosellier, J. S., and Cheresh, D. A., Integrins in cancer: biological implications and therapeutic opportunities. *Natl. Rev. Cancer*, **10**(1), pp. 9–22, 2010.

10. Pattabiraman, D. R., and Weinberg, R. A., Tackling the cancer stem cells — what challenges do they pose? *Natl. Rev. Drug. Discov.*, **13**(7), pp. 497–512, 2014.

11. Frantz, C., Stewart, K. M., and Weaver, V. M., The extracellular matrix at a glance. *J. Cell. Sci.*, **123**(24), pp. 4195–4200, 2010.

12. Cox, T. R., and Erler, J. T., Remodeling and homeostasis of the extracellular matrix: implications for fibrotic diseases and cancer. *Dis. Model. Mech.*, **4**(2), pp. 165–178, 2011.

13. Valastyan, S., and Weinberg, R. A., Tumor metastasis: molecular insights and evolving paradigms. *Cell*, **147**(2), pp. 275–292, 2011.

14. Leblond, C. P., and Inoue, S., Structure, composition, and assembly of basement membrane. *Am. J. Anat.*, **185**(4), pp. 367–390, 1989.

15. Askari, J. A. *et al.*, Linking integrin conformation to function. *J. Cell. Sci.*, **122**(2), pp. 165–170, 2009.

16. Finger, E. C., and Giaccia, A. J., Hypoxia, inflammation and the tumor microenvironment in metastatic disease. *Cancer Metastasis Rev.*, **29**(2), pp. 285–293, 2010.

17. Ridgway, P. F. *et al.*, Hypoxia increases reepithelialization via an alphavbeta6-dependent pathway. *Wound Repair Regen.*, **13**(2), pp. 158–164, 2005.

18. Berghoff, A. S. *et al.*, Alphavbeta3, alphavbeta5 and alphavbeta6 integrins in brain metastases of lung cancer. *Clin. Exp. Metastasis.*, **31**(7), pp. 841–851, 2014.

19. Chang, Q. *et al.*, Effect of antisense hypoxia-inducible factor 1alpha on progression, metastasis, and chemosensitivity of pancreatic cancer. *Pancreas*, **32**(3), pp. 297–305, 2006.

20. Rohwer, N. *et al.*, Hypoxia-inducible factor 1alpha mediates anoikis resistance via suppression of alpha5 integrin. *Cancer Res.*, **68**(24), pp. 10113–10120, 2008.

21. Lynch, C. C., and Matrisian, L. M., Matrix metalloproteinases in tumor-host cell communication. *Differentiation*, **70**(9, 10), pp. 561–573, 2002.

22. Brinckerhoff, C. E., and Matrisian, L. M., Matrix metalloproteinases: a *tail* of a frog that became a prince. *Nat. Rev. Mol. Cell. Biol.*, **3**(3), pp. 207–214, 2002.

23. Murphy, G., Tissue inhibitors of metalloproteinases. *Genome. Biol.*, **12**(11), p. 233, 2011.

24. Schmalfeldt, B. *et al.*, Increased expression of matrix metalloproteinases (MMP)-2, MMP-9, and the urokinase-type plasminogen activator is associated with progression from benign to advanced ovarian cancer. *Clin. Cancer Res.*, **7**(8), pp. 2396–2404, 2001.

25. Pulukuri, S. M. *et al.*, Epigenetic inactivation of the tissue inhibitor of metalloproteinase-2 (TIMP-2) gene in human prostate tumors. *Oncogene*, **26**(36), pp. 5229–5237, 2007.

26. Mohanam, S. *et al.*, Expression of tissue inhibitors of metalloproteinases: negative regulators of human glioblastoma invasion *in vivo*. *Clin. Exp. Metastasis.*, **13**(1), pp. 57–62, 1995.

27. Hua, H. *et al.*, Matrix metalloproteinases in tumorigenesis: an evolving paradigm. *Cell. Mol. Life Sci.*, **68**(23), pp. 3853–3868, 2011.

28. LeBleu, V. S., Macdonald, B., and Kalluri, R., Structure and function of basement membranes. *Exp. Biol. Med.* (Maywood), **232**(9), pp. 1121–1129, 2007.

29. Zeng, Z. S., Cohen, A. M. and Guillem, J.G. Loss of basement membrane type IV collagen is associated with increased expression of metalloproteinases 2 and 9 (MMP-2 and MMP-9) during human colorectal tumorigenesis. *Carcinogenesis*, **20**(5), pp. 749–755, 1999.

30. Davies, B. *et al.*, Activity of type IV collagenases in benign and malignant breast disease. *Br. J. Cancer.*, **67**(5), pp. 1126–1131, 1993.

31. Brown, P. D. *et al.*, Association between expression of activated 72-kilodalton gelatinase and tumor spread in non-small-cell lung carcinoma. *J. Natl. Cancer Inst.*, **85**(7), pp. 574–578, 1993.

32. Stearns, M. E., and Wang, M., Type IV collagenase (M(r) 72,000) expression in human prostate: benign and malignant tissue. *Cancer Res.*, **53**(4), pp. 878–883, 1993.

33. Zhu, S. *et al.*, Transcriptional upregulation of MT2-MMP in response to hypoxia is promoted by HIF-1alpha in cancer cells. *Mol. Carcinog.*, **50**(10), pp. 770–780, 2011.

34. Choi, J. Y. *et al.*, Overexpression of MMP-9 and HIF-1alpha in breast cancer cells under hypoxic conditions. *J. Breast Cancer*, **14**(2), pp. 88–95, 2011.
35. Shyu, K. G. *et al.*, Hypoxia-inducible factor 1alpha regulates lung adenocarcinoma cell invasion. *Exp. Cell. Res.*, **313**(6), pp. 1181–1191, 2007.
36. Petrella, B. L., Lohi, J., and Brinckerhoff, C. E., Identification of membrane type-1 matrix metalloproteinase as a target of hypoxia-inducible factor-2 alpha in von Hippel-Lindau renal cell carcinoma. *Oncogene*, **24**(6), pp. 1043–1052, 2005.
37. Choi, S. H. *et al.*, Effects of the knockdown of hypoxia inducible factor-1alpha expression by adenovirus-mediated shRNA on angiogenesis and tumor growth in hepatocellular carcinoma cell lines. *Korean J. Hepatol.*, **16**(3), pp. 280–287, 2010.
38. Xiao, Q., and Ge, G., Lysyl oxidase, extracellular matrix remodeling and cancer metastasis. *Cancer Microenviron.*, **5**(3), pp. 261–273, 2012.
39. Chang, J., and Erler, J., Hypoxia-mediated metastasis. *Adv. Exp. Med. Biol.*, **772**, pp. 55–81, 2014.
40. Trackman, P. C. *et al.*, Post-translational glycosylation and proteolytic processing of a lysyl oxidase precursor. *J. Biol. Chem.*, **267**(12), pp. 8666–8671, 1992.
41. Panchenko, M. V. *et al.*, Metalloproteinase activity secreted by fibrogenic cells in the processing of prolysyl oxidase. Potential role of procollagen C-proteinase. *J. Biol. Chem.*, **271**(12), pp. 7113–7119, 1996.
42. Csiszar, K., Lysyl oxidases: a novel multifunctional amine oxidase family. *Prog. Nucleic Acid Res. Mol. Biol.*, **70**, pp. 1–32, 2001.
43. Erler, J. T. *et al.*, Hypoxia-induced lysyl oxidase is a critical mediator of bone marrow cell recruitment to form the premetastatic niche. *Cancer Cell.*, **15**(1), pp. 35–44, 2009.
44. Cox, T. R. *et al.*, The hypoxic cancer secretome induces premetastatic bone lesions through lysyl oxidase. *Nature*, **522**(7554), pp. 106–110, 2015.
45. Kirschmann, D. A. *et al.*, A molecular role for lysyl oxidase in breast cancer invasion. *Cancer Res.*, **62**(15), pp. 4478–4483, 2002.
46. Erler, J. T. *et al.*, Lysyl oxidase is essential for hypoxia-induced metastasis. *Nature*, **440**(7088), pp. 1222–1226, 2006.
47. Barry-Hamilton, V. *et al.*, Allosteric inhibition of lysyl oxidase-like-2 impedes the development of a pathologic microenvironment. *Nat. Med.*, **16**(9), pp. 1009–1017, 2010.
48. Bennewith, K. L. *et al.*, The role of tumor cell-derived connective tissue growth factor (CTGF/CCN2) in pancreatic tumor growth. *Cancer Res.*, **69**(3), pp. 775–784, 2009.

49. de Winter, P., Leoni, P., and Abraham, D., Connective tissue growth factor: structure-function relationships of a mosaic, multifunctional protein. *Growth Factors*, **26**(2), pp. 80–91, 2008.

50. Abreu, J. G. *et al.*, Connective-tissue growth factor (CTGF) modulates cell signalling by BMP and TGF-beta. *Nat. Cell. Biol.*, **4**(8), pp. 599–604, 2002.

51. Inoki, I. *et al.*, Connective tissue growth factor binds vascular endothelial growth factor (VEGF) and inhibits VEGF-induced angiogenesis. *FASEB J.*, **16**(2), pp. 219–221, 2002.

52. Lipson, K. E. *et al.*, CTGF is a central mediator of tissue remodeling and fibrosis and its inhibition can reverse the process of fibrosis. Fibrogenesis *Tissue Repair*, **5**(1), p. S24, 2012.

53. Finger, E. C. *et al.*, CTGF is a therapeutic target for metastatic melanoma. *Oncogene*, **33**(9), pp. 1093–1100, 2014.

54. Braig, S. *et al.*, CTGF is overexpressed in malignant melanoma and promotes cell invasion and migration. *Br. J. Cancer.*, **105**(2), pp. 231–238, 2011.

55. Higgins, D. F. *et al.*, Hypoxic induction of Ctgf is directly mediated by Hif-1. *Am. J. Physiol. Renal Physiol.*, **287**(6), pp. F1223–1232, 2004.

56. Shimo, T. *et al.*, Connective tissue growth factor as a major angiogenic agent that is induced by hypoxia in a human breast cancer cell line. *Cancer Lett.*, **174**(1), pp. 57–64, 2001.

57. Chen, P. S. *et al.*, CTGF enhances the motility of breast cancer cells via an integrin-alphavbeta3-ERK1/2-dependent S100A4-upregulated pathway. *J. Cell. Sci.*, **120**(12), pp. 2053–2065, 2007.

58. Tsai, H. C. *et al.*, CTGF increases matrix metalloproteinases expression and subsequently promotes tumor metastasis in human osteosarcoma through down-regulating miR-519d. *Oncotarget*, **5**(11), pp. 3800–3812, 2014.

59. Esteban, M. A. *et al.*, Regulation of E-cadherin expression by VHL and hypoxia-inducible factor. *Cancer Res.*, **66**(7), pp. 3567–3575, 2006.

60. Lamouille, S., Xu, J., and Derynck, R., Molecular mechanisms of epithelial-mesenchymal transition. *Nat. Rev. Mol. Cell. Biol.*, **15**(3), pp. 178–196, 2014.

61. Hotz, B. *et al.*, Epithelial to mesenchymal transition: expression of the regulators snail, slug, and twist in pancreatic cancer. *Clin. Cancer Res.*, **13**(16), pp. 4769–4776, 2007.

62. Luo, D. *et al.*, Mouse snail is a target gene for HIF. *Mol. Cancer Res.*, **9**(2), pp. 234–245, 2011.

63. Zhang, Y., Fan, N., and Yang, J., Expression and clinical significance of hypoxia-inducible factor 1alpha, Snail and E-cadherin in human ovarian cancer cell lines. *Mol. Med. Rep.*, **12**(3), pp. 3393–3399, 2015.

64. Chen, J. *et al.*, Hypoxia potentiates Notch signaling in breast cancer leading to decreased E-cadherin expression and increased cell migration and invasion. *Br. J. Cancer.*, **102**(2), pp. 351–360, 2010.

65. Zhang, W. *et al.*, HIF-1alpha Promotes Epithelial-Mesenchymal Transition and Metastasis through Direct Regulation of ZEB1 in Colorectal Cancer. *PLoS One*, **10**(6), p. e0129603, 2015.

66. Zhe, X., Cher, M. L., and Bonfil, R. D., Circulating tumor cells: finding the needle in the haystack. *Am. J. Cancer Res.*, **1**(6), pp. 740–751, 2011.

67. Alix-Panabieres, C., and Pantel, K., Challenges in circulating tumour cell research. *Nat. Rev. Cancer*, **14**(9), pp. 623–631, 2014.

68. Gupta, G. P., and Massague, J., Cancer metastasis: building a framework. *Cell*, **127**(4), pp. 679–695, 2006.

69. Meng, S. *et al.*, Circulating tumor cells in patients with breast cancer dormancy. *Clin. Cancer Res.*, **10**(24), pp. 8152–8162, 2004.

70. Sun, L. *et al.*, Upregulation of BNIP3 mediated by ERK/HIF-1alpha pathway induces autophagy and contributes to anoikis resistance of hepatocellular carcinoma cells. *Future. Oncol.*, **10**(8), pp. 1387–1398, 2014.

71. Whelan, K. A. *et al.*, The oncogene HER2/neu (ERBB2) requires the hypoxia-inducible factor HIF-1 for mammary tumor growth and anoikis resistance. *J. Biol. Chem.*, **288**(22), pp. 15865–15877, 2013.

72. Whelan, K. A., and Reginato, M. J., Surviving without oxygen: hypoxia regulation of mammary morphogenesis and anoikis. *Cell Cycle*, **10**(14), pp. 2287–2294, 2011.

73. Kang, H. G. *et al.*, E-cadherin cell-cell adhesion in ewing tumor cells mediates suppression of anoikis through activation of the ErbB4 tyrosine kinase. *Cancer Res.*, **67**(7), pp. 3094–3105, 2007.

74. Wirtz, D., Konstantopoulos, K., and Searson, P. C., The physics of cancer: the role of physical interactions and mechanical forces in metastasis. *Nat. Rev. Cancer*, **11**(7), pp. 512–522, 2011.

75. Mitchell, M. J., and King, M. R., Fluid shear stress sensitizes cancer cells to receptor-mediated apoptosis via trimeric death receptors. *New. J. Phys.*, **15**, p. 015008, 2013.

76. Coussens, L. M., and Werb, Z., Inflammation and cancer. *Nature*, **420**(6917), pp. 860–867, 2002.

77. Labiano, S., Palazon, A., and Melero, I., Immune Response Regulation in the Tumor Microenvironment by Hypoxia. *Semin Oncol.*, **42**(3), pp. 378–386, 2015.

78. Kumar, V., and Gabrilovich, D. I., Hypoxia-inducible factors in regulation of immune responses in tumour microenvironment. *Immunology*, **143**(4), pp. 512–519, 2014.

79. Takeda, N. *et al.*, Differential activation and antagonistic function of HIF-{alpha} isoforms in macrophages are essential for NO homeostasis. *Genes. Dev.*, **24**(5), pp. 491–501, 2010.

80. Lewis, C. E. *et al.*, Cytokine regulation of angiogenesis in breast cancer: the role of tumor-associated macrophages. *J. Leukoc. Biol.*, **57**(5), pp. 747–751, 1995.

81. Luo, J. L. *et al.*, Inhibition of NF-kappaB in cancer cells converts inflammation- induced tumor growth mediated by TNFalpha to TRAIL-mediated tumor regression. *Cancer Cell*, **6**(3), pp. 297–305, 2004.

82. Landskron, G. *et al.*, Chronic inflammation and cytokines in the tumor microenvironment. *J. Immunol. Res.*, **2014**, p. 149185, 2014.

83. Bao, B. *et al.*, Hypoxia induced aggressiveness of prostate cancer cells is linked with deregulated expression of VEGF, IL-6 and miRNAs that are attenuated by CDF. *PLoS One*, **7**(8), p. e43726, 2012.

84. Hsing, C. H. *et al.*, Upregulated IL-19 in breast cancer promotes tumor progression and affects clinical outcome. *Clin. Cancer Res.*, **18**(3), pp. 713–725, 2012.

85. Shen, Z. *et al.*, IL10, IL11, IL18 are differently expressed in CD14+ TAMs and play different role in regulating the invasion of gastric cancer cells under hypoxia. *Cytokine*, **59**(2), pp. 352–357, 2012.

86. Sanguinetti, A. *et al.*, Interleukin-6 and pro inflammatory status in the breast tumor microenvironment. *World. J. Surg. Oncol.*, **13**, p. 129, 2015.

87. Zarogoulidis, P. *et al.*, Interleukin-8 and interleukin-17 for cancer. *Cancer Invest.*, **32**(5), pp. 197–205, 2014.

88. Schutyser, E. *et al.*, Hypoxia enhances CXCR4 expression in human microvascular endothelial cells and human melanoma cells. *Eur. Cytokine. Netw.*, **18**(2), pp. 59–70, 2007.

89. Martin, B. J., Inhibiting vasculogenesis after radiation: a new paradigm to improve local control by radiotherapy. *Semin. Radiat. Oncol.*, **23**(4), pp. 281–287, 2013.

90. Singh, R., Lillard, J. W., Jr., and Singh, S., Chemokines: key players in cancer progression and metastasis. *Front Biosci* (Schol Ed), **3**, pp. 1569–1582, 2011.

91. Muller, A. *et al.*, Involvement of chemokine receptors in breast cancer metastasis. *Nature*, **410**(6824), pp. 50–56, 2001.

92. Cavazos, D. A., and Brenner, A. J., Hypoxia in astrocytic tumors and implications for therapy. *Neurobiol Dis.*, **85**, pp. 227–233, 2015.

93. Albert, S. *et al.*, Focus on the role of the CXCL12/CXCR4 chemokine axis in head and neck squamous cell carcinoma. *Head Neck*, **35**(12), pp. 1819–1828, 2013.

94. Pitkin, L. *et al.*, Expression of CC chemokine receptor 7 in tonsillar cancer predicts cervical nodal metastasis, systemic relapse and survival. *Br. J. Cancer.*, **97**(5), pp. 670–677, 2007.

95. Tsuzuki, H. *et al.*, Oral and oropharyngeal squamous cell carcinomas expressing CCR7 have poor prognoses. *Auris Nasus Larynx.*, **33**(1), pp. 37–42, 2006.

96. Scala, S. *et al.*, Expression of CXCR4 predicts poor prognosis in patients with malignant melanoma. *Clin. Cancer Res.*, **11**(5), pp. 1835–1841, 2005.

97. Domanska, U. M. *et al.*, A review on CXCR4/CXCL12 axis in oncology: no place to hide. *Eur. J. Cancer.*, **49**(1), pp. 219–230, 2013.

98. Chatterjee, S., Behnam Azad, B., and Nimmagadda, S. The intricate role of CXCR4 in cancer. *Adv. Cancer. Res.*, **124**, pp. 31–82, 2014.

99. Gao, D. *et al.*, Microenvironmental regulation of epithelial-mesenchymal transitions in cancer. *Cancer Res.*, **72**(19), pp. 4883–4889, 2012.

100. Chaffer, C. L., Thompson, E. W., and Williams, E. D., Mesenchymal to epithelial transition in development and disease. *Cells Tissues Organs*, **185**(1–3), pp. 7–19, 2007.

101. Gurzu, S. *et al.*, Epithelial-mesenchymal, mesenchymal-epithelial, and endothelial-mesenchymal transitions in malignant tumors: An update. *World. J. Clin. Cases*, **3**(5), pp. 393–404, 2015.

102. Moen, I. *et al.*, Hyperoxic treatment induces mesenchymal-to-epithelial transition in a rat adenocarcinoma model. *PLoS One*, **4**(7), p. e6381, 2009.

103. Elloul, S. *et al.*, Mesenchymal-to-epithelial transition determinants as characteristics of ovarian carcinoma effusions. *Clin. Exp. Metastasis.*, **27**(3), pp. 161–172, 2010.

104. Pantel, K., and Alix-Panabieres, C., Circulating tumour cells in cancer patients: challenges and perspectives. *Trends Mol. Med.*, **16**(9), pp. 398–406, 2010.

105. Keith, B., and Simon, M. C., Hypoxia-inducible factors, stem cells, and cancer. *Cell*, **129**(3), pp. 465–472, 2007.

106. Lu, X., and Kang, Y., Hypoxia and hypoxia-inducible factors: master regulators of metastasis. *Clin. Cancer Res.*, **16**(24), pp. 5928–5935, 2010.

107. Harris, A. L., Hypoxia — a key regulatory factor in tumour growth. *Natl. Rev. Cancer*, **2**(1), pp. 38–47, 2002.

108. Yu, F. *et al.*, HGF expression induced by HIF-1alpha promote the proliferation and tube formation of endothelial progenitor cells. *Cell Biol. Int.*, **39**(3), pp. 310–317, 2015.

109. Mardilovich, K., and Shaw, L. M., Hypoxia regulates insulin receptor substrate-2 expression to promote breast carcinoma cell survival and invasion. *Cancer Res.*, **69**(23), pp. 8894–8901, 2009.

110. Ribatti, D., Judah Folkman, a pioneer in the study of angiogenesis. *Angiogenesis*, **11**(1), pp. 3–10, 2008.

111. Folkman, J., Long, D. M., Jr., and Becker, F. F., Growth and metastasis of tumor in organ culture. *Cancer*, **16**, pp. 453–467, 1963.

112. Nishida, N. *et al.*, Angiogenesis in cancer. *Vasc. Health Risk Manag.*, **2**(3), pp. 213–219, 2006.

113. Brahimi-Horn, M. C., Chiche, J., and Pouyssegur, J., Hypoxia and cancer. *J. Mol. Med. (Berl)*, **85**(12), pp. 1301–1307, 2007.

114. Dewhirst, M. W. *et al.*, Morphologic and hemodynamic comparison of tumor and healing normal tissue microvasculature. *Int. J. Radiat. Oncol. Biol. Phys.*, **17**(1), pp. 91–99, 1989.

115. Goel, S. *et al.*, Normalization of the vasculature for treatment of cancer and other diseases. *Physiol. Rev.*, **91**(3), pp. 1071–1121, 2011.

116. Kourembanas, S., Hannan, R. L., and Faller, D. V., Oxygen tension regulates the expression of the platelet-derived growth factor-B chain gene in human endothelial cells. *J. Clin. Invest.*, **86**(2), pp. 670–674, 1990.

117. Pichiule, P., Chavez, J. C., and LaManna, J. C., Hypoxic regulation of angiopoietin-2 expression in endothelial cells. *J. Biol. Chem.*, **279**(13), pp. 12171–12180, 2004.

118. Koong, A. C. *et al.*, Candidate genes for the hypoxic tumor phenotype. *Cancer Res.*, **60**(4), pp. 883–887, 2000.

119. Moens, S. *et al.*, The multifaceted activity of VEGF in angiogenesis — Implications for therapy responses. *Cytokine Growth Factor Rev.*, **25**(4), pp. 473–482, 2014.

120. Forsythe, J. A. *et al.*, Activation of vascular endothelial growth factor gene transcription by hypoxia-inducible factor 1. *Mol. Cell. Biol.*, **16**(9), pp. 4604–4613, 1996.

121. Liu, Y. *et al.*, Hypoxia regulates vascular endothelial growth factor gene expression in endothelial cells. Identification of a 5' enhancer. *Circ. Res.*, **77**(3), pp. 638–643, 1995.

122. Levy, A. P. *et al.*, Transcriptional regulation of the rat vascular endothelial growth factor gene by hypoxia. *J. Biol. Chem.*, **270**(22), pp. 13333–13340, 1995.

123. Olaso, E. *et al.*, Proangiogenic role of tumor-activated hepatic stellate cells in experimental melanoma metastasis. *Hepatology*, **37**(3), pp. 674–685, 2003.

124. Semenza, G. L., Cancer-stromal cell interactions mediated by hypoxia-inducible factors promote angiogenesis, lymphangiogenesis, and metastasis. *Oncogene*, **32**(35), pp. 4057–4063, 2013.

125. Thurston, G., Role of Angiopoietins and Tie receptor tyrosine kinases in angiogenesis and lymphangiogenesis. *Cell Tissue Res.*, **314**(1), pp. 61–68, 2003.

126. Simon, M. P., Tournaire, R., and Pouyssegur, J., The angiopoietin-2 gene of endothelial cells is up-regulated in hypoxia by a HIF binding site located in its first intron and by the central` factors GATA-2 and Ets-1. *J. Cell Physiol.*, **217**(3), pp. 809–818, 2008.

127. Laderoute, K. R. *et al.*, Opposing effects of hypoxia on expression of the angiogenic inhibitor thrombospondin 1 and the angiogenic inducer vascular endothelial growth factor. *Clin. Cancer Res.*, **6**(7), pp. 2941–2950, 2000.

128. McKeown, S. R., Defining normoxia, physoxia and hypoxia in tumours-implications for treatment response. *Br. J. Radiol.*, **87**(1035), p. 20130676, 2014.

129. Rockwell, S. *et al.*, Hypoxia and radiation therapy: past history, ongoing research, and future promise. *Curr. Mol. Med.*, **9**(4), pp. 442–458, 2009.

130. Teicher, B. A., Hypoxia and drug resistance. *Cancer Metastasis Rev.*, **13**(2), pp. 139–168, 1994.

131. Vaupel, P., and Harrison, L., Tumor hypoxia: causative factors, compensatory mechanisms, and cellular response. *Oncologist*, **9**(5), pp. 4–9, 2004.

132. Vaupel, P., Thews, O., and Hoeckel, M., Treatment resistance of solid tumors: role of hypoxia and anemia. *Med. Oncol.*, **18**(4), pp. 243–259, 2001.

133. Chi, J. T. *et al.*, Gene expression programs in response to hypoxia: cell type specificity and prognostic significance in human cancers. *PLoS Med*, **3**(3), pp. e47, 2006.

134. Kang, Y. *et al.*, A multigenic program mediating breast cancer metastasis to bone. *Cancer Cell*, **3**(6), pp. 537–549, 2003.

135. van 't Veer, L. J. *et al.*, Gene expression profiling predicts clinical outcome of breast cancer. *Nature*, **415**(6871), pp. 530–536, 2002.

136. Talks, K. L. *et al.*, The expression and distribution of the hypoxia-inducible factors HIF-1alpha and HIF-2alpha in normal human tissues, cancers, and tumor-associated macrophages. *Am. J. Pathol.*, **157**(2), pp. 411–421, 2000.

137. Moen, I., and Stuhr, L. E., Hyperbaric oxygen therapy and cancer — a review. *Target Oncol.*, **7**(4), pp. 233–242, 2012.

138. Daruwalla, J., and Christophi, C., Hyperbaric oxygen therapy for malignancy: a review. *World J. Surg.*, **30**(12), pp. 2112–2131, 2006.

139. Harisi, R., and Jeney, A., Extracellular matrix as target for antitumor therapy. *Onco. Targets Ther.*, **8**, pp. 1387–1398, 2015.

# Chapter 4

# Hypoxia and Cancer Stem Cell Regulation

Sofie Mohlin, Annika Jögi and Sven Påhlman*

*Translational Cancer Research,*
*Lund University Cancer Center at Medicon Village,*
*Building 406, Lund University,*
*SE-223 81 Lund, Sweden*
**Sven.Pahlman@med.lu.se*

## 1.  Introduction

The nature and existence of cancer stem cells have been discussed, questioned and researched upon for decades. The hypothesis that a defined small subpopulation of cancer stem cells within a given tumor solely is responsible for tumor initiation, metastatic progression, and drug resistance has been supported by studies in both hematological and solid malignancies. More recent data however highlights the influence of experimental variations (e.g. choice of mouse strain, presence or absence of certain immune cell populations, etc.) in determining the contribution of cancer stem cells to tumor initiation. In addition, it is becoming increasingly evident that tumor cells are highly dependent on, and influenced by, its microenvironment. There are examples of normal organ stem cells known to reside within hypoxic (i.e. low oxygenated) niches, and this seems to be the case also for cancer stem cells of at least some tumor types. Whether these stem cells and tumor stem cells are kept immature by the hypoxic milieu is largely an open question, but the promotion of immature cell phenotypes by hypoxia is well documented. The link between hypoxia, stem cell features and tumor initiation is further strengthened by the observations that many families with inheritable cancer have loss of genes or gain of function mutations in genes that leads to tumors with a pseudo-hypoxic phenotype and that tumor cells adjacent to blood vessels can have a gene expression pattern as if they were hypoxic. Arguing against a general role of hypoxia as a gatekeeper of adult organ stem cells is the notion that these cells are located in vascular niches in many tissues. In this chapter, we discuss the inhibitory effects of hypoxia on cell differentiation and the hypoxic and pseudo-hypoxic niches in relation to tumor aggressiveness and regulation and behavior of cancer cells.

## 2.  The Clonal versus Stem Cell Cancer Models

Adult or tissue stem cells are defined by two characteristics: capacity of self-renewal and asymmetric division resulting in multipotent progenitor cells with capacities to initiate the formation of distinct differentiation lineages. The notion that mature tissues originate from a tissue-specific, adult stem cell is widely accepted. One example of an adult stem cell that has been carefully identified and characterized in mouse and humans is the hematopoietic stem cell,[1-4] shown to be able to repopulate the entire blood- and immune system. In analogy, cancer stem cells should have self-renewal capacity and give rise to all malignantly transformed cell types of a given tumor. In search for the origin of cancer, two hypotheses have been established; the clonal evolution and the cancer stem cell model.

The term clonal evolution was first used by Peter Nowell in 1976, trying to summarize emerging data suggesting that cancer is the result of the neoplastic transformation of a single cell.[5] The clonal evolution model proposes that a normal cell malignantly transforms by induced genetic changes and that cancer develops by stepwise genetic variation and accumulation of events. Most cells exposed to a carcinogen with consequent acquired genetic variations will die from these changes due to e.g. metabolic disadvantages or immunological recognition. A few cells however will have a genetic advantage over their normal counterparts, and following exposure to new challenges, these cells will either be weakened and destroyed, or even more advantageous and eventually such a cell will give rise to a tumor mass. In the clonal evolution model, the acquired ability of a cancer cell to invade and metastasize distant organs as well as resistance to chemotherapy is conferred by the selection process.

The cancer stem cell model derives from observations by pathologists who recognized the similarities between tumor cells and embryonic cells already in the 1800s. The idea that cancer cells derive from embryo-like cells arose and was further fostered by the notion that tumor aggressiveness correlated positively to tumor cell immaturity. The identification of the first subpopulation of cells proven to have stem cell characteristics and an exclusive ability to form tumors did not occur until 1994, however, when John Dick and colleagues sorted acute myeloid leukemia (AML) cells by surface marker expression.[6] The cell population expressing CD34, but not CD38 ($CD34^+CD38^-$) was phenotypically immature and efficiently formed tumors when engrafted into severe combined immunodeficient (SCID) mice. $CD34^-$ or $CD34^+CD38^+$ cell populations were completely unable to propagate tumor growth *in vivo*. Since then, subpopulations of cells have been identified in many more tumor forms based on cell surface markers, growth characteristics (sphere-forming capacity) or drug resistance, and they all have in common their enhanced tumor-initiating capacity as compared to the remaining cells of the tumor.[7–16] The term cancer stem cell is restricted to cells able to initiate tumor growth, self-renew, and differentiate with multipotent capacity. However, it is not clear whether cells have gained these traits due to their progeny being a normal stem cell, via the process of dedifferentiation, or through somatic acquiring of such characteristics. In light of these unanswered questions, and the debate around using the term *cancer stem cell* for cells with an unknown origin, alternative terms, such as tumor-initiating or tumor-promoting cells, are being used. Considering relapsed tumors often gain novel mutations as compared to the primary tumor,[17] and the documented vast genetic heterogeneity in at least some tumors,[18] it seems likely that both the clonal and the stem cell models contribute to our understanding of how tumors evolve and become progressively more aggressive. With this notion in mind, we focus here on hypoxia, stem cells, cancer stem cells and the effects that oxygen might have on these cohorts of cells.

# 3.  The Stem Cell Niche

The search for adult stem cells has to some extent been a search for niches where these cell populations reside, based on the assumption that stem cells require defined conditions to stay immature and multipotent. Roy Schofield presented the first formulation of the existence of specified niches in a pioneering review article in the 1970s.[19] The niche hypothesis was based on the work by Till and McCulloch demonstrating that single cells were able to yield descendants of multiple lineages, while still preserving the multipotent feature of the mother cell.[20–22] The assay used in these studies, an *in vivo* spleen colony-forming (CFU-S) assay, is today known to rather measure multipotent progenitor cells than *bona fide* stem cells, but it was exactly this 'weakness' that made Schofield speculate that specialized bone marrow niches preserves or confers the reconstituting ability of stem cells.[19] The definition of a niche is dependent on anatomy and function[23] and can be described as a local tissue microenvironment directly regulating and maintaining a particular stem or progenitor cell population.[24]

As of today, the hematopoietic stem cell niche is the most well characterized niche, and early studies could map individual factors contributing to stem cell maintenance and hematopoiesis within the bone marrow.[25,26] The ability to define hematopoietic stem cells *in vivo* using cell surface markers[27] allowed for the discovery that these cells are five times more likely than other hematopoietic cells to reside in direct proximity to a sinusoid.[28] The frequent location adjacent to blood vessels suggested that hematopoietic stem cells reside within a perivascular niche maintained by endothelial or perivascular cells.[27,29] Despite the near-vascular location of hematopoietic stem cells, the bone marrow is often described as a hypoxic environment and studies have used positive pimonidazole and HIF-$1\alpha$ staining in these areas as evidence for hematopoietic stem cells residing within hypoxic niches.[30–32] However, and as discussed below, HIF-$1\alpha$ can be regulated by other factors than low oxygen levels *per se*, and a recent study using imaging of a nanoprobe more accurately determining the ambient oxygen found that the oxygen tensions in the bone marrow are in fact lowest around sinusoids,[33] elegantly connecting previous reports.

Embryonic stem cells seem to divide and give rise to differentiating progenies at hypoxic conditions during early embryogenesis.[34,35] As also adult stem cell niches (in e.g. bone marrow and kidney) have been reported to be hypoxic,[36-38] and dedifferentiation and promotion of a stem cell-like phenotype appear to be a general effect of hypoxia, one might assume that stem cells, embryonic and adult, require hypoxic conditions to maintain their phenotypes. However, perivascular stem cell niches have been described in several organs,[39] challenging hypoxia as a dominant stem cell-promoting factor.

## 4. Tissue Hypoxia

We know by now that vertebrate cells adapt to oxygen shortage by a dramatic change in their metabolic program and expression pattern of a large, but distinct, set of proteins. Due to variances in the response to hypoxia between affected tissues and the reasons causing hypoxia, there is no set oxygen tension defining it. Generally, the limit when the deficiency of oxygen becomes harmful to its surrounding is approximately 8–10 mmHg or 1% oxygen, and such oxygen tensions are considered hypoxic.[40]

Solid tumors frequently develop regions of hypoxia as they tend to outgrow the formation of new blood vessels within the tumor mass. The diffusion limit for oxygen is around 100–150 $\mu$m (around 5–10 cell layers), meaning that few tumor-associated vessels lead to cellular areas of little or no access to oxygen. In addition, tumor-associated vessels are often leaky and malfunctional, meaning that also tumor cells located adjacent to vascular structures may suffer from hypoxia. As a result, most parts of a solid tumor are less oxygenated than the adjacent non-malignant tissue[40,41] and one can conclude that tumor cells both survive and divide under hypoxic conditions. Normal and tumor cells alike adapt to oxygen deficiency by shifting their transcriptional program away from energy consuming processes such as protein translation, DNA repair and cell differentiation. This transcriptional shift constitutes the increased therapy resistant phenotype possessed by hypoxic tumors and have great implications in the tumor-treatment regime required.

## 4.1. Hypoxia inducible factors

The cellular adaptation to hypoxia is mainly mediated by the hypoxia inducible transcription factors (HIF)-1 and HIF-2. HIFs are part of the basic helix-loop-helix-PAS (Per-Arnt-Sim) family of proteins and are transcriptionally active only as complexes of one alpha and one beta subunit. The regulation of the three HIF alpha subunits (HIF-1$\alpha$,[42–44] HIF-2$\alpha$,[45,46] and HIF-3$\alpha$[47]) is oxygen dependent as the proteins become degraded at oxygenated conditions. The beta subunit (HIF-1$\beta$ or aryl hydrocarbon receptor nuclear translocator (ARNT)) is ubiquitously expressed independently of oxygen tensions. HIF-1$\alpha$ and HIF-2$\alpha$ share 48% primary amino acid sequence homology,[45] with the most conserved regions being the DNA binding (bHLH) and ARNT interaction (PAS) domains. Apart from the bHLH and PAS domains, the two alpha subunits also contain two transactivation domains (TADs) responsible for cofactor interactions, and one oxygen-dependent degradation domain (ODD) (Fig. 1). HIF-3$\alpha$ is less studied but is known to exist in splice variants lacking the C-terminal TAD, and is believed to mainly negatively regulate HIF-1 and HIF-2 by sequestering and thereby block hypoxia response element (HRE)-binding of the other two alpha subunits.[47,48]

## 4.2. Oxygen-dependent regulation of the HIFs

The regulation of HIF-1$\alpha$ and HIF-2$\alpha$ has historically been described to occur mainly at a post-translational level. The mRNA of the HIFs is continuously translated, but in the presence of oxygen, the HIF-$\alpha$ subunits are targeted for ubiquitination and subsequent proteasomal degradation. This

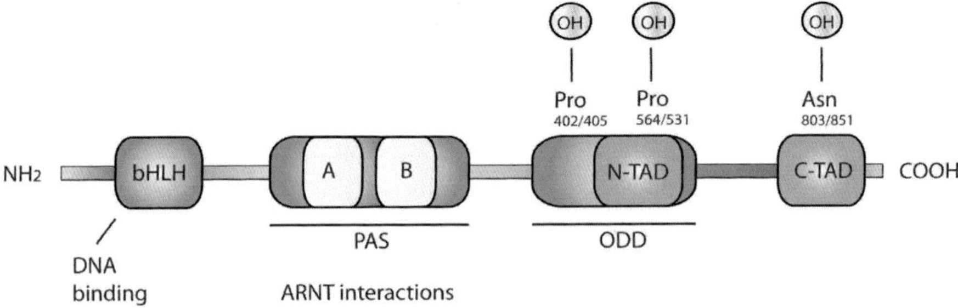


Fig. 1.   Domain structure of HIF alpha. HIF-1$\alpha$ and HIF-2$\alpha$ contain a DNA-binding bHLH domain, an ODD and two TADs. In presence of oxygen, the HIF alpha subunit is hydroxylated at two proline residues (Pro-402 and Pro-564 in HIF-1$\alpha$, and Pro-405 and Pro-531 in HIF-2$\alpha$) or at an asparagine residue (Asn-803 in HIF-1$\alpha$ or Asn-851 in HIF-2$\alpha$). (Adapted from Ref. 54.)

process is mediated by the von Hippel–Lindau (VHL) protein that binds to hydroxylated residues on the HIF-$\alpha$ proteins, a process carried out by prolyl hydroxylases (PHDs). The HIF-$\alpha$ subunits can also be modified via hydroxylation by factor inhibiting HIF-1 (FIH1) at specific asparagine residues (Asn-803 in HIF-1$\alpha$ and Asn-851 in HIF-2$\alpha$).[49,50] Due to the location of the Asn-hydroxylation site, the interaction of HIF-$\alpha$ with its cofactors CREB-binding protein (CBP) and p300 is hindered, disrupting proper HIF complex formation and transcriptional activity. Although FIH1 can target both HIF-1$\alpha$ and HIF-2$\alpha$, a single conserved amino acid substitution immediate to the hydroxylation site in HIF-2$\alpha$ seems to confer it less sensitive to FIH1 targeting and thereby regulation through this pathway.[51] In the absence of oxygen however, hydroxylation of the alpha subunits can no longer take place, and the HIF-$\alpha$ proteins are free to form transcriptional complexes together with ARNT and cofactors, regulating the expression of hundreds of target genes involved in various cellular processes (Fig. 2).

It is becoming increasingly evident, however, that the HIFs are regulated also by other mechanisms, including at the transcriptional level, both under hypoxic conditions and via e.g. growth factor-induced signaling

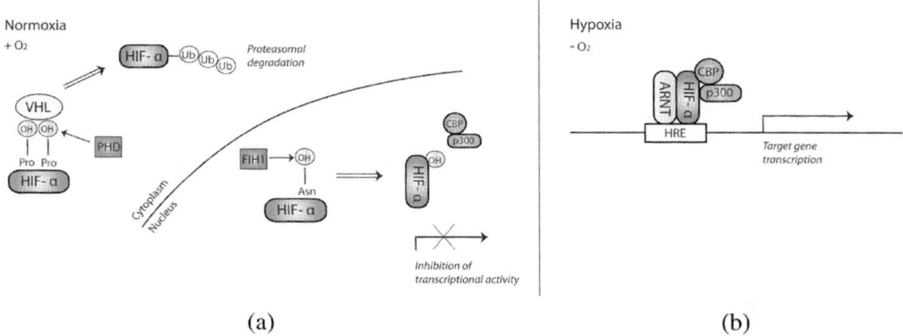


Fig. 2.    Oxygen-dependent regulation of HIF activity. At normoxia (2a), oxygen-dependent PHD proteins hydroxylate HIF alpha, leading to recognition of the alpha subunit by the VHL protein. In turn, this causes ubiquitination and proteasomal degradation of the HIF alpha protein. In the nucleus, oxygen-dependent protein FIH1 hydroxylates HIF alpha at a distinguished asparagine residue, leading to prevention of physical interaction between HIF alpha and cofactors. At low oxygen levels (2b), PHD proteins and FIH1 are unable to hydroxylate HIF-$\alpha$, allowing the HIF-$\alpha$ subunit to bind ARNT and cofactors to form a transcriptionally active HIF complex. (Adapted from Ref. 54.)

pathways.[52–55] Indeed, the HIF pathway and the HIFs themselves are tightly regulated at several different levels. For example, the PHD proteins are induced at hypoxia, suggesting a self-regulatory feedback loop.[56] In addition, hypoxia initiates a switch in the protein synthesis machinery governed by a complex consisting of HIF-2$\alpha$, RNA binding protein RBM4 and cap binding eIF4E2.[57] The complex is recruited to a large, but defined, set of mRNAs at hypoxia, promoting active translation at polysomes and thereby evasion of the otherwise hypoxia-induced repression of protein synthesis. The list of target genes include *HIF2A* itself, *ARNT*, *PHD2/EGLN1*, and *FIH1*, indicating continuous selective expression of HIF-2$\alpha$, while HIF-1$\alpha$ is suppressed as hypoxia persists, possibly explaining the downregulation of HIF-1$\alpha$ after acute hypoxic phases, observed in e.g. neuroblastoma and breast cancer cells.[58,59]

## 4.3. Oxygen-independent regulation of the HIFs

Although the surrounding oxygen levels normally determine the fate of the HIF alpha subunits, HIF-1$\alpha$ and HIF-2$\alpha$ can also be regulated by oxygen-independent mechanisms. Growth factor-induced signaling has been shown to induce expression of the HIF-1$\alpha$ protein, likely as part of a preventive program to prepare for subsequent increased oxygen requirements.[60] The majority of studies on growth factor-induced HIF expression have focused on HIF-1$\alpha$, and while all hypoxic cells have increased HIF-1$\alpha$ expression at least in acute phases, the induction of HIF-1$\alpha$ by growth factor-stimulation is cell type- and context specific. Several different growth factors and their cognate receptors have been shown to regulate HIF-1$\alpha$ translation (e.g. IGF-I,[61,62] insulin,[63] vascular endothelial growth factor (VEGF),[64] and EGF,[65] and effects are generally transduced via the PI3K- and/or Ras/MAPK pathways.[65,66] Individual proteins part of these signaling pathways are commonly deregulated in human cancers, leading to aberrant HIF transcriptional activity and initiated target gene expression also in oxygenated environments, a so-called pseudohypoxic state. Although less studied, HIF-2$\alpha$ levels can be regulated by growth factor receptor activation at non-hypoxic and hypoxic conditions, as in the case of cultured neuroblastoma cells.[55,67] Of interest, HIF-2$\alpha$ mRNA, protein and activity in HeLa and 786-0 cells were only recently described to be regulated in an oxygen- and proteasomal degradation-independent fashion by direct binding of E2F1.[65] In turn, E2F1 was tightly regulated by the deubiquitinase Cezanne, showing that HIF-2$\alpha$ can be controlled cell cycle dependently and in response to oncogenic signaling.[68]

## 4.4. HIFs and cancer aggressiveness

Hypoxia has for long been recognized as an independent factor predicting poor outcome in many tumor forms,[40] and although the mechanisms conferring the aggressive phenotype are not completely determined, resistance to chemotherapy, insensitivity to ionization, immature phenotypes, increased invasive capacity and decreased DNA repair are factors believed to contribute. The expression of *HIF1A* and *HIF2A* is frequent in solid tumors[69] and the respective contributions of HIF-1$\alpha$ and HIF-2$\alpha$ to tumor development and progression have been debated, but seem to be tumor-specific and in some cases even patient subgroup-specific. One illustrative example is breast cancer, where early studies correlated HIF-1$\alpha$ expression with reduced disease-free survival,[70–75] however, most of these studies used small materials and correlations were only observed in subsets of patients, such as lymph-node positive or T1/T2 tumors. Later studies have rather correlated HIF-1$\alpha$ expression with favorable outcome.[76,77] The predictive role of HIF-2$\alpha$ has been less studied, but two reports have suggested that high expression correlates with nodal and distal metastasis and poor patient outcome, respectively.[76,78]

Another interesting cancer form from a HIF point of view is clear cell renal cell carcinomas. These tumors are often characterized by their loss of VHL expression, leading to constitutive HIF alpha protein expression and increased vascularization.[79,80] Despite VHL targeting both HIF-1$\alpha$ and HIF-2$\alpha$ for degradation, a large proportion of VHL deficient tumors and cell lines express HIF-2$\alpha$ exclusively, and HIF-2$\alpha$ seems to play a major role in tumor progression.[81–85] These findings might be explained by two distinct single nucleotide polymorphisms (SNPs) in the *HIF2A* gene that have been identified in a large clinical material, associating with renal cell carcinoma susceptibility.[86]

# 5. Hypoxia Promotes Immature, Stem Cell-Like Phenotypes

HIF-2$\alpha$ is expressed distinctly and transiently during murine[87,88] and human[55,89] sympathetic nervous system development, and studies on the influence by hypoxia on cells of the sympathetic neuronally derived tumor neuroblastoma is therefore of interest. Hypoxia induces a dedifferentiation program in neuroblastoma cells.[87] Low stage of neuroblastoma cell differentiation correlates to poor prognosis and advanced clinical stage[90] and in line with these observations, intense HIF-2$\alpha$ expression in tumor specimens correlates to distant metastasis and poor prognosis.[59] Similar data were reported in breast cancer where hypoxic cancer cells showed an immature phenotype and downregulation of estrogen receptor in receptor positive tumors.[58] Immunohistochemical staining for HIF-2$\alpha$ revealed a positive association to distant metastasis and unfavorable outcome.[76] The negative effect of hypoxia on cell differentiation is not restricted to malignant cells as normal human breast epithelial precursor cells with capacity to form differentiated, acini-like structures in 3D-cultures at normoxia, fail to do so when grown under hypoxic conditions.[91] Interestingly, the hypoxic, immature and non-polarized cells continue to proliferate slowly, while cells forming the differentiated acini-like structures at normoxia stopped to proliferate. A link between stem cell traits in breast epithelial precursor cells and HIF was further indicated during post-lactational mammary involution, a process characterized by selective death of differentiated epithelial cells, but rescue of stem cell pools for re-building the breast ductal network. In the involuting breast tissue, a population of cells expressing HIF-2$\alpha$ and the stem/basal marker CK14 was detected, suggesting selective survival of HIF-2$\alpha$ positive epithelial stem cells.[92]

# 6. Pseudohypoxia

Assuming that the primary role of HIFs is to adapt cells to hypoxic conditions, one might ask if non-hypoxic mechanisms regulating HIF expression and HIF activities are biologically relevant. Today, we know of at least two apparently different mechanisms in tumors where non-hypoxic activation of HIFs can be linked to tumor aggressiveness and even tumorigenesis. One mechanism involves the activation of HIF-2, but not HIF-1, under physiological oxygen conditions as observed in neuroblastoma and glioma cells.[53,59] Neuroblastoma cells cultured at 5% oxygen to mimic physiological end capillary oxygen levels express active HIF-2, transcribing bona fide hypoxia-driven genes, and thus defining a pseudohypoxic phenotype.[59] In neuroblastoma and glioblastoma tissues, HIF-$2\alpha$ is highly expressed in tumor cells located in perivascular niches,[53,93] and in the case of neuroblastoma, these tumor cells display an immature and cancer stem cell-like phenotype. As presence of highly HIF-$2\alpha$ expressing cells in neuroblastoma correlates to metastasizing disease, we have proposed that these immature, mesenchymal-like tumor cells have cancer stem cell features and are pseudohypoxic.[93,94]

The second mechanism involves genetic activation of pathways leading to a pseudohypoxic phenotype. VHL deletions in clear cell renal cell carcinomas and other tumor forms lead to constitutively high levels of HIF alpha subunits due to impaired oxygen-dependent proteasomal degradation of these proteins.[95] As described above, HIF-$2\alpha$ seems to be the oncogenic HIF form in these VHL negative clear cell renal cell carcinomas, suggesting that HIF-2 is the common denominator of the pseudohypoxic phenotype as will be discussed below. Two other tumor forms that also associate with the VHL disease are paraganglioma and pheochromocytoma. These tumors are particularly interesting when discussing pseudohypoxia and cancer as they frequently carry deletions of VHL or mutations in other genes (*SDHA, SDHB, SDHC, SDHD, FH*) resulting in a pseudohypoxic phenotype by stabilization of the HIF alpha subunits.[96,97] The succinyl dehydrogenase (SDH) subunits form complex II in the mitochondrial citric acid cycle and electron transport chain, catalyzing the conversion of succinate into fumarate (Fig. 3). The mutations in SDH subunits and fumarate hydroxylase (FH) impair SDH and FH activities with increased cellular succinate and fumarate levels as a result. These molecules compete with $\alpha$-ketoglutarate for binding to PHDs. While $\alpha$-ketoglutarate is required for PHD activity, succinate and fumarate inhibit the PHDs, resulting in stabilization of HIFs as their proline residues are no longer hydroxylated, and they therefore cannot be recognized for VHL-mediated proteasomal degradation. Thus, in paraganglioma and pheochromocytoma several modes of genetic aberrations lead to

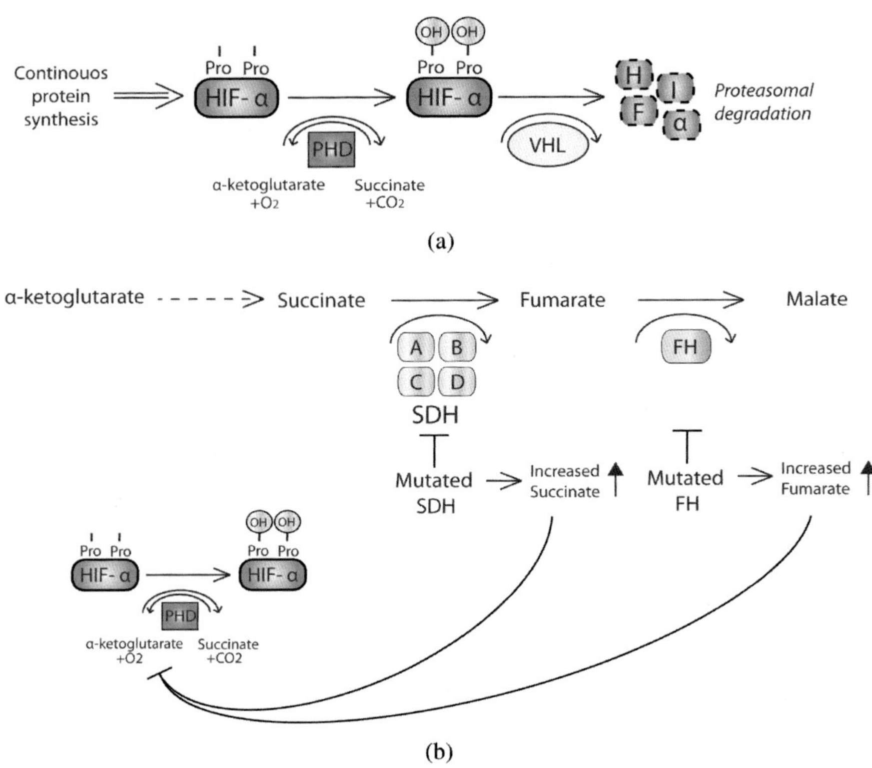



Fig. 3.    The roles of α-ketoglutarate, succinate and fumarate in PHD-driven hydroxylation and degradation of HIF-α subunits. (a) The PHDs require molecular oxygen and α-ketoglutarate (2-oxoglutarate) to hydroxylate the two proline residues on HIF alpha subunits, rendering them susceptible for VHL-dependent proteasomal degradation. (b) In mitochondria, α-ketoglutarate is degraded to succinate, which in turn is converted to fumarate by SDH and malate by FH. Each of the four SDH subunits (A–D) and FH can be mutated in cancer, resulting in elevated levels of succinate and fumarate, respectively. Succinate and fumarate blocks the interaction of α-ketoglutarate with PHDs and thus results in stabilization of HIF-α subunits also in an oxygenated setting.

a pseudohypoxic phenotype and as several of these mutations associate with various syndromes and thus are inherited, we conclude that the pseudohypoxic phenotype is oncogenic. Gene expression analysis of these two tumor forms reveals two clusters of tumors based on the expression signatures. Tumors with the VHL and SDHx mutations belong to the cluster of more malignant tumors,[96] emphasizing the tumorigenic power of the pseudohypoxic phenotype.

The first identified mutations (gain-of-function) in any of the HIF alpha subunits themselves in cancer were recently reported, suggesting a direct HIF-dependent mechanism to reach pseudohypoxic conditions in cancer. These mutations hit *HIF2A* and were first reported in two patients with paraganglioma with associated erythrocytosis.[98] Both mutations occurred in exon 12, resulting in amino acid substitutions in proximity to the PHD hydroxylation site in HIF-2$\alpha$. The substitution most likely induces conformational changes resulting in reduced affinity for PHD and VHL binding as a result, and indeed leads to increased protein half-life and HIF-2$\alpha$ activity.[98] The findings are in agreement with previous identification of *HIF2A* gain-of-function mutations in familial erythrocytosis,[99] and have later been followed by the identification of additional mutations in the *HIF2A* gene in pheochromocytoma and paraganglioma patients without erythrocytosis,[100] and two novel mutations in somatostatinomas and paragangliomas.[101] Interestingly, paraganglioma, pheochromocytomas and the childhood tumor neuroblastoma all originate from trunk neural crest-derived, sympathoadrenal precursor cells and are thus closely related. We conclude that all three tumor forms can create pseudohypoxic conditions by activating HIF-2, although by different mechanisms, events that correlate to aggressive disease.

The identification of tumor cells that have an activated HIF response under oxygenated conditions creating a pseudohypoxic phenotype show that at least HIF degradation can be regulated by as yet unknown mechanisms. This phenomenon is not a feature restricted to tumor cells. During normal development, HIF-2$\alpha$ is detected in embryonic human sympathetic chain ganglia[55] and later in fetal human and embryonic mouse paraganglia.[88,89] In tumor tissue, macrophages are frequently HIF-2$\alpha$ positive, also in tumor areas that are well oxygenated without HIF-1$\alpha$ protein expression. These observations, and the link between pseudohypoxia and HIF-2$\alpha$ in clear cell renal cell carcinoma, neuroblastoma, glioma, paraganglioma and pheochromocytoma strongly suggest that this state is primarily defined by non-hypoxia-induced activation of HIF-2. A cornerstone in this mechanism must involve impaired or reduced degradation of HIF-2$\alpha$ at physiological oxygen tension as demonstrated in neuroblastoma and breast carcinoma.[59,76]

The negative regulation of HIFs by FIH1 is probably also altered in order to create a HIF driven pseudohypoxic response. The association between HIF-2 and pseudohypoxia might be partly explained by the preferential targeting of HIF-1$\alpha$ over HIF-2$\alpha$ for FIH1,[51] a protein still expressed in for instance oxygenated VHL negative renal cell carcinoma cells.

## 6.1. The hypoxic and pseudohypoxic cancer stem cell niches

Cultured neuroblastoma cells express HIF-2$\alpha$, but not HIF-1$\alpha$, at near-physiological oxygen tensions (5% oxygen) and HIF-2$\alpha$ forms an active transcription complex together with cofactors under these conditions.[59] In neuroblastoma tissues, most tumor cells lack, or express low levels of HIF-2$\alpha$, but infrequent tumor cells with high HIF-2$\alpha$ protein expression can be detected. These HIF-2$\alpha$ positive tumor cells are mainly located adjacent to blood vessels and they express HIF-2 downstream target genes such as VEGF, suggesting HIF-2 transcriptional activity also *in vivo*.[93] Further characterization revealed that these cells lack or express low levels of sympathetic neuronal differentiation markers such as tyrosine hydroxylase and neuron-specific enolase, but instead express neural crest-associated vimentin, Notch, and HES-1. We concluded that these tumor cells (identified by their MYCN amplification) present with a mesenchymal and cancer stem cell-like phenotype and postulated that they are indeed neuroblastoma stem cells.[93] High HIF-2$\alpha$ expression associates with poor outcome also in glioblastoma[53] and HIF-2$\alpha$ is expressed in isolated glioblastoma stem cell populations.[102] Interestingly, in glioma specimens, HIF-2$\alpha$ is expressed in perivascularly located glioma cells that coexpress cancer stem cell markers.[53] Thus, in both neuroblastoma and glioblastoma, a small fraction of putative cancer stem cells reside in a niche that appears to be pseudohypoxic *in lieu* of their high HIF-2$\alpha$ protein levels but lack of HIF-1$\alpha$ protein expression (Fig. 4).[53,93]

Several human myeloid malignancies, including chronic myelogenous leukemia (CML), myelodysplastic syndromes (MDSs), AML and blast crisis CML originate from transformed hematopoietic stem or precursor cells. These different leukemic cells have been shown to hijack

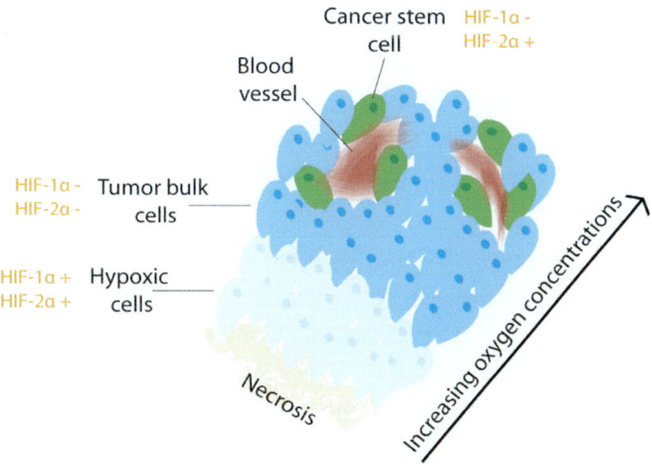


Fig. 4. Perivascular location of cancer stem cells (such as in neuroblastoma and glioma) with high HIF-2$\alpha$, but low HIF-1$\alpha$, expression.

the bone marrow niche used by normal hematopoietic stem cells by exploiting factors known to be important for proper homing.[103] For example, the hematopoietic stem cell niche appears to promote HIF-2$\alpha$ expression, as HIF-2$\alpha$ protects AML and human hematopoietic stem cells from cell death induced by endoplasmic reticulum stress.[104] Leukemic stem cells are however less dependent on, and less sensitive to, the surrounding factors constituting the bone marrow niche, and it has become increasingly clear that the niche is remodeled into a self-reinforcing malignant bone marrow niche supporting continuous disease development.[105]

The presence and nature of cancer stem cell niches in solid tumors has not been established for most tumor forms and the biochemical cues that constitute these putative niches are not known in detail. In both neuroblastoma and glioma, HIF-2$\alpha$ seems to link to the immature stem cell-like phenotype[93] and HIF-2 driven genes like VEGF might be factors contributing to the formation of the niche in close proximity to blood vessels.[53,93,106] It is not yet established whether these cells express HIF-2$\alpha$ due to their spatial distribution or if their location depends on this expression pattern. We hypothesize that targeting HIF-2 in at least glioma and neuroblastoma would potentially drive the immature stem cell-like tumor cells into more differentiated bulk tumor cell that can be targeted by conventional cytotoxic drugs. An alternative or additional approach would be to directly target the niche once molecular patterns creating these niches have been delineated.

## Acknowledgments

This work was supported by the Swedish Cancer Society, the Children's Cancer Foundation of Sweden, the Swedish Research Council, Fru Berta Kamprads stiftelse, the SSF Strategic Center for Translational Cancer Research — CREATE Health, VINNOVA, BioCARE, a Strategic Research Program at Lund University, Hans von Kantzows Stiftelse, Gunnar Nilsson's Cancer Foundation, the Crafoord foundation, and the research funds of Malmö University Hospital.

## References

1. Baum, C. M., Weissman, I. L., Tsukamoto, A. S., Buckle, A. M., and Peault, B., Isolation of a candidate human hematopoietic stem-cell population. *Proc. Natl. Acad. Sci. USA*, **89**, pp. 2804–2808, 1992.
2. Morrison, S. J., and Weissman, I. L., The long-term repopulating subset of hematopoietic stem cells is deterministic and isolatable by phenotype. *Immunity*, **1**, pp. 661–673, 1994.
3. Osawa, M., Hanada, K., Hamada, H., and Nakauchi, H., Long-term lympho-hematopoietic reconstitution by a single CD34-low/negative hematopoietic stem cell. *Science*, **273**, pp. 242–245, 1996.
4. Spangrude, G. J., Heimfeld, S., and Weissman, I. L., Purification and characterization of mouse hematopoietic stem cells. *Science*, **241**, pp. 58–62, 1988.
5. Nowell, P. C. The clonal evolution of tumor cell populations. *Science*, **194**, pp. 23–28, 1976.
6. Lapidot, T., Sirard, C., Vormoor, J., Murdoch, B., Hoang, T., Caceres-Cortes, J., Minden, M., Paterson, B., Caligiuri, M. A., and Dick, J. E., A cell initiating human acute myeloid leukaemia after transplantation into SCID mice. *Nature*, **367**, pp. 645–648, 1994.
7. Al-Hajj, M., Wicha, M. S., Benito-Hernandez, A., Morrison, S. J., and Clarke, M. F., Prospective identification of tumorigenic breast cancer cells. *Proc. Natl. Acad. Sci. USA*, **100**, pp. 3983–3988, 2003.

8. Eramo, A., Lotti, F., Sette, G., Pilozzi, E., Biffoni, M., Di Virgilio, A., Conticello, C., Ruco, L., Peschle, C., and De Maria, R., Identification and expansion of the tumorigenic lung cancer stem cell population. *Cell Death Differ.*, **15**, pp. 504–514, 2008.

9. Hermann, P. C., Huber, S. L., Herrler, T., Aicher, A., Ellwart, J. W., Guba, M., Bruns, C. J., and Heeschen, C., Distinct populations of cancer stem cells determine tumor growth and metastatic activity in human pancreatic cancer. *Cell Stem Cell*, **1**, pp. 313–323, 2007.

10. O'Brien, C. A., Pollett, A., Gallinger, S., and Dick, J. E., A human colon cancer cell capable of initiating tumour growth in immunodeficient mice. *Nature*, **445**, pp. 106–110, 2007.

11. Patrawala, L., Calhoun, T., Schneider-Broussard, R., Li, H., Bhatia, B., Tang, S., Reilly, J. G., Chandra, D., Zhou, J., Claypool, K. *et al.*, Highly purified CD44+ prostate cancer cells from xenograft human tumors are enriched in tumorigenic and metastatic progenitor cells. *Oncogene*, **25**, pp. 1696–1708, 2006.

12. Read, T. A., Fogarty, M. P., Markant, S. L., McLendon, R. E., Wei, Z., Ellison, D. W., Febbo, P. G., and Wechsler-Reya, R. J., Identification of CD15 as a marker for tumor-propagating cells in a mouse model of medulloblastoma. *Cancer Cell*, **15**, pp. 135–147, 2009.

13. Ricci-Vitiani, L., Lombardi, D. G., Pilozzi, E., Biffoni, M., Todaro, M., Peschle, C., and De Maria, R., Identification and expansion of human colon-cancer-initiating cells. *Nature*, **445**, pp. 111–115, 2007.

14. Schatton, T., Murphy, G. F., Frank, N. Y., Yamaura, K., Waaga-Gasser, A. M., Gasser, M., Zhan, Q., Jordan, S., Duncan, L. M., Weishaupt, C. *et al.*, Identification of cells initiating human melanomas. *Nature*, **451**, pp. 345–349, 2008.

15. Singh, S. K., Hawkins, C., Clarke, I. D., Squire, J. A., Bayani, J., Hide, T., Henkelman, R. M., Cusimano, M. D., and Dirks, P. B., Identification of human brain tumour initiating cells. *Nature*, **432**, pp. 396–401, 2004.

16. Taylor, M. D., Poppleton, H., Fuller, C., Su, X., Liu, Y., Jensen, P., Magdaleno, S., Dalton, J., Calabrese, C., Board, J. *et al.*, Radial glia cells are candidate stem cells of ependymoma. *Cancer Cell*, **8**, pp. 323–335, 2005.

17. Eleveld, T. F., Oldridge, D. A., Bernard, V., Koster, J., Daage, L. C., Diskin, S. J., Schild, L., Bentahar, N. B., Bellini, A., Chicard, M. *et al.*, Relapsed neuroblastomas show frequent RAS-MAPK pathway mutations. *Nat. Genet.*, **47**, pp. 864–871, 2015.

18. Gerlinger, M., Rowan, A. J., Horswell, S., Larkin, J., Endesfelder, D, Gronroos, E., Martinez, P., Matthews, N., Stewart, A., Tarpey, P. *et al.*, Intratumor heterogeneity and branched evolution revealed by multiregion sequencing. *New Engl. J. Med.*, **366**, pp. 883–892, 2012.

19. Schofield, R., The relationship between the spleen colony-forming cell and the haemopoietic stem cell. *Blood Cells*, **4**, pp. 7–25, 1978.

20. Siminovitch, L., McCulloch, E. A., and Till, J. E., The Distribution of Colony-Forming Cells among Spleen Colonies. *J. Cell. Physiol.*, **62**, pp. 327–336, 1963.

21. Siminovitch, L., Till, J. E., and McCulloch, E. A., Decline in Colony-Forming Ability of Marrow Cells Subjected to Serial Transplantation into Irradiated Mice. *J. Cell. Physiol.*, **64**, pp. 23–31, 1964.

22. Till, J. E., and McCulloch, E. A., A direct measurement of the radiation sensitivity of normal mouse bone marrow cells. *Radiat. Res*, **14**, pp. 213–222, 1961.

23. Scadden, D. T., The stem-cell niche as an entity of action. *Nature*, **441**, pp. 1075–1079, 2006.

24. Morrison, S. J., and Scadden, D. T., The bone marrow niche for haematopoietic stem cells. *Nature*, **505**, pp. 327–334, 2014.

25. Dexter, T. M., Allen, T. D., and Lajtha, L. G., Conditions controlling the proliferation of haemopoietic stem cells *in vitro*. *J. Cell. Phys.*, **91**, pp. 335–344, 1977.

26. Lord, B. I., Testa, N. G., and Hendry, J. H., The relative spatial distributions of CFUs and CFUc in the normal mouse femur. *Blood*, **46**, pp. 65–72, 1975.

27. Kiel, M. J., Yilmaz, O. H., Iwashita, T., Yilmaz, O. H., Terhorst, C., and Morrison, S. J., SLAM family receptors distinguish hematopoietic stem and progenitor cells and reveal endothelial niches for stem cells. *Cell*, **121**, pp. 1109–1121, 2005.

28. Kiel, M. J., Radice, G. L., and Morrison, S. J., Lack of evidence that hematopoietic stem cells depend on N-cadherin-mediated adhesion to osteoblasts for their maintenance. *Cell Stem Cell*, **1**, pp. 204–217, 2007.

29. Sugiyama, T., Kohara, H., Noda, M., and Nagasawa, T., Maintenance of the hematopoietic stem cell pool by CXCL12-CXCR4 chemokine signaling in bone marrow stromal cell niches. *Immunity*, **25**, pp. 977–988, 2006.

30. Nombela-Arrieta, C., Pivarnik, G., Winkel, B., Canty, K. J., Harley, B., Mahoney, J. E., Park, S. Y., Lu, J., Protopopov, A., and Silberstein, L. E., Quantitative imaging of haematopoietic stem and progenitor cell localization and hypoxic status in the bone marrow microenvironment. *Nat. Cell Biol.*, **15**, pp. 533–543, 2013.

31. Parmar, K., Mauch, P., Vergilio, J. A., Sackstein, R., and Down, J. D., Distribution of hematopoietic stem cells in the bone marrow according to regional hypoxia. *Proc. Natl. Acad. Sci. USA*, **104**, pp. 5431–5436, 2007.

32. Takubo, K., Goda, N., Yamada, W., Iriuchishima, H., Ikeda, E., Kubota, Y., Shima, H., Johnson, R. S., Hirao, A., Suematsu, M., and Suda, T., Regulation of the HIF-1alpha level is essential for hematopoietic stem cells. *Cell Stem Cell*, **7**, pp. 391–402, 2010.

33. Spencer, J. A., Ferraro, F., Roussakis, E., Klein, A., Wu, J., Runnels, J. M., Zaher, W., Mortensen, L. J., Alt, C., Turcotte, R. *et al.*, Direct measurement of local oxygen concentration in the bone marrow of live animals. *Nature*, **508**, pp. 269–273, 2014.

34. Burton, G. J., Oxygen, the Janus gas; its effects on human placental development and function. *J. Anat.*, **215**, pp. 27–35, 2009.

35. Mohyeldin, A., Garzon-Muvdi, T., and Quinones-Hinojosa, A., Oxygen in stem cell biology: a critical component of the stem cell niche. *Cell Stem Cell*, **7**, pp. 150–161, 2010.

36. Gezer, D., Vukovic, M., Soga, T., Pollard, P. J., and Kranc, K. R., Concise review: genetic dissection of hypoxia signaling pathways in normal and leukemic stem cells. *Stem Cells*, **32**, pp. 1390–1397, 2014.

37. Oliver, J. A., Maarouf, O., Cheema, F. H., Martens, T. P., and Al-Awqati, Q., The renal papilla is a niche for adult kidney stem cells. *J. Clin. Invest.*, **114**, pp. 795–804, 2004.

38. Zhang, W., and Edwards, A., Oxygen transport across vasa recta in the renal medulla. *Am. J. Physiol. — Heart C.*, **283**, pp. H1042–1055, 2002.

39. Putnam, A. J., The Instructive Role of the Vasculature in Stem Cell Niches. *Biomater. Sci.*, **2**, pp. 1562–1573, 2014.

40. Höckel, M., and Vaupel, P., Tumor hypoxia: definitions and current clinical, biologic, and molecular aspects. *J. Natl. Cancer Inst.*, **93**, pp. 266–276, 2001.

41. Brown, J. M., and Wilson, W. R., Exploiting tumour hypoxia in cancer treatment. *Nat. Rev. Cancer*, **4**, pp. 437–447, 2004.

42. Semenza, G. L., and Wang, G. L., A nuclear factor induced by hypoxia via de novo protein synthesis binds to the human erythropoietin gene enhancer at a site required for transcriptional activation. *Mol. Cell. Biol*, **12**, pp. 5447–5454, 1992.

43. Wang, G. L., Jiang, B. H., Rue, E. A., and Semenza, G. L., Hypoxia-inducible factor 1 is a basic-helix-loop-helix-PAS heterodimer regulated by cellular O2 tension. *Proc. Natl. Acad. Sci. USA*, **92**, pp. 5510–5514, 1995.

44. Wang, G. L., and Semenza, G. L., Purification and characterization of hypoxia-inducible factor 1. *J. Biol. Chem.*, **270**, pp. 1230–1237, 1995.

45. Tian, H., McKnight, S. L., and Russell, D. W., Endothelial PAS domain protein 1 (EPAS1), a transcription factor selectively expressed in endothelial cells. *Genes & Dev.*, **11**, pp. 72–82, 1997.

46. Wiesener, M. S., Turley, H., Allen, W. E., Willam, C., Eckardt, K. U., Talks, K. L., Wood, S. M., Gatter, K. C., Harris, A. L., Pugh, C. W. *et al.*, Induction of endothelial PAS domain protein-1 by hypoxia: characterization and comparison with hypoxia-inducible factor-1alpha. *Blood.*, **92**, pp. 2260–2268, 1998.

47. Makino, Y., Cao, R., Svensson, K., Bertilsson, G., Asman, M., Tanaka, H., Cao, Y., Berkenstam, A., and Poellinger, L., Inhibitory PAS domain protein is a negative regulator of hypoxia-inducible gene expression. *Nature*, **414**, pp. 550–554, 2001.

48. Maynard, M. A., Evans, A. J., Shi, W., Kim, W. Y., Liu, F. F., and Ohh, M., Dominant-negative HIF-3 alpha 4 suppresses VHL-null renal cell carcinoma progression. *Cell Cycle*, **6**, pp. 2810–2816, 2007.

49. Lando, D., Peet, D. J., Gorman, J. J., Whelan, D. A., Whitelaw, M. L., and Bruick, R. K., FIH-1 is an asparaginyl hydroxylase enzyme that regulates the transcriptional activity of hypoxia-inducible factor. *Genes & Dev.*, **16**, pp. 1466–1471, 2002.

50. Lando, D., Peet, D. J., Whelan, D. A., Gorman, J. J., and Whitelaw, M. L., Asparagine hydroxylation of the HIF transactivation domain a hypoxic switch. *Science*, **295**, pp. 858–861, 2002.

51. Bracken, C. P., Fedele, A. O., Linke, S., Balrak, W., Lisy, K., Whitelaw, M. L., and Peet, D. J., Cell-specific regulation of hypoxia-inducible factor (HIF)-1alpha and HIF-2alpha stabilization and transactivation in a graded oxygen environment. *J. Biol. Chem.*, **281**, pp. 22575–22585, 2006.

52. Hamidian, A., von Stedingk, K., Munksgaard Thorén, M., Mohlin, S., and Påhlman, S., Differential regulation of HIF-1alpha and HIF-2alpha in neuroblastoma: Estrogen-related receptor alpha (ERRalpha) regulates HIF2A transcription and correlates to poor outcome. *Biochem. Biophys. Res. Comm.*, **461**, pp. 560–567, 2015.

53. Li, Z., Bao, S., Wu, Q., Wang, H., Eyler, C., Sathornsumetee, S., Shi, Q., Cao, Y., Lathia, J., McLendon, R. E. *et al.*, Hypoxia-inducible factors regulate tumorigenic capacity of glioma stem cells. *Cancer Cell*, **15**, pp. 501–513, 2009.

54. Mohlin, S., IGF, PI3K and HIF-2 in Normal and Tumor Development. (Doctoral Dissertation). Lund University, 2013.

55. Mohlin, S., Hamidian, A., and Påhlman, S., HIF2A and IGF2 expression correlates in human neuroblastoma cells and normal immature sympathetic neuroblasts. *Neoplasia.*, **15**, pp. 328–334, 2013.

56. Aprelikova, O., Chandramouli, G. V., Wood, M., Vasselli, J. R., Riss, J., Maranchie, J. K., Linehan, W. M., and Barrett, J. C., Regulation of HIF

prolyl hydroxylases by hypoxia-inducible factors. *J. Cell. Biochem.*, **92**, pp. 491–501, 2004.

57. Uniacke, J., Holterman, C. E., Lachance, G., Franovic, A., Jacob, M. D., Fabian, M. R., Payette, J., Holcik, M., Pause, A., and Lee, S., An oxygen-regulated switch in the protein synthesis machinery. *Nature*, **486**, pp. 126–129, 2012.

58. Helczynska, K., Kronblad, A., Jogi, A., Nilsson, E., Beckman, S., Landberg, G., and Pahlman, S., Hypoxia promotes a dedifferentiated phenotype in ductal breast carcinoma in situ. *Cancer Res.*, **63**, pp. 1441–1444, 2003.

59. Holmquist-Mengelbier, L., Fredlund, E., Löfstedt, T., Noguera, R., Navarro, S., Nilsson, H., Pietras, A., Vallon-Christersson, J., Borg, A., Gradin, K. *et al.*, Recruitment of HIF-1alpha and HIF-2alpha to common target genes is differentially regulated in neuroblastoma: HIF-2alpha promotes an aggressive phenotype. *Cancer Cell*, **10**, pp. 413–423, 2006.

60. Semenza, G. L., Targeting HIF-1 for cancer therapy. *Nat. Rev. Cancer*, **3**, pp. 721–732, 2003.

61. Beppu, K., Nakamura, K., Linehan, W. M., Rapisarda, A., and Thiele, C. J., Topotecan blocks hypoxia-inducible factor-1alpha and vascular endothelial growth factor expression induced by insulin-like growth factor-I in neuroblastoma cells. *Cancer Res.*, **65**, pp. 4775–4781, 2005.

62. Fukuda, R., Hirota, K., Fan, F., Jung, Y. D., Ellis, L. M., and Semenza, G. L., Insulin-like growth factor 1 induces hypoxia-inducible factor 1-mediated vascular endothelial growth factor expression, which is dependent on MAP kinase and phosphatidylinositol 3-kinase signaling in colon cancer cells. *J. Biol. Chem.*, **277**, pp. 38205–38211, 2002.

63. Treins, C., Giorgetti-Peraldi, S., Murdaca, J., Semenza, G. L., and Van Obberghen, E., Insulin stimulates hypoxia-inducible factor 1 through a phosphatidylinositol 3-kinase/target of rapamycin-dependent signaling pathway. *J. Biol. Chem.*, **277**, pp. 27975–27981, 2002.

64. Calvani, M., Trisciuoglio, D., Bergamaschi, C., Shoemaker, R. H., and Melillo, G., Differential involvement of vascular endothelial growth factor in the survival of hypoxic colon cancer cells. *Cancer Res.*, **68**, pp. 285–291, 2008.

65. Zhong, H., Chiles, K., Feldser, D., Laughner, E., Hanrahan, C., Georgescu, M. M., Simons, J. W., and Semenza, G. L., Modulation of hypoxia-inducible factor 1alpha expression by the epidermal growth factor/phosphatidylinositol 3-kinase/PTEN/AKT/FRAP pathway in human prostate cancer cells: implications for tumor angiogenesis and therapeutics. *Cancer Res.*, **60**, pp. 1541–1545, 2000.

66. Blancher, C., Moore, J. W., Robertson, N., and Harris, A. L., Effects of ras and von Hippel-Lindau (VHL) gene mutations on hypoxia-inducible factor (HIF)-1alpha, HIF-2alpha, and vascular endothelial growth factor expression and their regulation by the phosphatidylinositol 3′-kinase/Akt signaling pathway. *Cancer Res.*, **61**, pp. 7349–7355, 2001.

67. Mohlin, S., Hamidian, A., von Stedingk, K., Bridges, E., Wigerup, C., Bexell, D., and Påhlman, S., PI3K-mTORC2 but not PI3K-mTORC1 regulates transcription of HIF2A/EPAS1 and vascularization in neuroblastoma. *Cancer Res.*, **75**(21), pp. 4617–4628, 2015.

68. Moniz, S., Bandarra, D., Biddlestone, J., Campbell, K. J., Komander, D., Bremm, A., and Rocha, S., Cezanne regulates E2F1-dependent HIF2alpha expression. *J. Cell Sci.*, **15**, pp. 3082–3093, 2015.

69. Talks, K. L., Turley, H., Gatter, K. C., Maxwell, P. H., Pugh, C. W., Ratcliffe, P. J., and Harris, A. L., The expression and distribution of the hypoxia-inducible factors HIF-1alpha and HIF-2alpha in normal human tissues, cancers, and tumor-associated macrophages. *Am. J. Pathol.*, **157**, pp. 411–421, 2000.

70. Bos, R., van der Groep, P., Greijer, A. E., Shvarts, A., Meijer, S., Pinedo, H. M., Semenza, G. L., van Diest, P. J., and van der Wall, E., Levels of hypoxia-inducible factor-1alpha independently predict prognosis in patients with lymph node negative breast carcinoma. *Cancer*, **97**, pp. 1573–1581, 2003.

71. Dales, J. P., Garcia, S., Meunier-Carpentier, S., Andrac-Meyer, L., Haddad, O., Lavaut, M. N., Allasia, C., Bonnier, P., and Charpin, C., Overexpression of hypoxia-inducible factor HIF-1alpha predicts early relapse in breast cancer: retrospective study in a series of 745 patients. *Int. J. Cancer*, **116**, pp. 734–739, 2005.

72. Generali, D., Berruti, A., Brizzi, M. P., Campo, L., Bonardi, S., Wigfield, S., Bersiga, A., Allevi, G., Milani, M., Aguggini, S. *et al.*, Hypoxia-inducible factor-1alpha expression predicts a poor response to primary chemoendocrine therapy and disease-free survival in primary human breast cancer. *Clin. Cancer Res.*, **12**, pp. 4562–4568, 2006.

73. Gruber, G., Greiner, R. H., Hlushchuk, R., Aebersold, D. M., Altermatt, H. J., Berclaz, G., and Djonov, V., Hypoxia-inducible factor 1 alpha in high-risk breast cancer: an independent prognostic parameter? *Breast Cancer Res.*, **6**, pp. R191–198, 2004.

74. Kronblad, A., Jirström, K., Rydén, L., Nordenskjöld, B., and Landberg, G., Hypoxia inducible factor-1alpha is a prognostic marker in premenopausal patients with intermediate to highly differentiated breast cancer but

not a predictive marker for tamoxifen response. *Int. J. Cancer*, **118**, pp. 2609–2616, 2006.

75. Schindl, M., Schoppmann, S. F., Samonigg, H., Hausmaninger, H., Kwasny, W., Gnant, M., Jakesz, R., Kubista, E., Birner, P., Oberhuber, G. *et al.*, Overexpression of hypoxia-inducible factor 1alpha is associated with an unfavorable prognosis in lymph node-positive breast cancer. *Clin. Cancer Res.*, **8**, pp. 1831–1837, 2002.

76. Helczynska, K., Larsson, A. M., Holmquist Mengelbier, L., Bridges, E., Fredlund, E., Borgquist, S., Landberg, G., Påhlman, S., and Jirström, K., Hypoxia-inducible factor-2alpha correlates to distant recurrence and poor outcome in invasive breast cancer. *Cancer Res.*, **68**, pp. 9212–9220, 2008.

77. Tan, E. Y., Campo, L., Han, C., Turley, H., Pezzella, F., Gatter, K. C., Harris, A. L., and Fox, S. B., BNIP3 as a progression marker in primary human breast cancer; opposing functions in in situ versus invasive cancer. *Clin. Cancer Res.*, **13**, pp. 467–474, 2007.

78. Giatromanolaki, A., Sivridis, E., Fiska, A., and Koukourakis, M. I., Hypoxia-inducible factor-2 alpha (HIF-2 alpha) induces angiogenesis in breast carcinomas. *Appl. Immunohisto. M. M.*, **14**, pp. 78–82, 2006.

79. Gnarra, J. R., Tory, K., Weng, Y., Schmidt, L., Wei, M. H., Li, H., Latif, F., Liu, S., Chen, F., Duh, F. M. *et al.*, Mutations of the VHL tumour suppressor gene in renal carcinoma. *Nat. Genet.*, **7**, pp. 85–90, 1994.

80. Herman, J. G., Latif, F., Weng, Y., Lerman, M. I., Zbar, B., Liu, S., Samid, D., Duan, D. S., Gnarra, J. R., Linehan, W. M. *et al.*, Silencing of the VHL tumor-suppressor gene by DNA methylation in renal carcinoma. *Proc. Natl. Acad. Sci. USA*, **91**, pp. 9700–9704, 1994.

81. Kondo, K., Kim, W. Y., Lechpammer, M., and Kaelin, W. G., Jr., Inhibition of HIF2alpha is sufficient to suppress pVHL-defective tumor growth. *PLoS Biol.*, **1**, p. E83, 2003.

82. Krieg, M., Haas, R., Brauch, H., Acker, T., Flamme, I., and Plate, K. H., Up-regulation of hypoxia-inducible factors HIF-1alpha and HIF-2alpha under normoxic conditions in renal carcinoma cells by von Hippel-Lindau tumor suppressor gene loss of function. *Oncogene*, **19**, pp. 5435–5443, 2000.

83. Maxwell, P. H., Wiesener, M. S., Chang, G. W., Clifford, S. C., Vaux, E. C., Cockman, M. E., Wykoff, C. C., Pugh, C. W., Maher, E. R., and Ratcliffe, P. J., The tumour suppressor protein VHL targets hypoxia-inducible factors for oxygen-dependent proteolysis. *Nature*, **399**, pp. 271–275, 1999.

84. Raval, R. R., Lau, K. W., Tran, M. G., Sowter, H. M., Mandriota, S. J., Li, J. L., Pugh, C. W., Maxwell, P. H., Harris, A. L., and Ratcliffe, P. J., Contrasting

properties of hypoxia-inducible factor 1 (HIF-1) and HIF-2 in von Hippel-Lindau-associated renal cell carcinoma. *Mol. Cell. Biol.*, **25**, pp. 5675–5686, 2005.

85. Zimmer, M., Doucette, D., Siddiqui, N., and Iliopoulos, O., Inhibition of hypoxia-inducible factor is sufficient for growth suppression of VHL-/-tumors. *Mol. Cancer Res.*, **2**, pp. 89–95, 2004.

86. Purdue, M. P., Johansson, M., Zelenika, D., Toro, J. R., Scelo, G., Moore, L. E., Prokhortchouk, E., Wu, X., Kiemeney, L. A., Gaborieau, V. *et al.*, Genome-wide association study of renal cell carcinoma identifies two susceptibility loci on 2p21 and 11q13.3. *Nat. Genet.*, **43**, pp. 60–65, 2011.

87. Jögi, A., Øra, I., Nilsson, H., Lindeheim, A., Makino, Y., Poellinger, L., Axelson, H., and Påhlman, S., Hypoxia alters gene expression in human neuroblastoma cells toward an immature and neural crest-like phenotype. *Proc. Natl. Acad. Sci. USA*, **99**, pp. 7021–7026, 2002.

88. Tian, H., Hammer, R. E., Matsumoto, A. M., Russell, D. W., and McKnight, S. L., The hypoxia-responsive transcription factor EPAS1 is essential for catecholamine homeostasis and protection against heart failure during embryonic development. *Genes & Dev.*, **12**, pp. 3320–3324, 1998.

89. Nilsson, H., Jögi, A., Beckman, S., Harris, A. L., Poellinger, L., and Påhlman, S., HIF-2alpha expression in human fetal paraganglia and neuroblastoma: relation to sympathetic differentiation, glucose deficiency, and hypoxia. *Exp. Cell Res.*, **303**, pp. 447–456, 2005.

90. Fredlund, E., Ringner, M., Maris, J. M., and Påhlman, S., High Myc pathway activity and low stage of neuronal differentiation associate with poor outcome in neuroblastoma. *Proc. Natl. Acad. Sci. USA*, **105**, pp. 14094–14099, 2008.

91. Vaapil, M., Helczynska, K., Villadsen, R., Petersen, O. W., Johansson, E., Beckman, S., Larsson, C., Påhlman, S., and Jögi, A., Hypoxic conditions induce a cancer-like phenotype in human breast epithelial cells. *PloS One*, **7**, p. e46543, 2012.

92. Påhlman, S., Lund, L. R., and Jögi, A., Differential HIF-1alpha and HIF-2alpha Expression in Mammary Epithelial Cells during Fat Pad Invasion, Lactation, and Involution. *PloS One*, **10**, p. e0125771, 2015.

93. Pietras, A., Gisselsson, D., Øra, I., Noguera, R., Beckman, S., Navarro, S., and Påhlman, S., High levels of HIF-2alpha highlight an immature neural crest-like neuroblastoma cell cohort located in a perivascular niche. *J. Pathol.*, **214**, pp. 482–488, 2008.

94. Pietras, A., Hansford, L. M., Johnsson, A. S., Bridges, E., Sjölund, J., Gisselsson, D., Rehn, M., Beckman, S., Noguera, R., Navarro, S. *et al.*, HIF-2alpha maintains an undifferentiated state in neural crest-like human

neuroblastoma tumor initiating cells. *Proc. Natl. Acad. Sci. USA*, **106**, pp. 16805–16810, 2009.

95. Kaelin, W. G., Jr., The von Hippel-Lindau tumour suppressor protein: O2 sensing and cancer. *Nat. Rev. Cancer*, **8**, pp. 865–873, 2008.

96. Dahia, P. L., Pheochromocytoma and paraganglioma pathogenesis: learning from genetic heterogeneity. *Nat. Rev. Cancer*, **14**, pp. 108–119, 2014.

97. Jochmanova, I., Yang, C., Zhuang, Z., and Pacak, K., Hypoxia-inducible factor signaling in pheochromocytoma: turning the rudder in the right direction. *J. Natl. Cancer Inst.*, **105**, pp. 1270–1283, 2013.

98. Zhuang, Z., Yang, C., Lorenzo, F., Merino, M., Fojo, T., Kebebew, E., Popovic, V., Stratakis, C. A., Prchal, J. T., and Pacak, K., Somatic HIF2A gain-of-function mutations in paraganglioma with polycythemia. *New Engl. J. Med.*, **367**, pp. 922–930, 2012.

99. Percy, M. J., Furlow, P. W., Lucas, G. S., Li, X., Lappin, T. R., McMullin, M. F., and Lee, F. S., A gain-of-function mutation in the HIF2A gene in familial erythrocytosis. *New Engl. J. Med.*, **358**, pp. 162–168, 2008.

100. Comino-Mendez, I., de Cubas, A. A., Bernal, C., Alvarez-Escola, C., Sanchez-Malo, C., Ramirez-Tortosa, C. L., Pedrinaci, S., Rapizzi, E., Ercolino, T., Bernini, G. *et al.*, Tumoral EPAS1 (HIF2A) mutations explain sporadic pheochromocytoma and paraganglioma in the absence of erythrocytosis. *Hum. Mol. Gen.*, **22**, pp. 2169–2176, 2013.

101. Yang, C., Sun, M. G., Matro, J., Huynh, T. T., Rahimpour, S., Prchal, J. T., Lechan, R., Lonser, R., Pacak, K., and Zhuang, Z., Novel HIF2A mutations disrupt oxygen sensing, leading to polycythemia, paragangliomas, and somatostatinomas. *Blood*, **121**, pp. 2563–2566, 2013.

102. McCord, A. M., Jamal, M., Shankavaram, U. T., Lang, F. F., Camphausen, K., and Tofilon, P. J., Physiologic oxygen concentration enhances the stem-like properties of CD133+ human glioblastoma cells in vitro. *Mol. Cancer Res.*, **7**, pp. 489–497, 2009.

103. Sipkins, D. A., Wei, X., Wu, J. W., Runnels, J. M., Cote, D., Means, T. K., Luster, A. D., Scadden, D. T., and Lin, C. P., In vivo imaging of specialized bone marrow endothelial microdomains for tumour engraftment. *Nature*, **435**, pp. 969–973, 2005.

104. Rouault-Pierre, K., Lopez-Onieva, L., Foster, K., Anjos-Afonso, F., Lamrissi-Garcia, I., Serrano-Sanchez, M., Mitter, R., Ivanovic, Z., de Verneuil, H., Gribben, J. *et al.*, HIF-2alpha protects human hematopoietic stem/progenitors and acute myeloid leukemic cells from apoptosis induced by endoplasmic reticulum stress. *Cell Stem Cell*, **13**, pp. 549–563, 2013.

          *Tumor Hypoxia*

105. Schepers, K., Campbell, T. B., and Passegue, E., Normal and leukemic stem cell niches: insights and therapeutic opportunities. *Cell Stem Cell*, **16**, pp. 254–267, 2015.
106. Calabrese, C., Poppleton, H., Kocak, M., Hogg, T. L., Fuller, C., Hamner, B., Oh, E. Y., Gaber, M. W., Finklestein, D., Allen, M. *et al.*, A perivascular niche for brain tumor stem cells. *Cancer Cell*, **11**, pp. 69–82, 2007.

# Chapter 5

# Hypoxia and Senescence

Yashi Gupta and Scott M. Welford*

*Department of Radiation Oncology,
Case Western Reserve University School of Medicine,
Cleveland, OH, USA*
**scott.welford@case.edu*

## 1. Introduction

Cellular aging and the inability of cells to divide indefinitely was first elucidated by Hayflick in the 1960s, and led to subsequent strides in the standardization of cell culture experimentation.[1] Hayflick noticed that normal human fibroblast cells could perform a limited number of cell divisions before arresting, and remained unable to re-enter cell cycle. Additionally, it was observed that the number of divisions normal cells could accomplish depended on the age of the donor. The limit on cell divisions of cultured cells became known as the Hayflick Limit, and cells that reach the limit were termed senescent. In contrast, however, cells were found to be able to overcome the limit when transformed into malignant cells, allowing for infinite proliferation and an explanation for cells such as HeLa cells that did not exhibit senescence.[2] Senescent cells were soon defined as metabolically active cells, which experience mitogenic arrest in response to a variety of extracellular and intracellular stressors. Unlike quiescent cells arrested in G0, senescent cells are irreversibly cell cycle

127

arrested. Together, Hayflick's observations initiated a field of cell biology that has had profound effects on the understanding of aging and cancer, and has reinforced the need to maintain physiological parameters when designing and interpreting biological model systems. While revealed initially from *in vitro* experiments, it is thought that senescence is fundamentally an evolutionary process derived for the function of preventing transmission of genetic damage to daughter cell generations, thereby hindering malignant transformations.

## 2.  Phenotypes of Senescent Cells

Visually, cells entering senescence appear to be enlarged and vacuolated.[1,3] Metabolically, senescent cells experience increase in glycolysis, as reported in human senescent skin and lung fibroblasts,[4,5] as well as an increase in uncoupled respiration[6]; the increase in oxidative phosphorylation is hypothesized to compensate for deficiencies associated with proton leakage (OXPHOS) that accompany aging. In spite of the increased proton leakage, adenosine triphosphate/adenosine diphosphate (ATP/ADP) ratios remain unchanged in senescent skin fibroblasts[5]; however, ATP turnover decreases.[7] Furthermore, changes in phospholipid metabolism have also been observed: glycerophosphocholine (GPC) levels increase, while phosphocholine (PC) levels decrease in the senescent state, regardless of the trigger for senescence.[8] In tumorous cells, however, the GPC to PC ratio is decreased,[9] providing a contrast between cancer and senescence. Perhaps differences in metabolic profiles between tumor and senescent cells can lend a clue to malignant transformation.

Senescent cells also display gross changes in chromatin structure. The chromatin structure of senescent cells is markedly affected, as cells become populated with a heterochromatin phenotype due to vast gene silencing in the arrested state. In 2003, Narita *et al.* discovered the abundance of foci termed senescence-associated heterochromatic foci (SAHF) in senescent cells. The formation of SAHF is accompanied with the recruitment of many proteins, including Rb, to E2F promoter regions, resulting in silencing of E2F target genes.[10] The importance of the Rb pathway is highlighted by evidence that shows an essential role for Rb in the induction of senescence; cells deficient in Rb and related proteins fail to senesce.[11,12] Changes in chromatin structure can be visualized through 4'6-diamindino-2-phenylindole (DAPI) staining and antibodies to macroH2A, HP1$\gamma$ and H3K9Me2/3.[13] Although SAHF can be a phenotype of senescence, the two are not always coupled. For example, loss of tumor suppressor phosphatase and tensin homolog (PTEN) and subsequent AKT activation can lead to senescence without SAHF.[14] Nonetheless, major chromatin changes are prevalent.

Finally, senescent cells do not exist in a vacuum, and in fact directly affect surrounding cells. A hallmark of senescence induced by DNA damage is the senescence-associated secretory phenotype (SASP). SASP involves the secretion of a wide variety of cytokines, chemokines, growth factors and proteases. SASP can steer neighboring cells in either direction of senescence or proliferation. Grouped as soluble factors, shed receptors/ligands, non-protein soluble factors, and extracellular matrix/non-soluble factors, some of the secreted factors induce senescence, while others potentiate cell survival and proliferative signals.[3,15] p53 induced senescence in hepatic stellate cells gives rise to a characteristic extra cellular matrix and SASP profile that inhibits transformation to hepatocellular carcinoma, a trend not observed in p53 proficient cells.[16] At the opposing end, tumor-promoting secreted factors include IL1, IL6, IL8, IGF binding protein family members, GRO$\alpha$ and MIF.[15] Although, similar secretory phenotypes are not observed in cases of senescence initiated via overexpression of cell cycle inhibitors p16 and p21, as DNA damage is necessary for SASP,[15] loss of p53 function greatly enhances SASP.[17] Activation of p53/p21 and p16/pRB function to inhibit tumor formation, but the SASP that accompanies the senescent phase of cells can have an opposing effect. The juxtaposition of tumor suppressive and tumorigenic responses makes the relationship between cancer and senescence intriguing in the context of evolutionary processes.

## 3. Markers of Senescent Cells

One of the major markers for senescent cells, known as senescence-associated $\beta$-gal (SA-$\beta$-gal), is the gold standard for detection of senescence (Fig. 1). Resulting from an increase in lysosomal $\beta$-gal enzymatic activity and increase in lysosome structure, blue $\beta$-gal staining has been

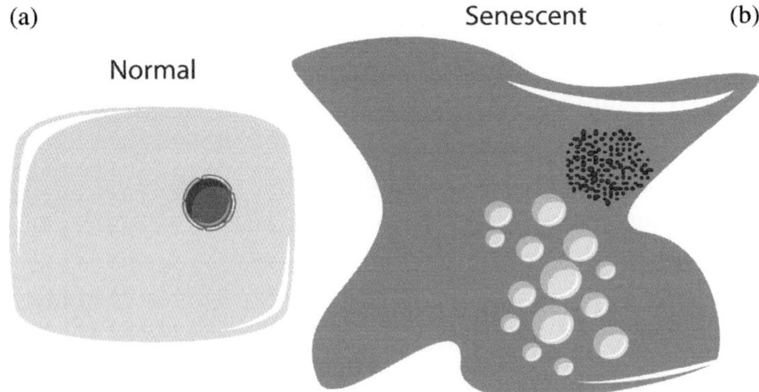


Fig. 1.   Markers and phenotypes of senescent cells. Normal cell (a) versus senescent cell (b). Enlarged and vacuolated senescent cells stain blue with SA-$\beta$-Gal as well as having a punctate like staining pattern in the nucleus when stained for SAHF molecular markers. Although markers for senescence exist, their individual specificity is low and multiple markers are needed to confirm the senescent stage of a cell. Figure produced with the aid of Servier Medical Art with modifications: retrieved from http://www.servier.com/Powerpoint-image-bank.

observed in tissue culture cells, animal models, and in aging cells in people. Interestingly, the biological function of SA-$\beta$-gal is not fully understood regarding its role in the induction or maintenance of senescence.[18,19] It has been shown however, that aging fibroblasts from patients with recessive G(M1)-gangliosidosis and defective lysosomal $\beta$-galactosidase, can still enter replicative senescence.[19] Further, cells in which the GLB1 gene encoding lysosomal $\beta$-galactosidase is depleted can be induced to senesce.[19] Thus, while SA-$\beta$-gal remains a defining feature of senescent cells, it appears to be more of a passenger than a driver of the phenotype. Additionally, SA-$\beta$-gal is prone to false positives, as over confluence and hydrogen peroxide ($H_2O_2$) can also induce SA-$\beta$-gal signal.[20] As a result, while SA-$\beta$-gal is widely used, a preponderance of markers has become requisite to convincingly demonstrate that senescence has occurred.

When stained for DNA, normal cells appear uniform and continuous; senescent cells, however, have punctate like patterns of DNA in the form of SAHF.[10] It is thought senescence associated gene silencing is responsible for the punctate like appearance, as gene silencing involves tightening of chromatin structure via chromatin modifications. Chromatin and genetic regulation is moderated by a series of acetylation and methylation events of histones; acetylation is generally involved in gene upregulation, but methylation can be either activating or repressing, depending on the site of methylation. Chromatin markers including DAPI along with H3K9me3, HP1γ staining, and macroH2A, all of which are components of SAHF and involved in transcriptional repression, can be used to identify SAHF. Methylation at histone 3 lysine 9 (H3K9me) has a repressive function and is upregulated in senescent cells. HP1γ, or histone binding protein 1 γ, localizes to methylated lys9 and is also involved in transcriptional repression[21]; HP1γ levels dissipate from mitotic chromosomes.[22] MacroH2A is a histone variant of the H2A family that has been shown to be involved in the repression of the inactivated X chromosome, and is downregulated in pluripotent stem cells compared to their differentiated cells.[23] Like SA-β-gal, SAHF are not a reliable method for detection of senescence; SAHF may not be necessary for development of senescence, and are dependent on cell type and the senescence trigger.[24] Thus the need for using multiple chromatin markers to accurately identify senescent cells is further perpetuated.

The last category of senescence markers is a group of molecular markers. Proteins elevated or activated in senescence include p21, p16, p15, DCR2, and NOTCH3.[25] Recently, Althubiti *et al.* have performed proteomic analysis of proteins associated with the plasma membrane in senescent cells and found 107 proteins specific to senescent cells. Proteins including DEP1, STX4, VAMP3, VPS26A, PLD3, NTAL, ARMCX3, LANCL1, B2MG, and EBP50 have the potential to preferentially mark for senescence.[25] Currently, there is no specific molecule that is expressed solely in senescent cells that is sufficient to define a senescent cell on its own. However, in conjunction with physical and enzymatic markers, senescent cells can be identified.

## 4. Molecular Pathways Driving Senescence

When cells experience irreparable levels of stress-induced damage, cells have three programed options for resolution: senescence, apoptosis (or other programed death), or autophagy. How cells determine which of these response pathways to pursue is incompletely understood, but crosstalk at the level of p53 has been hypothesized.[26] Two major pathways have been implicated in the regulation of senescence: p53/p21, and p16[INK4a]/pRb. The activation of these canonical tumor suppressor pathways is thought to protect from malignant transformations as they lead to cell cycle arrest. Malignant cells need to overcome the activation of these pathways to become carcinogenic. p53 is well known as a crucial DNA damage response (DDR) protein and tumor suppressor; Li-Fraumeni patients, who are heterozygous mutants for p53, have increased susceptibility to cancer occurrence due to the presence of only one wild type p53 allele.[27] Roles of p53 are vast and not limited to tumor suppression, with known functions in metabolism, fertility, neurodegenerative diseases, apoptosis, and promotion of aging, p53 regulation is critical in many aspects of cellular function.[28] The activation of p53 following damage is initiated by signaling-induced phosphorylation that interrupts interaction with its inhibitor, MDM2, or via downregulation of MDM2 or other inhibitory binding partners.[29] Once activated, p53 drives expression of a host of cell cycle regulatory and apoptotic proteins such as p21, PUMA, NOXA, and GADD45.[28] p16 is a transcript of the INK4/ARF locus and has a dichotomous role in cancer and senescence; while levels of p16[INK4a] are downregulated in a majority of cancers, they have been shown to be upregulated in several tumors.[30] Like p53, p16[INK4a] promotes cell cycle arrest. By binding to CDK4/6, p16[INK4a] inhibits phosphorylation of pRB, leading to cycle arrest.[31] ARF, a transcript from an alternate reading frame in the INK4/ARF locus, functions to inhibit MDM2 and induce senescence by increasing p53 activity.[31] Furthermore, autophagy was found to be required for efficient establishment of senescence.[32] Several autophagy related genes were found to be upregulated in the senescent phase; upregulation of these genes induced autophagy and senescence, while inhibition delayed the senescent phenotype.[33] Thus integration of signaling networks in various contexts result in senescent or death responses.

## 5. Stresses that Induce Senescence

Stresses that can provoke entrance into senescence include: telomeric dysfunction, mitochondrial deterioration, oxidative stress, severe genotoxic stress, and oncogene expression (Fig. 2).[15] Telomeric dysfunction leads to

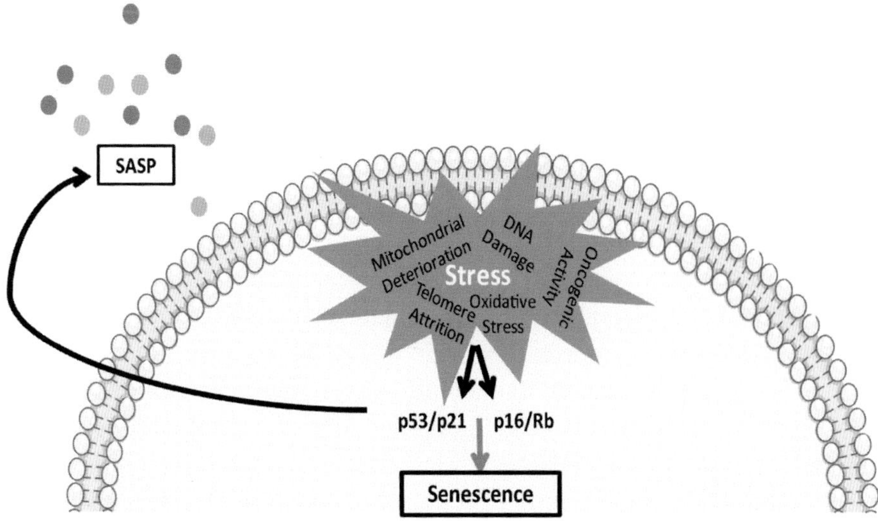


Fig. 2. Inducers of senescence. A myriad of stressors activate p53/p21 and p16/RB signaling which are required for induction of senescence. The process of senescence induction can lead to a SASP, which can further perpetuate senescence or help cells in overcoming the senescent fate. Figure produced with the aid of Servier Medical Art: retrieved from http://www.servier.com/Powerpoint-image-bank.

replicative senescence, and results from the decapping of telomeres with each cell division cycle. Functioning to distinguish the end of chromosomes from that of DNA double stranded breaks and to prevent nucleolytic attack, telomeres shorten due to the nature of lagging strand replication. Since DNA replication occurs 5′–3′, the replication of the complementary (lagging) strand, occurs through the use of Okazaki fragments, which require placement of RNA primers for 5′–3′ replication in segments. RNA nuclease then removes the primers, and DNA polymerase and DNA ligase fill in the primer gaps and connect the individual segments. This RNA to DNA conversion only takes place if there is a DNA segment preceding the RNA primer, so in the case of the last primer, this conversion does not take place and the RNA is degraded, leading to progressive telomere shortening known as the "end replication problem." The correlation between proliferative ability and the length of the guanine rich chromosome ends was discovered in the early 1990s; Allsopp *et al.* found that telomere length, rather than donor age, determined the replication limit of cells.[34] Replicative senescence is also thought to involve improper telomere cap formation. The cap, which consists of duplex loops called t-loops, along with its coat of protective proteins known as telomeric repeat binding factors (TRFs), play a role in preventing end-to-end fusion of chromosomes, and the subsequent activation of the DNA damage-p53 pathway and cell cycle arrest.[35] It is clear that telomeres play a crucial role in the induction of senescence, but the exact mechanism(s) have yet to be fully elucidated.

In addition to genomic degradation, with age comes a wide variety of changes to the mitochondria. Increased disorganization of mitochondrial structure, decline in OXPHOS function, accumulation of mitochondrial DNA (mtDNA) mutations, and increased mitochondrial production of reactive oxygen species (ROS) are all forms of mitochondrial stress that accompany the process of aging.[36] Mitochondrion copy numbers decrease, mitochondrial size increases, and the number of cristae decrease. Disorganization of mitochondrial quantity and structure leads to increased proton leakage and respiratory decoupling, which can result in damaging increases in ROS and oxidative stress induced damage. An increase in ROS and oxidative stress can lead to cellular and mtDNA damage. The majority of ROS within the cell are mitochondria generated, and can lead to increased DNA, protein, and lipid damage. As mutations to cellular and mtDNA increase and accumulate with age, mitochondrial structure is further compromised, proton leakage increased, and the cycle is perpetuated leading to further increase in ROS and DDR. Cellular responses to damage may include activation of DDR pathways or cell cycle exit via induction of senescence through activation p53 and p16 pathways, apoptosis, or autophagy. The role of the mitochondria as the powerhouse of the cell lends it to be a crucial player in aging and senescence.

In addition to telomere degradation and mitochondrial stress, molecular/genetic changes of the cell can also induce senescence. Specifically, oncogene-induced-senescence (OIS) is initiated when tumor suppressors are functionally lost or oncogenes are activated. In order to suppress cancer development, OIS induces the activation of the p53 and p16 pathways to induce senescence.[37] The list of oncogenes that induce senescence is abundant and lends to a myriad of mechanisms for how they induce senescence. Hyperproliferation, cell signaling, metabolic shifts, and SASP profiles have all been implicated in OIS. For example, increased levels of oncogenic proteins can lead to an initial induction of hyperproliferation, resulting in replicative stress and DNA damage sensing, and subsequently activate tumor suppressor pathways and senescence.[38] Indeed, senescence associated with H-RAS$^{V12}$ is accompanied with increased replication as evidenced by an increase in active replicons, as well as increased number of alterations in DNA replication fork progression.[39] Inhibition of the DDR in the H-RAS$^{V12}$ model abrogates induction of senescence,[39] suggesting the importance of DDR in oncogene induced hyperproliferation. A study of multiple major oncogenes confirmed that expression of the oncogenes was accompanied with an abundance of double stranded breaks, while inhibition of double strand break repair via ATM knockdown led to suppression of senescence induction and increased tumor size and invasiveness *in vivo*.[40] Akt signaling has been long associated with cell survival and uncontrolled cell cycle progression. In the case of the oncogenic RAS, Akt was found to be required for susceptibility to RAS induced senescence.[41] Along with affecting RAS induced senescence, Akt was also found to protect from ROS induced apoptosis.[41] Furthermore, a 2013 study by Kaplon *et al.* provides a link between senescence and metabolism. Oncogenic BRAF$^{V600E}$ induced senescence was found to correlate with an increase in pyruvate dehydrogenase (PDH) levels via inhibition of pyruvate dehydrogenase kinase 1 (PDK1), along with activation of pyruvate dehydrogenase phosphatase 2 (PDP2); depletion of PKD1 resulted in regression of existing melanomas and subpopulations resistant to targeted BRAF inhibition.[42] In another study, secreted factor IGFBP7, implicated in SASP, inhibited BRAF/MEK/ERK signaling and induced senescence and apoptosis in human melanoma cell line.[43] Notably, the SASP profile increase in IGFBP7 has a prosenescent function in melanoma. Yet another SASP factor, PAI-1, was found to be an important downstream factor to p53 signaling and senescence. PAI-1 knockdown was associated with escape from senescence, while ectopic expression of PAI-1 induced a senescent phenotype.[44] It is evident that the classic pathways involved in carrying out senescence are crucial, regardless of the source of initiation. Although functioning as a different mode to induce senescence, OIS is identified by biomarkers such as SA-$\beta$-gal and has a similar senescent phenotype to replicative senescence.

# 6. Senescent Cells and the Hypoxic Microenvironment

Just as senescent cells are now known to influence neighboring cells through their secretory phenotypes, it is also quite apparent that tissue microenvironments can directly influence the fates of would-be senescent cells. Hypoxia has a well-established role in normal development through its influence of angiogenesis, cell fate decisions, and organ development. In aging, hypoxia is known to increase in tissues due to depressed responsiveness of the hypoxia inducible transcription factors (HIFs), and correlates with the appearance of senescence cells.[18,45] Furthermore, the link of senescence to oxidative stress regulation places oxygen directly in the center of environmental factors that control senescence.[46] It has been shown that hypoxic environments slow down onset of senescence and elongate the lifespan of cells.[47,48] Accordingly, hyperoxic conditions result in an increase in oxidative stress via increased mitochondrial ROS and induce senescence. Indeed, addition of $H_2O_2$ results in an induction of senescence,[49] while addition of N-acetyl cysteine (NAC) inhibits senescence.[50] These results demonstrate the anti-tumor suppressive nature of hypoxia on a cell autonomous nature. In contrast, severe hypoxia has recently been linked to the conversion of quiescent cells to a senescent state.[51] Thus, the current data suggests a two-sided relationship between hypoxia and senescence that can be complicated by the tissue and cell types involved.

Hypoxic environments affect the senescence phenotype in a multifaceted manner, a prime example being regulation of the cell cycle (Fig. 3). Cell cycle progression mediated by HIF-1$\alpha$ is a result of targets involved in regulating the cell cycle, such as p21,[52] p27[53] and CSC25A.[54] Depending on the oxygen content and cell type, HIF mediated affects can be arresting or proliferative. Decreases in oxygen from atmospheric levels initiate a hyperproliferative state, yet induce cell cycle arrest at levels below physiologically tolerable in primary fibroblasts.[48,55] HIF-1$\alpha$ can act directly on gene promoters in a sequence specific manner or indirectly through protein — protein interactions. For example, HIF-1$\alpha$ has been shown to bind MDM2 stabilizing p53 and to displace Myc upregulating p21,[52,56] both of which result in cell cycle arrest. Due to the multitude of

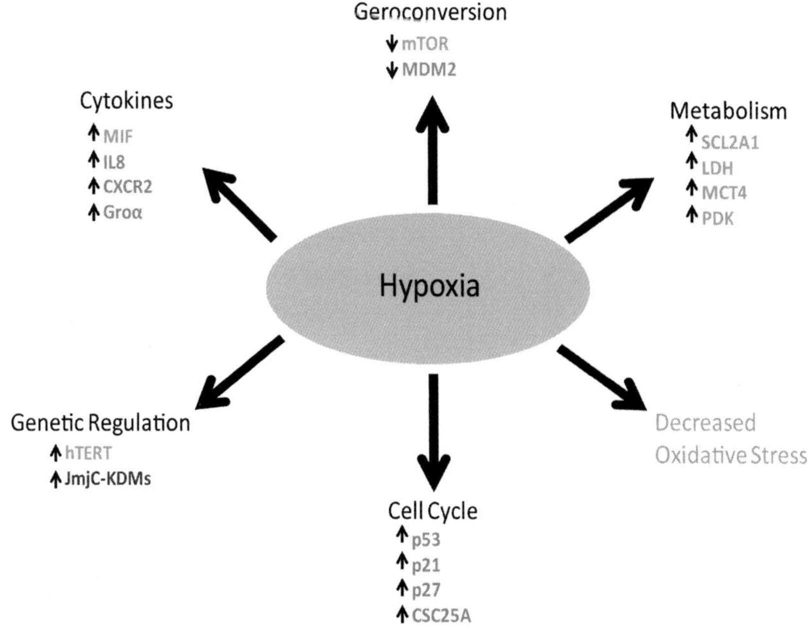



Fig. 3. Interactions of hypoxia and the senescent phenotype. Hypoxia results in many cellular changes that are coincident (black), antagonistic (ovals), or drivers of senescence (rectangles).

mechanisms through which HIF can affect protein expression, differences in expression profiles can contribute to the dual nature of cell cycle progression mediated by oxygen content.

Hypoxia of course has a noted effect on metabolism. The senescence phenotype is interestingly also accompanied by a metabolic shift towards increased glycolysis, which is also common in tumor cells where it is known as the Warburg effect. It is known that targets of HIF-1$\alpha$ include mostly all of the genes involved in the glycolytic pathway, attributing lower oxygen content to the switch to a more anaerobic pathway. In clear cell renal cell carcinoma (ccRCC), for example, a malignancy that simulates a constitutive hypoxic environment by loss of function of the von Hippel–Lindau (VHL) tumor suppressor that negatively regulates HIF, genes including glucose transporter 1 (SLC2A1), lactate dehydrogenase

(LDH), monocarboxylate transporter 4 (MCT4), and pyruvate dehydrogenase kinase (PDK) are all upregulated.[57] Furthermore, inhibitors of glycolysis (e.g. PDK inhibitors) in ccRCC tumors in animal models grow notably slower.[58] Coincidentally, VHL loss has been shown to induce OIS in an oxygen dependent manner, such that in the normal oxygen conditions of the mouse kidney, OIS is suppressed.[59] Use of the anaerobic pathway for ATP production helps reduce ROS generation, thereby attenuating oxidative stress that can induce senescence in primary cells. Thus, natural hypoxia in the kidney helps avert senescent induction. It has also been noted in model systems that glycolytic enzymes such as phosphoglucose isomerase (PGI)[60] and phosphoglycerate mutase (PGM)[61] have been identified as genes able to bypass senescence. Thus the metabolic switch and reduction of mitochondrial ROS correlate with the hypoxic suppression of senescence in several models.

Imperative to the induction of senescence, the p53 tumor suppressor is also activated by hypoxia, though only at severely low levels of oxygen (<0.5%).[62] Oxygen levels required for HIF-$1\alpha$ induction are considerably milder, in the range of 2–5% oxygen, depending on the basal level of the tissue of interest. However, in cases where genotoxic stress occurs in cells exposed to hypoxia, where HIF-$1\alpha$ and p53 are both activated, it is of note that several reports indicate direct and indirect interaction between HIF-$1\alpha$ and p53, which can either promote p53 stabilization or HIF-$1\alpha$ degradation, and thereby act to facilitate senescence induction.[56,63–67] Several HIF-$1\alpha$ targets have been implicated in regulating senescence or p53 directly, including p21, MIF, and PAI-1.

Interestingly, a variety of secreted factors that regulate senescence are HIF target genes, adding another layer of complexity to the SASP. MIF is upregulated and effects a cell survival and a proliferative state,[68] and is part of the SASP. IL8, also in the SASP, is a HIF-$1\alpha$ target as well as the IL8 receptor, CXCR2; and GRO$\alpha$ expression is upregulated in hypoxic pulmonary arteries.[69] As chemokines, IL8 and GRO$\alpha$ have been shown to reinforce the senescent phenotype in human fibroblasts.[69,70] Thus again conflicting hypoxic effector proteins lead to opposing senescent phenotypes which have been shown to be induced by SASP and alter neighboring non-senescent cells.[71]

Recently, a process termed geroconversion was described to involve the transition of cells from reversible, quiescent state, to irreversible senescent state.[51] A key regulator of geroconversion, mTOR, has been identified. Interestingly, mTOR is hypoxia inhibited.[72] Inhibition of mTOR via hypoxia is found to suppress geroconversion and prolong cellular lifespan in a p53 and HIF-1$\alpha$ independent manner.[73] In one study, turnover of MDM2 was required for geroconversion by inhibition of CDK4.[74] As HIF-1$\alpha$ has been shown to interact with MDM2 and attenuate p53 degradation,[64] hypoxia has an additional layer of regulation in geroconversion.

A major regulator of proliferative senescence is the HIF-1$\alpha$ target, human telomerase reverse transcriptase (hTERT). hTERT is the catalytic unit of the telomerase complex which plays a role in telomere extension and the prolonging of senescence induction. One way cells can transform and avoid regulation by senescence is through upregulation of hTERT in a hypoxic fashion. Indeed, fibroblast population doublings were increased by 10 under hypoxia induced hTERT upregulation, by delaying replicative senescence.[75] Furthermore, mutations in the TERT promoter have been found in gliomas, leading to increased transcriptional activity of TERT under hypoxia and poor responses to temozolomide, corresponding to poor prognosis of glioma patients.[76] Thus hTERT is an example of hypoxia-mediated suppression of senescence that has implications beyond primary cell transformation into tumor cells.

Finally, transcriptional regulation and chromatin remodeling have a recurring role in the induction of senescence; from the silencing of genes that lead to SAHF to the aberrant regulation of oncogenes, gene regulation is at the core of senescence. Several studies have linked hypoxia to changes in epigenetic topography.[77–80] JmjC-domain containing histone lysine demethylases (JmjC–KDMs) are members of the 2-oxoglutarate (2OG) dependent oxygenase family that regulate methylation levels of histones. Several JmjC–KDMs are in fact transcriptional targets of HIF targets.[80–82] Some of these HIF target KDMs have been implicated in numerous cancers and have been shown to be involved in cell cycle and proliferation, yet again linking hypoxia to senescence. So while the HIF-mediated epigenetic regulators have not yet been explicitly linked to senescence regulation, it stands to reason that the final layer of coincidence is likely to have biological overlap.

# References


1. Hayflick, L., The limited in vitro lifetime of human diploid cell strains. *Exp. Cell Res.*, **37**, pp. 614–636, 1965.
2. Shay, J. W., and Wright, W. E., Hayflick, his limit, and cellular ageing. *Nat. Rev. Mol. Cell. Biol.*, **1**(1), pp. 72–76, 2000.
3. Campisi, J., and Robert, L., Cell senescence, role in aging and age-related diseases. *Interdisciplinary Topics in Gerontol.*, **39**, pp. 45–61, 2014.
4. Bittles, A. H., and Harper, N., Increased glycolysis in ageing cultured human diploid fibroblasts. *Biosc; Rep.*, **4**(9), pp. 751–756, 1984. Epub 1984/09/01.
5. Goldstein, S., Ballantyne, S. R., Robson, A. L., and Moerman, E. J., Energy metabolism in cultured human fibroblasts during aging *in vitro*. *J. Cell. Physiol.*, **112**(3), pp. 419–424, 1982.
6. Hutter, E., Renner, K., Pfister, G., Stöckl, P., Jansen-Dürr, P., and Gnaiger, E., Senescence-associated changes in respiration and oxidative phosphorylation in primary human fibroblasts. *Biochem., J.*, **380**(Pt 3), pp. 919–928, 2004.
7. Muggleton-Harris, A. L., and Defuria, R., Age-dependent metabolic changes in cultured human fibroblasts. *In Vitro Cell. Dev. Biol.*, **21**(5), pp. 271–276, 1985.
8. Gey, C., and Seeger, K., Metabolic changes during cellular senescence investigated by proton NMR-spectroscopy. *Mechanisms Ageing dev.*, **134**(3–4), pp. 130–138, 2013.
9. Iorio, E., Mezzanzanica, D., Alberti, P., Spadaro, F., Ramoni, C., D'Ascenzo, S. et al., Alterations of choline phospholipid metabolism in ovarian tumor progression. *Cancer Res.*, **65**(20), pp. 9369–9376, 2005. Epub 2005/10/19.
10. Narita, M., Nunez, S., Heard, E., Narita, M., Lin, A. W., Hearn, S.A. et al., Rb-mediated heterochromatin formation and silencing of E2F target genes during cellular senescence. *Cell.*, **113**(6), pp. 703–716, 2003. Epub 2003/06/18.
11. Dannenberg, J. H., van Rossum, A., Schuijff, L., and te Riele, H., Ablation of the retinoblastoma gene family deregulates G(1) control causing immortalization and increased cell turnover under growth-restricting conditions. *Genes Dev.*, **14**(23), pp. 3051–3064, 2000. Epub 2000/12/15.
12. Sage, J., Mulligan, G. J., Attardi, L. D., Miller, A., Chen, S., Williams, B. et al., Targeted disruption of the three Rb-related genes leads to loss of G(1) control and immortalization. *Genes Dev.*, **14**(23), pp. 3037–3050, 2000. Epub 2000/12/15.
13. Aird, K. M., and Zhang, R., Detection of senescence-associated heterochromatin foci (SAHF). *Methods in molecular biology,* (Clifton, NJ). **965**, pp. 185–196, 2013.
14. Kennedy, A. L., Morton, J. P., Manoharan, I., Nelson, D. M., Jamieson, N. B., Pawlikowski, J.S. et al., Activation of the PIK3CA/AKT pathway suppresses

senescence induced by an activated RAS oncogene to promote tumorigenesis. *Mol. Cell.*, **42**(1), pp. 36–49, 2011.

15. Coppe, J. P., Desprez, P. Y., Krtolica, A., and Campisi, J., The senescence-associated secretory phenotype: the dark side of tumor suppression. *Annu. Rev. Pathol.*, **5**, pp. 99–118, 2010. Epub 2010/01/19.

16. Lujambio, A., Akkari, L., Simon, J., Grace, D., Tschaharganeh Darjus, F., Bolden Jessica, E. *et al.*, Non-Cell-Autonomous Tumor Suppression by p53. *Cell*, **153**(2), pp. 449–460, 2013.

17. Coppe, J. P., Patil, C. K., Rodier, F., Sun, Y., Munoz, D. P., Goldstein, J. *et al.*, Senescence-associated secretory phenotypes reveal cell-nonautonomous functions of oncogenic RAS and the p53 tumor suppressor. *PLoS Biol.*, **6**(12), pp. 2853–2868, 2008.

18. Dimri, G. P., Lee, X., Basile, G., Acosta, M., Scott, G., Roskelley, C. *et al.*, A biomarker that identifies senescent human cells in culture and in aging skin *in vivo*. *Proc. Natl. Acad. Sci. USA*, **92**(20), pp. 9363–9367, 1995.

19. Lee, B. Y., Han, J. A., Im, J. S., Morrone, A., Johung, K., Goodwin, E. C. *et al.* Senescence-associated $\beta$-galactosidase is lysosomal $\beta$-galactosidase. *Aging Cell.*, **5**(2), pp. 187–195, 2006. Epub 2006/04/22.

20. Yang, N. C., and Hu, M. L., The limitations and validities of senescence associated-$\beta$-galactosidase activity as an aging marker for human foreskin fibroblast Hs68 cells. *Experimental Gerontology.*, **40**(10), pp. 813–819, 2005. Epub 2005/09/13.

21. Nishibuchi, G., and Nakayama, J., Biochemical and structural properties of heterochromatin protein 1: understanding its role in chromatin assembly. *J. biochem.*, **156**(1), pp. 11–20, 2014. Epub 2014/05/16.

22. Jacobs, S. A., Taverna, S. D., Zhang, Y., Briggs, S. D., Li, J., Eissenberg, J. C. *et al.*, Specificity of the HP1 chromo domain for the methylated N-terminus of histone H3. *EMBO J.* **20**(18), pp. 5232–5241, 2001. Epub 2001/09/22.

23. Gaspar-Maia, A., Qadeer, Z. A., Hasson, D., Ratnakumar, K., Leu, N. A., Leroy, G. *et al.*, MacroH2A histone variants act as a barrier upon reprogramming towards pluripotency. *Nature Comm.*, **4**, p. 1565, 2013. Epub 2013/03/07.

24. Kosar, M., Bartkova, J., Hubackova, S., Hodny, Z., Lukas, J., and Bartek, J., Senescence-associated heterochromatin foci are dispensable for cellular senescence, occur in a cell type- and insult-dependent manner and follow expression of p16(ink4a). *Cell Cycle.*, **10**(3), pp. 457–468, 2011. Epub 2011/01/21.

25. Althubiti, M., Lezina, L., Carrera, S., Jukes-Jones, R., Giblett, S. M., Antonov, A. *et al.*, Characterization of novel markers of senescence and their prognostic potential in cancer. *Cell death & disease.*, **5**: p. e1528, 2014. Epub 2014/11/21.

26. Vicencio, J. M., Galluzzi, L., Tajeddine, N., Ortiz, C., Criollo, A., Tasdemir, E. *et al.*, Senescence, apoptosis or autophagy? When a damaged cell must decide its path — a mini-review. *Gerontology.*, **54**(2), pp. 92–99, 2008. Epub 2008/05/03.

27. Merino, D., and Malkin, D., p53 and hereditary cancer. *Subcellular Biochem.*, **85**, pp. 1–16, 2014. Epub 2014/09/10.

28. Meek, D. W. Regulation of the p53 response and its relationship to cancer. *Biochem. J.*, **469**(3), pp. 325–346, 2015. Epub 2015/07/25.

29. Hu, W., Feng, Z., and Levine, A. J., The Regulation of Multiple p53 Stress Responses is Mediated through MDM2. *Genes Cancer.*, **3**(3–4), pp. 199–208, 2012. Epub 2012/11/15.

30. Romagosa, C., Simonetti, S., Lopez-Vicente, L., Mazo, A., Lleonart, M. E., Castellvi, J. *et al.*, p16(Ink4a) overexpression in cancer: a tumor suppressor gene associated with senescence and high-grade tumors. *Oncogene.*, **30**(18), pp. 2087–2097, 2011. Epub 2011/02/08.

31. Serrano, M., The tumor suppressor protein p16INK4a. *Exp. Cell. Res.*, **237**(1), pp. 7–13, 1997. Epub 1998/01/07.

32. White, E., and Lowe, S. W., Eating to exit: autophagy-enabled senescence revealed. *Genes Dev.*, **23**(7), pp. 784–787, 2009. Epub 2009/04/03.

33. Young, A. R., Narita, M., Ferreira, M., Kirschner, K., Sadaie, M., Darot, J. F. *et al.*, Autophagy mediates the mitotic senescence transition. *Genes Dev.*, **23**(7), pp. 798–803, 2009. Epub 2009/03/13.

34. Allsopp, R. C., Vaziri, H., Patterson, C., Goldstein, S., Younglai, E. V., Futcher, A.B. *et al.*, Telomere length predicts replicative capacity of human fibroblasts. *Proc. Natl. Acad. Sci. USA,* **89**(21), pp. 10114–10118, 1992. Epub 1992/11/01.

35. Karlseder, J., Smogorzewska, A., and de Lange, T., Senescence induced by altered telomere state, not telomere loss. *Science.*, **295**(5564), pp. 2446–2449, 2002. Epub 2002/03/30.

36. Lee, H. C., and Wei, Y. H., Mitochondria and aging. *Adv. Exp. Medi. Biol.*, **942**, pp. 311–327, 2012. Epub 2012/03/09.

37. Xu, Y., Li, N., Xiang, R., and Sun, P., Emerging roles of the p38 MAPK and PI3K/AKT/mTOR pathways in oncogene-induced senescence. *Trends. Biochem. Sci.*, **39**(6), pp. 268–276, 2014.

38. Kilbey, A., Terry, A., Cameron, E. R., and Neil, J. C., Oncogene-induced senescence: an essential role for Runx. *Cell cycle,* (Georgetown, Tex). **7**(15), pp. 2333–2340, 2008.

39. Di Micco, R., Fumagalli, M., Cicalese, A., Piccinin, S., Gasparini, P., Luise, C. *et al.*, Oncogene-induced senescence is a DNA damage response triggered by DNA hyper-replication. *Nature,* **444**(7119), pp. 638–642, 2006.

40. Bartkova, J., Rezaei, N., Liontos, M., Karakaidos, P., Kletsas, D., Issaeva, N. *et al.*, Oncogene-induced senescence is part of the tumorigenesis barrier imposed by DNA damage checkpoints. *Nature*, **444**(7119), pp. 633–637, 2006.

41. Nogueira, V., Park, Y., Chen, C. C., Xu, P. Z., Chen, M. L., Tonic, I. *et al.*, Akt determines replicative senescence and oxidative or oncogenic premature senescence and sensitizes cells to oxidative apoptosis. *Cancer Cell.*, **14**(6), pp. 458–470, 2008.

42. Kaplon, J., Zheng, L., Meissl, K., Chaneton, B., Selivanov, V. A., Mackay, G. *et al.*, A key role for mitochondrial gatekeeper pyruvate dehydrogenase in oncogene-induced senescence. *Nature*, **498**(7452), pp. 109–112, 2013. Epub 2013/05/21.

43. Wajapeyee, N., Serra, R. W., Zhu, X., Mahalingam, M., and Green, M. R., Oncogenic BRAF Induces Senescence and Apoptosis through Pathways Mediated by the Secreted Protein IGFBP7. *Cell*, **132**(3), pp. 363–374, 2008.

44. Kortlever, R. M., Higgins, P. J., and Bernards, R., Plasminogen activator inhibitor-1 is a critical downstream target of p53 in the induction of replicative senescence. *Nat. Cell. Biol.*, **8**(8), pp. 877–884, 2006.

45. Hoenig, M. R., Bianchi, C., Rosenzweig, A., and Sellke, F. W., Decreased vascular repair and neovascularization with ageing: mechanisms and clinical relevance with an emphasis on hypoxia-inducible factor-1. *Curr. Mol. Med.*, **8**(8), pp. 754–767, 2008. Epub 2008/12/17.

46. Lu, T., and Finkel, T., Free radicals and senescence. *Exp Cell Res.*, **314**(9), pp. 1918–1922, 2008. Epub 2008/02/20.

47. von Zglinicki, T., Saretzki, G., Docke, W., and Lotze, C., Mild hyperoxia shortens telomeres and inhibits proliferation of fibroblasts: a model for senescence? *Exp. Cell. Res.*, **220**(1), pp. 186–193, 1995.

48. Packer, L., and Fuehr, K., Low oxygen concentration extends the lifespan of cultured human diploid cells. *Nature*, **267**(5610), pp. 423–425, 1977.

49. Chen, Q., and Ames, B. N., Senescence-like growth arrest induced by hydrogen peroxide in human diploid fibroblast F65 cells. *Proc. Natl. Acad. Sci. USA*, **91**(10), pp. 4130–4134, 1994.

50. Lee, A. C., Fenster, B. E., Ito, H., Takeda, K., Bae, N. S., Hirai, T. *et al.*, Ras proteins induce senescence by altering the intracellular levels of reactive oxygen species. *J. Biol. Chem.*, **274**(12), pp. 7936–7940, 1999.

51. Blagosklonny, M. V., Geroconversion: irreversible step to cellular senescence. *Cell. Cycle.*, **13**(23), pp. 3628–3635, 2014. Epub 2014/12/09.

52. Koshiji, M., Kageyama, Y., Pete, E. A., Horikawa, I., Barrett, J. C., and Huang, L. E., HIF-1alpha induces cell cycle arrest by functionally counteracting Myc. *EMBO J.*, **23**(9), pp. 1949–1956, 2004.

53. Gardner, L. B., Li, Q., Park, M. S., Flanagan, W. M., Semenza, G. L., and Dang, C. V., Hypoxia inhibits G1/S transition through regulation of p27 expression. *J. Biol. Chem.*, **276**(11), pp. 7919–7926, 2001.

54. Hammer, S., To, K. K., Yoo, Y. G., Koshiji, M., and Huang, L. E., Hypoxic suppression of the cell cycle gene CDC25A in tumor cells. *Cell Cycle.*, **6**(15), 1919–1926, 2007.

55. Parrinello, S., Samper, E., Krtolica, A., Goldstein, J., Melov, S., and Campisi, J., Oxygen sensitivity severely limits the replicative lifespan of murine fibroblasts. *Nat. Cell. Biol.*, **5**(8), pp. 741–747, 2003.

56. An, W. G., Kanekal, M., Simon, M. C., Maltepe, E., Blagosklonny, M. V., and Neckers, L. M., Stabilization of wild-type p53 by hypoxia-inducible factor 1[alpha]. *Nature*, **392**(6674), pp. 405–408, 1998.

57. Pinthus, J. H., Whelan, K. F., Gallino, D., Lu, J. P., and Rothschild, N., Metabolic features of clear-cell renal cell carcinoma: mechanisms and clinical implications. *Can. Urol. Assoc. Journal, Journal de l'Association des urologues du Canada*, **5**(4), pp. 274–282, 2011. Epub 2011/08/02.

58. Kinnaird, A., Dromparis, P., Saleme, B., Gurtu, V., Watson, K., Paulin, R. *et al.*, Metabolic modulation of clear-cell renal cell carcinoma with dichloroacetate, an inhibitor of pyruvate dehydrogenase kinase. *Eur. Urol.*, **69**(4), pp. 734–744, 2016.

59. Welford, S. M., Dorie, M. J., Li, X., Haase, V. H., and Giaccia, A. J., Renal oxygenation suppresses VHL loss-induced senescence that is caused by increased sensitivity to oxidative stress. *Mol. Cell. Biol.*, **30**(19), 4595–4603, 2010.

60. Funasaka, T., Hu, H., Yanagawa, T., Hogan, V., and Raz, A., Down-regulation of phosphoglucose isomerase/autocrine motility factor results in mesenchymal-pp. to-epithelial transition of human lung fibrosarcoma cells. *Cancer Res.*, **67**(9), pp. 4236–4243, 2007. Epub 2007/05/08.

61. Kondoh, H., Lleonart, M. E., Gil, J., Wang, J., Degan, P., Peters, G. *et al.*, Glycolytic enzymes can modulate cellular life span. *Cancer. Res.*, **65**(1), pp. 177–185, 2005.

62. Hammond, E. M., Denko, N. C., Dorie, M. J., Abraham, R. T., and Giaccia, A. J., Hypoxia links ATR and p53 through replication arrest. *Mol. Cell. Biol.*, **22**(6), pp. 1834–1843, 2002.

63. Ravi, R., Mookerjee, B., Bhujwalla, Z. M., Sutter, C. H., Artemov, D., Zeng, Q. *et al.*, Regulation of tumor angiogenesis by p53-induced degradation of hypoxia-inducible factor 1alpha. *Genes Dev.*, **14**(1), pp. 34–44, 2000.

64. Chen, D., Li, M., Luo, J., and Gu, W., Direct interactions between HIF-1 alpha and Mdm2 modulate p53 function. *J. Biol. Chem.*, **278**(16), pp. 13595–13598, 2003.

65. Blagosklonny, M. V., An, W. G., Romanova, L. Y., Trepel, J., Fojo, T., and Neckers, L., p53 inhibits hypoxia-inducible factor-stimulated transcription. *J. Biol. Chem.*, **273**(20), pp. 11995–11998, 1998.

66. Sánchez-Puig, N., Veprintsev, D. B., and Fersht, A. R., Binding of Natively Unfolded HIF-1α ODD Domain to p53. *Mol. Cell.*, **17**(1), pp. 11–21, 2005.

67. Hansson, L. O., Friedler, A., Freund, S., Rüdiger, S., and Fersht, A. R., Two sequence motifs from HIF-1α bind to the DNA-binding site of p53. *Proc. Nat. Acad. Sci.*, **99**(16), pp. 10305–10309, 2002.

68. Welford, S. M., Bedogni, B., Gradin, K., Poellinger, L., Broome, Powell, M., and Giaccia, A. J., HIF1alpha delays premature senescence through the activation of MIF. *Genes Dev.*, **20**(24), pp. 3366–3671, 2006.

69. Acosta, J. C., O'Loghlen, A., Banito, A., Guijarro, M. V., Augert, A., Raguz, S. *et al.*, Chemokine signaling via the CXCR2 receptor reinforces senescence. *Cell.*, **133**(6), pp. 1006–1018, 2008.

70. Kuilman, T., Michaloglou, C., Vredeveld, L. C., Douma, S., van Doorn, R., Desmet, C. J. *et al.*, Oncogene-induced senescence relayed by an interleukin-dependent inflammatory network. *Cell*, **133**(6), pp. 1019–1031, 2008.

71. Canino, C., Mori, F., Cambria, A., Diamantini, A., Germoni, S., Alessandrini, G. *et al.*, SASP mediates chemoresistance and tumor-initiating-activity of mesothelioma cells. *Oncogene*, pp. **31**(26), 3148–3163, 2012. Epub 2011/10/25.

72. Brugarolas, J., Lei, K., Hurley, R. L., Manning, B. D., Reiling, J. H., Hafen, E. *et al.*, Regulation of mTOR function in response to hypoxia by REDD1 and the TSC1/TSC2 tumor suppressor complex. *Genes Dev.*, **18**(23), pp. 2893–2904, 2004. Epub 2004/11/17.

73. Leontieva, O. V., Natarajan, V., Demidenko, Z. N., Burdelya, L. G., Gudkov, A. V., and Blagosklonny, M. V. Hypoxia suppresses conversion from proliferative arrest to cellular senescence. *Proc. Natl. Acad. Sci. USA*, **109**(33), pp. 13314–13318, 2012. Epub 2012/08/01.

74. Kovatcheva, M., Liu, D. D., Dickson, M. A., Klein, M. E., O'Connor, R., Wilder, F. O. *et al.*, MDM2 turnover and expression of ATRX determine the choice between quiescence and senescence in response to CDK4 inhibition. *Oncotarget.*, **6**(10), pp. 8226–8243, 2015. Epub 2015/03/25.

75. Bell, E. L., Klimova, T. A., Eisenbart, J., Schumacker, P. T., and Chandel, N. S., Mitochondrial reactive oxygen species trigger hypoxia-inducible factor-dependent extension of the replicative life span during hypoxia. *Mol. Cell. Biol.*, **27**(16), pp. 5737–5745, 2007.

76. Chen, C., Han, S., Meng, L., Li, Z., Zhang, X., and Wu, A., TERT promoter mutations lead to high transcriptional activity under hypoxia and

temozolomide treatment and predict poor prognosis in gliomas. *PLoS One*, **9**(6), p. e100297, 2014. Epub 2014/06/18.

77. Salminen, A., Kauppinen, A., and Kaarniranta, K., 2-Oxoglutarate-dependent dioxygenases are sensors of energy metabolism, oxygen availability, and iron homeostasis: potential role in the regulation of aging process. *Cell. Mol. Life. Sci.*, (CMLS), **72**(20), pp. 3897–3914, 2015. Epub 2015/06/30.

78. Ponnaluri, V. K., Vadlapatla, R. K., Vavilala, D. T., Pal, D., Mitra, A. K., and Mukherji, M., Hypoxia induced expression of histone lysine demethylases: implications in oxygen-dependent retinal neovascular diseases. *Biochem. Biophys. Res. Commun.*, **415**(2), pp. 373–377, 2011. Epub 2011/11/01.

79. Tausendschon, M., Dehne, N., and Brune, B., Hypoxia causes epigenetic gene regulation in macrophages by attenuating Jumonji histone demethylase activity. *Cytokine.*, **53**(2), pp. 256–262, 2011. Epub 2010/12/07.

80. Beyer, S., Kristensen, M. M., Jensen, K. S., Johansen, J. V., and Staller, P., The histone demethylases JMJD1A and JMJD2B are transcriptional targets of hypoxia-inducible factor HIF. *J. Biol. Chem.*, **283**(52), pp. 36542–36552, 2008. Epub 2008/11/06.

81. Pollard, P. J., Loenarz, C., Mole, D. R., McDonough, M. A., Gleadle, J. M., Schofield, C. J. *et al.*, Regulation of Jumonji-domain-containing histone demethylases by hypoxia-inducible factor (HIF)-1alpha. *Biochem. J.*, **416**(3), pp. 387–394, 2008. Epub 2008/08/21.

82. Hancock, R. L., Dunne, K., Walport, L. J., Flashman, E., and Kawamura, A., Epigenetic regulation by histone demethylases in hypoxia. *Epigenomics.*, **7**(5), pp. 791–811, 2015. Epub 2015/04/03.

# Chapter 6

# Hypoxic Reprograming of Tumor Metabolism, Matching Environmental Supply with Biosynthetic Demand

Betina McNeil, Ioanna Papandreou and Nicholas C. Denko*

*Department of Radiation Oncology, Ohio State University Wexner Medical Center and Comprehensive Cancer Center, Columbus OH 43210, USA*
**Nicholas.denko@osumc.edu*

## 1. Introduction

Tumor cells can detect and respond to changes in their microenvironment. Nutrients and oxygen exist in a state of supply and demand within the tumor, and oxygen supply that does not meet the demand establishes a condition of hypoxia. Hypoxia is frequently found in human tumors and clinical studies have identified it as a predictor of poor patient outcome. Cells respond to hypoxia with a series of adaptive changes in gene expression and function. Many gene expression changes in hypoxia are due to activation of the hypoxia inducible factor or HIF-1. This transcription factor regulates many changes in intermediate metabolism that supports cell growth in hypoxia. HIF contributes to hypoxic reprogramming of glucose, pyruvate and glutamine metabolism as well as oxidative phosphorylation, and glycogen and lipid metabolism. Hypoxic reprogramming has been shown experimentally to be critical for the growth of model tumors by several groups. This chapter will provide an outline of the identified mechanisms of hypoxic reprogramming, and attempt to provide a context explaining how these adaptive changes fill the metabolic requirements for cell growth when molecular oxygen is limiting.

## 2.  Genesis of Tumor Hypoxia

Hypoxia exists when the supply of oxygen does not meet the demand of the tissue. This can occur in a variety of physiological and pathophysiological conditions. One example is the hypoxic zone that develops downstream of a damaged blood vessel. In this case, hypoxia-induced responses promote reduction in oxygen consumption and restoration of blood flow (and oxygen delivery) during the healing process. When blood flow is restored, oxygen levels return to normal, and hypoxia is resolved. This is an example of how blood flow can play a relatively acute or transient role initiating hypoxia, with the adaptive process resolving it.[1,2]

Conversely, in pathophysiological settings such as cancer, hypoxia can persist in the tumors likening them to "wounds that do not heal".[3,4] A chronic form of diffusion-limited hypoxia has been observed in solid tumors.[5] In this case, oxygen is consumed by tumor cells, establishing gradients along feeding blood vessels as well as parallel to blood vessels.[6] Rapidly dividing tumor cells multiply faster than their oxygen support can develop, and therefore become chronically hypoxic, initiating a cellular response that does not resolve.[7] In this case, the tumor mass continues to grow and demand more oxygen from the limited vasculature that cannot keep pace with the tumor growth. It is hypothesized that in prolonged hypoxia, it is the resultant adaptive response that promotes tumor cell survival and allow proliferation. One central component of the cellular adaptation to hypoxia is through altered intermediate metabolism. **The driving goal of hypoxic cell metabolic adaptation is to reduce the consumption of oxygen while still supplying the metabolites necessary for biosynthetic processes.**

# 3. Hypoxia-Inducible Factor (HIF) is a Key Regulator of Hypoxic Adaptation

Hypoxia-inducible factors HIF-1$\alpha$, HIF-2$\alpha$, and HIF-3$\alpha$, are transcription factors that are highly inducible in low oxygen tension and stimulate transcription of dozens of target genes. HIF-1 was first identified as responsible for the induction of the erythropoietin gene in low oxygen conditions.[8] HIF-$\alpha$s are proteolytically degraded rapidly in normoxia, but become stabilized in hypoxia.[9] HIF-1 is a heterodimeric transcription factor consisting of one molecule of HIF-1$\alpha$ and one of the constitutive HIF-1$\beta$/ARNT.[10] Together these proteins bind to the hypoxia-responsive element (HRE) found in many promoters and stimulate gene transcription in response to low oxygen.[8]

The major molecular mechanism that regulates HIF-1$\alpha$ protein destruction in normoxia is oxygen dependent hydroxylation and proteolysis. Briefly, in normal oxygen conditions, HIF-$\alpha$ proteins are hydroxylated on two target proline residues by a family of hydroxylases.[11–13] Prolyl hydroxylases (PHD 1–3) are responsible for residue-specific hydroxylation of HIF-1$\alpha$ on residues 402 and 564.[14] After hydroxylation, the modified HiF-$\alpha$ protein is recognized by the tumor suppressor/E3 ligase von Hippel–Lindau (VHL). HIF-1$\alpha$ is poly-ubiquitinated by VHL (in a complex with elongins B and C and cullin) and marked for proteasomal degradation.[15] The substrates for the enzymatic hydroxylation reaction are $\alpha$-ketoglutarate and molecular oxygen (with iron [Fe+2] as a cofactor).[16] Therefore, when oxygen is not present for the hydroxylase reaction, HIF-$\alpha$ is not modified and is not marked for destruction. The molecular oxygen sensor is therefore also responsible for HIF-$\alpha$ destruction.

HIF-1 activity can also be stimulated to some degree by oncogenic activation. Activation of oncogenes such as RAS,[17] HER2[18], and AKT/MTOR,[19] as well as loss of the tumor suppressor phosphatase and tensin homolog (PTEN)[20] have all been reported to stimulate HIF-1 activity. There are various mechanisms reported for the relative stimulations, but the consensus is that cancer cells have a pronounced HIF response, and this may contribute to an exaggerated level of HIF target gene activation and adaptive responses in tumors. Comparative immunohistochemistry supports the model that HIF-1 is highly expressed in human cancers.[21] This analysis of pathological specimens provided evidence that HIF-1$\alpha$ impacts human cancer progression. HIF therefore contributes to many aspects of cancer biology in model as well as spontaneous human tumors. This chapter is focused on the mechanisms of hypoxic reprogramming of tumor cell metabolism and its impact on cell and tumor growth. Hypoxia has been extensively studied and implicated in many aspects of glycolysis, glutaminolysis, mitochondrial biogenesis and function, pH regulation, lipogenesis and glycogen metabolism (Table 1).

Table 1. Metabolic adaptations in hypoxia.

| Metabolic Process | Hypoxic Response | Effect | References |
|---|---|---|---|
| Glycolysis | ↑ glucose transporters<br>↑ glycolytic enzymes | ↑ glycolytic flux<br>↑ pyruvate<br>↑ NADH | 28, 29, 35–38 |
| Pyruvate Metabolism | ↑ LDHA and MCTs | ↑ lactate<br>NADH → NAD+ | 45–47 |
| | ↑ PDHK1 and PDHK3 | ↓ PDH activity<br>↓ pyruvate oxidation | 51, 53 |
| | ↑ NDRG3 | ↑ ERK activity | 49 |
| Electron Transport | ↑ COXVa and ↓ COXVb<br>↑ NDUFA4L2 | Efficient oxygen consumption<br>↓ ETC activity | 60, 62 |
| Glutamine Metabolism | ↑ SIAH2 ↓ OGDH2 | ↑ reductive carboxylation<br>↑ lipogenesis from glutamine | 70, 73–76 |
| Fatty acid synthesis | ↑ HILPDA<br>↑ CPT1c | ↑ lipid droplets<br>↑ fatty acid oxidation | 80, 82<br>87, 90, 91 |
| Glycogen Metabolism | ↑ glycogen synthase (early) | ↑ glycogen | 78, 79 |
| | ↑ glycogen phosphorylase (late) | ↓ glycogen | 78 |
| Extracelluar acidification | ↑ CAIX | ↓ pHe<br>↑ pHi | 49, 50 |

Abbreviations: lactate dehydrogenase (LDH), monocarboxylate transporters(MCT), pyruvate dehydrogenase kinase(PDHK), cytochrome oxidase(COX), seven in abstentia homology 2(SIAH2), oxoglutarate dehydrogenase(OGDH), hypoxia inducible lipid droplet associated protein(HILPDA), carnitine palmitoyl transferase(CPT), carbonic anhydrase 9(CAIX).

# 4. Reprogramming of Glucose Metabolism

Glucose is the major fuel for cellular growth, energy production and homeostasis. Cancer cells are highly reliant on glucose for both anabolic processes and production of ATP. However, cancer cells that consume glucose also generate high levels of lactate that is secreted into the extracellular space. The process of uptake of large amounts of glucose and production of lactate even when oxygen is present is termed "aerobic glycolysis." This cancer-specific phenomenon was recognized in the 1920's and 30's by Otto Warburg[22] and is termed the "Warburg Effect."[23] The clinical application of the FDG-PET scan indicates that many human tumors are highly glucose avid when compared to the corresponding normal tissue.[24] The reason for the increased uptake of glucose by tumor cells is poorly understood, but is thought to support a highly proliferative state that requires large amounts of macromolecular synthesis.[25] The Warburg effect therefore describes enhanced breakdown of glucose to pyruvate by tumor cells, but also reduced mitochondrial oxidation of pyruvate. The combination of enhanced glucose uptake, but also production of lactate due to reduced mitochondrial activity is promoted by oncogenic transformation,[26] but greatly enhanced by HIF activation.[27]

Uptake of glucose by the cell requires facilitated transport by a family of glucose transporters (GLUT1-4 or SLC2A1-4). There is widespread expression of GLUTs throughout the various tissues of the body. However, GLUT1 and 3 are in some ways the highest capacity and most widely expressed transports in cancers, accounting for the majority of glucose uptake there. Interestingly, these genes are also transcriptional targets of HIF-1.[28,29] Functionally, hypoxia has been shown to increase glucose uptake in cell lines *in vitro*, and in model tumors.[30,31] Likewise, cells engineered to overexpress GLUTs also show enhanced glucose uptake. GLUT1 and 3 have been used in numerous clinical studies to identify sections from tumors with regions of hypoxia, and have shown that patients with high GLUT1 or 3 expressing tumors have an unfavorable clinical outcome.[32–34]

After entry into the cell, glucose is phosphorylated by hexokinase to produce a charged molecule (glucose 6-phosphate) which is trapped within the cell. The fate of the glucose-6P and the Warburg effect is strongly influenced by HIF activation. Almost every enzyme in the glycolytic pathway has been reported to be hypoxia/HIF inducible. HIF-dependent mRNA induction has been reported for *Hexokinase 2 (HK2), phosphofructose kinase, fructose 1,6 bisphosphatase, glyceraldehyde 3-phosphate dehydrogenase, phosphoglycerokinase 1 (Pgk1), aldolase, enolase, trisphosphate isomerase, phosphoenolpyruvate kinase, and pyruvate kinase.*[35–38] The concerted induction of these enzymes indicates that hypoxia stimulates an enhanced flux from glucose to pyruvate. This high rate of glycolysis generates 2 molecules each of ATP and NADH per molecule of glucose. The significance of hexokinase 2,[39] fructose 1–6 bisphosphatase[40] and pyruvate kinase[41] has been elegantly described to support cancer metabolism in model tumors and human pathological specimens. Interestingly, several glycolytic enzymes have also been shown to be important for model tumor growth through non-metabolic mechanisms.[42,43] However, the cancer cell must also direct the fate of the large amount of pyruvate that is produced by glycolysis, and HIF activation has a significant impact on this as well.

## 5. Pyruvate Metabolism in Hypoxia

The two primary directions for pyruvate metabolism are either through the activity of lactate dehydrogenase to lactate or oxidation in the mitochondria. Either of these pathways will regenerate NAD+ from the NADH produced at GAPDH, supporting additional glycolysis. Therefore, the cellular decision that regulates pyruvate metabolism is contingent on other requirements. It has been hypothesized that the shift to lactate production away from mitochondrial function is in part driven by the need to reduce oxygen consumption.[27–44] Because the mitochondria are the major sink for oxygen consumption within the cell, it appears logical that in conditions of reduced environmental oxygen, mitochondrial activity would be actively reduced.

Hypoxia-responsive gene expression promotes both the elevated lactate production and the reduced mitochondrial function. In order to stimulate lactate production, HIF activates expression of LDHA and MCT4.[45,46] These enzymes are responsible for conversion of pyruvate to lactate and the export of lactate to the extracellular space, respectively. Genetic knockdown of LDHA expression suppresses the growth of model breast cancers.[47] Interestingly, a recent report described an additional function for lactate within the hypoxic cell. Hypoxia-induced protein NDRG3 is degraded in a PHD2/VHL-dependent manner under normoxic conditions. However, in low oxygen, reduced PHD2 activity stabilizes NDRG3. At the same time, high levels of lactate within the cell bind to NDRG3. Lactate-bound NRDG3 has been implicated in raf-ERK activation to stimulate tumor cell growth in a hypoxia and lactate-dependent manner.[48] Extracellular lactic acid produces protons and reduced pH contributing to the acidotic microenvironment. These protons can be trapped in the extracellular space by the activity of the HIF-inducible carbonic anhydrase IX,[49–50] there by the low extracellular pH helps to maintain a physiological intracellular pH.

In normoxic tissue, pyruvate is converted to Acetyl-CoA by the pyruvate dehydrogenase complex (PDC). PDC resides in the mitochondrial matrix and serves as the first committed step of glucose oxidation. Pyruvate-derived acetyl-CoA is used for the production of citrate by citrate synthase within the TCA cycle. Subsequent oxidative phosphorylation produces up to 36 ATP per molecule of glucose and is far more efficient than the 2 ATP generated by substrate-level based phosphorylation in glycolysis.

HIF-1 activation reduces PDC activity, pyruvate flux into the TCA cycle, and oxygen consumption. Several years ago, it was observed that HIF-1 induces expression of pyruvate dehydrogenase kinase 1 and 3 genes (PDHK1 and PDHK3).[51–53] These related kinases are highly conserved and are thought to phosphorylate only one target protein, the pyruvate dehydrogenase E1$\alpha$ subunit.[54] Pyruvate dehydrogenase is a conserved E1, E2, E3 multisubunit dehydrogenase complex.[55] The E1 subunit of PDH is composed of E1$\alpha$ and E1-$\beta$ subunits that form the E1$\alpha_2$E1$\beta_2$ heterotetramer. Phosphorylation of any one of the three PDHK target serine residues in E1a is sufficient to inactivate recombinant PDC.[54] All PDHKs can phosphorylate Ser293 (site 1) and Ser300 (site 2) but PDHK1 is unique in its ability to phosphorylate Ser232 (site 3), suggesting a unique functional significance to PDHK1.[56] Hyperphosphorylation of PDH E1$\alpha$ has been observed in hypoxia in a PDHK1-dependent manner, and loss of PDHK1 compromises the growth of model tumors.[57] The hypoxic downregulation of mitochondrial function appears to enhance the oncogene-dependent Warburg effect. Tyrosine kinase signaling mechanisms have also been implicated in controlling PDHK1 activity. Site-specific phosphorylation of PDHK1 at Tyr136, Tryr243, and Tyr244 by FGFR enhanced PDHK1 activity and subsequent decrease in mitochondrial glucose oxidation.[58,59]

## 6. Regulation of Mitochondrial Biogenesis and Function in Hypoxia

Several other mechanisms have also been reported to reduce mitochondrial function in a hypoxia- and HIF-dependent manner. Hypoxia has been reported to inhibit mitochondrial biogenesis, modify the activity of cytochrome oxidase, and of complex 1 of the electron transport chain (ETC). In 2007, Semenza and colleagues proposed a model in which HIF-dependent expression of myc interacting protein Mxi decreased myc activity and the result was decreased mitochondrial biogenesis. Later that year, the same group published a report that hypoxia also regulated the expression of subunits of cytochorme oxidase,[60] similar to what is found in yeast after a shift to growth in anoxia.[61] A more recent report has identified the NDUFA4L2 gene as a hypoxia-inducible HIF target gene.[62] The NDUFA4L2 protein associates as a part of complex 1 of the electron transport chain, and its expression inhibits complex 1 activity, reducing mitochondrial function and oxygen consumption.

The turnover of mitochondria has also been proposed to be regulated by hypoxia. Several groups have suggested that the hypoxia-inducible mitochondrial proteins BNIP3 and BNIP3L participate in the process of mitophagy, or autophagic destruction of mitochondria.[63,64] While the concept has intuitive appeal, the primary data supporting a decrease in mitochondrial biomass is limited. Due to the dynamic nature of mitochondrial lifespan, it is difficult to follow the fate of individual mitochondria. The molecular interactions that regulate mitochondrial turnover need to be more clearly defined, because other reports indicate that hypoxic mitophagy is dependent on AMPK but not HIF.[65,66]

# 7. Reprogramming of Glutamine Metabolism

Blood levels of free glutamine are up to 20 times greater than that of other free amino acids, indicating a role for more than protein synthesis.[67,68] In fact, glutamine can be used in several metabolic pathways ranging from energy production to glutathione synthesis and lipogenesis.[69] It has been recognized since tissue culture began that addition of glutamine greatly enhanced the growth of cells *in vitro*. In the last several years, it has become apparent that growth of cells in hypoxia is even more dependent on glutamine as an anabolic substrate.[70]

Glutamine metabolism in cancer cells has been highlighted by the recognition that activation of the myc oncogene can stimulate glutamine metabolism.[71] Glutamine entry into the cell requires one of several amino acid transporters. ASCT2 (SLC1a5) and SNAT5 (SLC28a5) are thought to be major contributors to glutamine uptake and both genes are transcriptional targets of deregulated myc.[71] However, no reports have implicated HIF in the expression of glutamine transporters. Upon entry into the cell, glutamine is most commonly broken down by a two-step process by glutaminase and glutamate dehydrogenase to generate $\alpha$-ketoglutarate ($\alpha$KG), also known as 2-oxoglutarate. Alternative pathways for glutamine catabolism exist,[72] but the result generates $\alpha$KG for entry into the TCA cycle.

In growing cancer cells, glutamine takes on an anabolic role as a carbon source to replenish TCA cycle intermediates. This process is termed anaplerosis, which is taken from the Greek and can be translated as to "refill oneself." This is necessary in hypoxia because there is reduced carbon flow from glucose into the TCA cycle due to phosphorylation of $E1\alpha$ and reduced PDC activity (see pyruvate metabolism above). However, cells continue to synthesize fatty acids *de novo* using citrate as a major source to make acetyl-CoA. Citrate is an intermediate in the TCA cycle and can be transported to the cytoplasm, used to make acetyl CoA and oxaloacetate by ATP citrate lyase, and oxaloacetate returned to the TCA cycle minus two carbons. In order to replenish the removed carbons, glutamine-derived $\alpha$KG enters the TCA cycle at $\alpha$KGDH where oxidative metabolism produces succinyl-CoA.

Several years ago, it was recognized that mitochondrial glutamine metabolism had a profound shift in hypoxia. Tracer studies showed very clearly that instead of following the well-established path of $\alpha$KG oxidation to succinyl-CoA, glutamine derived $\alpha$KG took the reductive path in the "reverse" direction through isocitrate dehydrogenase. In hypoxic cells, or in VHL negative cells, much of the citrate used to make fatty acids came from glutamine and went through the reductive IDH cycle.[70,73–75] However, it was not until 2014 that Sun and Denko reported on the mechanism responsible.[76] They observed a decrease in the activity of the $\alpha$KGDH complex and this decrease was due to the proteolysis of a splice variant of the E1 subunit. The E3 ubiquitin ligase SIAH2 was activated in a HIF-dependent manner and polyubiquitinated OGDH2, marking it for proteolysis. Glutamine-derived $\alpha$KG built up in the mitochondrial, and flowed in the reverse direction to make citrate. Surprisingly, expression of a point mutant of OGDH2 that removed the ubiquitination site was resistant to destruction and blocked the growth of model tumors. *In vitro* experiments suggested that reductive carboxylation is necessary for fatty acid synthesis, underlying the importance of reductive glutamine metabolism in hypoxic tumors.

Summarizing hypoxic mitochondrial function, we find that hypoxia reduces glucose flux into the TCA cycle through phosphorylation of PDH. However, growth of hypoxic cells requires citrate and *de novo* fatty acid synthesis, so glutamine is used instead. In environmental conditions when oxygen is limiting, the cell uses a reductive pathway to generate the citrate from glutamine-derived $\alpha$KG, reducing oxygen consumption while maintaining redox balance and macromolecular biosynthesis (Fig. 1).

## 8. Reprogramming of Glycogen Metabolism

The most common subtype of renal cancer is the "clear cell" histology. This tumor is most commonly associated with loss of the VHL tumor suppressor and constitutive HIF-1 activation.[77] Interestingly, the "clear cell" morphology comes during processing for paraffin embedding. Dehydration of the tissue through various organic solvents results in the dissolving of non-polar compounds in the cell. In renal clear cell cancers, there is often a large single vesicle in the cell that is dissolved during processing,

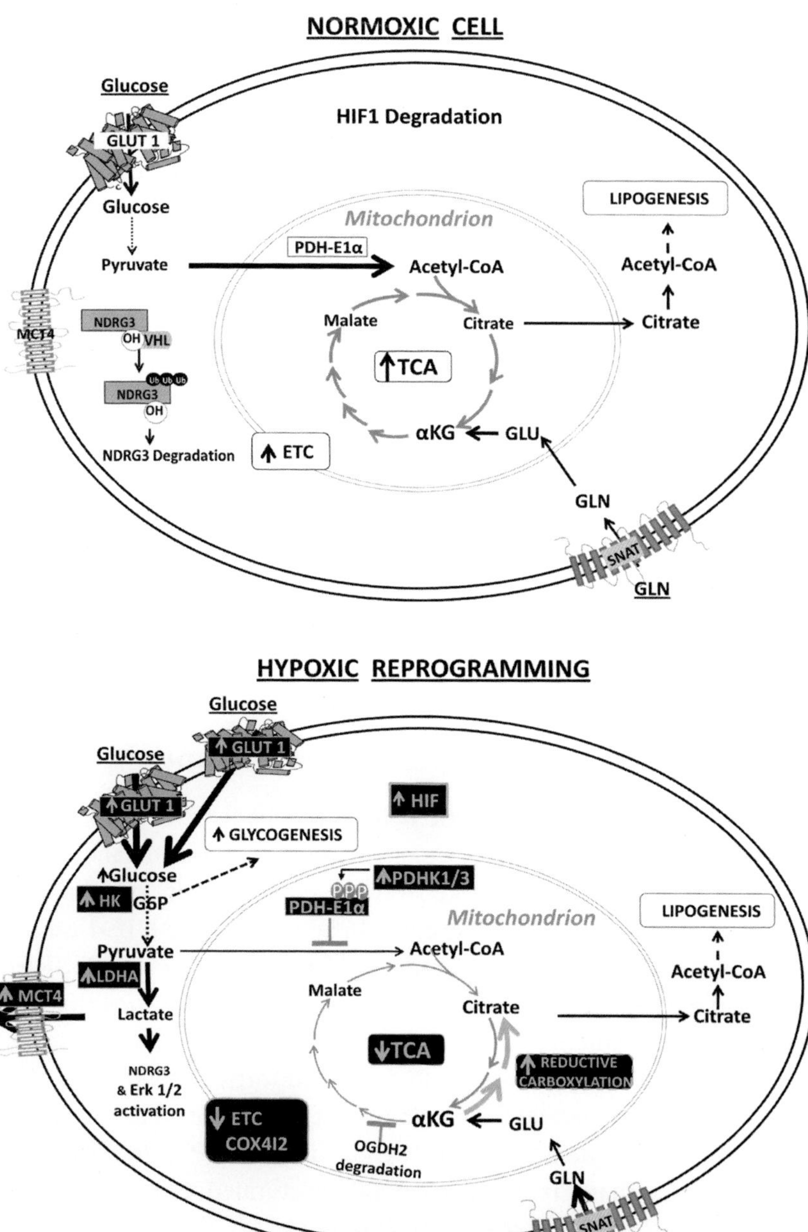


Fig. 1.  Schematic representation of major metabolic changes occuring in cells exposed to hypoxia. Glucose uptake is increased in hypoxia, pyruvate flux into the mitochondria decreased, lactate secretion increased, glutamine metabolism in the mitochondria shifts from oxidative to reductive.

resulting in the clear appearance. This vesicle is typically filled with either neutral lipids or glycogen, both of which can accumulate during chronic HIF-1 activation. These findings indicate that both glycogen and lipid storage are stimulated by HIF-1 activation.

Glycogen is an effective way for the cell to store glucose for retrieval at a later time and its metabolism relies upon four primary enzymes. Glycogen synthase and branching enzyme are responsible for synthesis and glycogen phosphorylase and debranching enzyme for breakdown. Favaro *et al.* showed that both glycogen synthase and glycogen phosphorylase can be hypoxia-inducible genes.[78] Interestingly, glycogen accumulates in acute hypoxia and gradually decreases over time. These changes appeared to protect cancer cells from senescence and damage by reactive oxygen species by promoting increased flux through the pentose phosphate pathway and production of NADPH. The significance of these pathways is apparent because knockdown of PGYL had a profound inhibitory effect on the growth of model tumors.[78] HIF2a has been implicated in this process, as activation of it alone can lead to accumulation of glycogen in renal tubule cells.[79]

## 9. Lipid Metabolism and Storage in Hypoxia

Accumulation of lipids in hypoxic cells is mechanistically more complicated because there are many species of lipids that are metabolized, and both *de novo* synthesis and uptake from the environment contribute to the accumulation of lipids in hypoxic cells. In addition to the HIF-1 transcription factor, the sterol response element binding proteins 1 and 2 (SREBP1 and 2) also regulate lipid homeostasis in hypoxia. SREBP was first shown to be hypoxia responsive in fission yeast.[80] This inducible transcription factor is proteolytically processed to the active form in conditions of lipid stress. Target genes encode for enzymes that are responsible for fatty acid synthesis (SREBP1) and cholesterol synthesis (SREBP2). In conditions of severe hypoxia, there is a decrease in unsaturated fatty acids due to reduced activity of the sterol CoA desaturase (SCD1), at least in part because molecular oxygen is a substrate for its enzymatic activity.[81] Reduced levels of unsaturated fatty acids produce endoplasmic reticulum (ER) stress,[82,83] and stimulates uptake of unsaturated lysophospholipids from the environment.[84]

There is some debate as to the importance of *de novo* lipogenesis versus uptake of fatty acids from the environment to supply the demands of the cell. There has also been a debate as to the metabolic precursor for lipogenesis. In normoxic conditions, glucose predominates as the substrate of choice, cycling through citrate in the mitochondria to produce acetyl-CoA. In hypoxia, with HIF-1 activation and OGDH2 destroyed, glutamine appears to follow a reductive path to citrate. However, recent reports have identified a role for free acetate to be used by acetyl-CoA synthase to directly produce acetyl-CoA.[85,86] Whichever substrate is used, *de novo* lipogenesis appears to be important for the growth of model tumors.

Interestingly, hypoxic lipogenesis contributes to storage of lipids, rather than catabolism. While there is some suggestion that lipid breakdown may be stimulated by the HIF-1 dependent induction of Cpt1c,[87] lipid can be visualized and stored in large lipid droplets in hypoxic cells. The poorly understood lipid droplet is the cellular depot for neutral lipids.[88] These large droplets contain a neutral lipid core, a phospholipid monolayer and are decorated by a number of lipid droplet proteins. The mechanism of lipid droplet formation is also poorly understood, but cells treated with hypoxia produce or enlarge lipid droplets. Several hypoxia-inducible proteins play a part in lipid droplet formation such as hSulf1,[89] fatty acid binding proteins 1 and 3,[90] and HILPDA.[91] Some reports have suggested that the benefit of the lipid droplet is not necessarily during hypoxia, but upon reoxygenation.[90]

## 10. Hypoxia Induced miRNAs Add an Additional Layer to Regulate Metabolism

There have been several reports of hypoxia-responsive micro RNAs.[92] These short non-coding RNAs can act as regulators of mRNA stability and translation. They can target numerous mRNAs and fine tune their expression. The miRNA cluster around 199a[93] and 210[94] have both been reported as HIF-responsive, and capable of modulating the hypoxic expression of many genes. Mir 210 has been specifically implicated in regulating hypoxic mitochondrial function,[95] and mirs 132 and 155 have been implicated in the hypoxic regulation of Hexokinase ll.[96] However, it has also been reported that DICER is downregulated in hypoxia and this attenuates miRNA processing. DICER is a necessary component of the miRNA system, so its reduction results in decreased global levels of miR-NAs. In hypoxia, reduced DICER appears to be important for the maximal induction of several HIF target genes that participate in metabolic remodeling, including GLUT1 and BNIP3L.[97]

## 11. Conclusions

The fundamental biochemical reactions that comprise intermediate metabolism have been understood at the enzymatic level for many years. However, it now appears that the ability to regulate these processes in response to environmental signals is an essential component that allows the cell to adapt to suboptimal growth conditions. The hypoxic response is an evolutionarily conserved response that can be found in early metazoans as evolutionarily distant as *C elegans*.[98] The ability of cancer cells to adapt to hypoxia is perhaps most apparent in the case of chronic hypoxia found in the solid tumor. Genetic ablation of the adaptive circuits regulating hypoxic glucose metabolism (such as hexokinase or pyruvate dehydrogenase kinase 1) have profound inhibitory effects on the growth of model tumors. Likewise, forced stability of mutant OGDH2 blocks hypoxic adaptation of glutamine metabolism and also inhibits growth of model tumors. Similarly, loss of Cpt1c deregulates hypoxic lipid oxidation and also compromises growth of model tumors. These examples all show that it is the plasticity of intermediate metabolism that is necessary for the growth of tumors. In this way, it may be possible to develop therapies that are designed to interfere with the hypoxic regulation of metabolism and not necessarily the basic metabolic processes that are essential for the growth of well-oxygenated normal cells.

## References


1. Hong, W. X. *et al.*, The Role of Hypoxia-Inducible Factor in Wound Healing. *Adv. Wound Care*, (New Rochelle), **3**(5), pp. 390–399, 2014.
2. Semenza, G. L., Vascular responses to hypoxia and ischemia. *Arterioscler Thromb. Vasc. Biol.*, **30**(4), pp. 648–652, 2010.

3. Dvorak, H. F., Tumors: wounds that do not heal. Similarities between tumor stroma generation and wound healing. *N. Engl. J. Med.*, **315**(26), pp. 1650–1659, 1986.

4. Dvorak, H. F., Tumors: wounds that do not heal-redux. *Cancer Immunol. Res.*, **3**(1), pp. 1–11, 2015.

5. Coleman, C. N., Hypoxia in tumors: a paradigm for the approach to biochemical and physiologic heterogeneity. *J. Natl Cancer Inst.*, **80**(5), pp. 310–317, 1988.

6. Helmlinger, G. *et al.*, Interstitial pH and pO2 gradients in solid tumors *in vivo*: high-resolution measurements reveal a lack of correlation. *Nat. Med.*, **3**(2), pp. 177–182, 1997.

7. Moeller, B. J. *et al.*, The relationship between hypoxia and angiogenesis. *Semin. Radiat. Oncol.*, **14**(3), pp. 215–221, 2004.

8. Wang, G. L., and Semenza, G. L., General involvement of hypoxia-inducible factor 1 in transcriptional response to hypoxia. *Proc. Natl. Acad. Sci. USA.*, **90**(9), pp. 4304–4308, 1993.

9. Maxwell, P. H. *et al.*, The tumour suppressor protein VHL targets hypoxia-inducible factors for oxygen-dependent proteolysis. *Nature*, **399**(6733), pp. 271–275, 1999.

10. Wang, G. L., and Semenza, G. L. Purification and characterization of hypoxia-inducible factor 1. *J. Biol. Chem.*, **270**(3), pp. 1230–1237, 1995.

11. Jaakkola, P. *et al.*, Targeting of HIF-alpha to the von Hippel-Lindau ubiquitylation complex by O2-regulated prolyl hydroxylation. *Science*, **292**(5516), pp. 468–472, 2001.

12. Epstein, A. C. *et al.*, C. elegans EGL-9 and mammalian homologs define a family of dioxygenases that regulate HIF by prolyl hydroxylation. *Cell*, **107**(1), pp. 43–54, 2001.

13. Bruick, R. K., and McKnight, S. L., A conserved family of prolyl-4-hydroxylases that modify HIF. *Science*, **294**(5545), pp. 1337–1340, 2001.

14. Myllyharju, J., and Koivunen, P., Hypoxia-inducible factor prolyl 4-hydroxylases: common and specific roles. *Biol. Chem.*, **394**(4), pp. 435–448, 2013.

15. Tanimoto, K. *et al.*, Mechanism of regulation of the hypoxia-inducible factor-1 alpha by the von Hippel-Lindau tumor suppressor protein. *EMBO J.*, **19**(16), pp. 4298–4309, 2000.

16. Hirsila, M. *et al.*, Characterization of the human prolyl 4-hydroxylases that modify the hypoxia-inducible factor. *J. Biol. Chem.*, **278**(33), pp. 30772–30780, 2003.

17. Mazure, N. M. *et al.*, Induction of vascular endothelial growth factor by hypoxia is modulated by a phosphatidylinositol 3-kinase/Akt signaling pathway in Ha-ras-transformed cells through a hypoxia inducible factor-1 transcriptional element. *Blood*, **90**(9), pp. 3322–3331, 1997.

18. Laughner, E. *et al.*, HER2 (neu) signaling increases the rate of hypoxia-inducible factor 1alpha (HIF-1alpha) synthesis: novel mechanism for HIF-1-mediated vascular endothelial growth factor expression. *Mol. Cell. Biol.*, **21**(12), pp. 3995–4004, 2001.

19. Brugarolas, J. B. *et al.*, TSC2 regulates VEGF through mTOR-dependent and -independent pathways. *Cancer Cell*, **4**(2), pp. 147–158, 2003.

20. Zundel, W. *et al.*, Loss of PTEN facilitates HIF-1-mediated gene expression. *Genes Dev.*, **14**(4), pp. 391–396, 2000.

21. Zhong, H. *et al.*, Overexpression of hypoxia-inducible factor 1alpha in common human cancers and their metastases. *Cancer Res.*, **59**(22), pp. 5830–5835, 1999.

22. Warburg, O., Wind, F., and Negelein, E., The metabolism of tumors in the body. *J. Gen. Physiol.*, **8**(6), pp. 519–530, 1927.

23. Warburg, O., On respiratory impairment in cancer cells. *Science*, **124**(3215), pp. 269–270, 1956.

24. Ohno, Y. *et al.*, Three-way comparison of whole-body MR, coregistered whole-body FDG PET/MR, and integrated whole-body FDG PET/CT imaging: TNM and stage assessment capability for non-small cell lung cancer patients. *Radiology*, **275**(3), pp. 849–961, 2015.

25. Cairns, R. A., Harris, I. S., and Mak, T. W., Regulation of cancer cell metabolism. *Nat. Rev. Cancer*, **11**(2), pp. 85–95, 2011.

26. DeBerardinis, R. J. *et al.*, The biology of cancer: metabolic reprogramming fuels cell growth and proliferation. *Cell Metab.*, **7**(1), pp. 11–20, 2008.

27. Denko, N. C., Hypoxia, HIF1 and glucose metabolism in the solid tumour. *Nat. Rev. Cancer*, **8**(9), pp. 705–713, 2008.

28. O'Rourke, J. F. *et al.*, Identification of hypoxically inducible mRNAs in HeLa cells using differential-display PCR. Role of hypoxia-inducible factor-1. *Eur. J. Biochem.*, **241**(2), pp. 403–410, 1996.

29. Gleadle, J .M., and Ratcliffe, P. J., Induction of hypoxia-inducible factor-1, erythropoietin, vascular endothelial growth factor, and glucose transporter-1 by hypoxia: evidence against a regulatory role for Src kinase. *Blood*, **89**(2), pp. 503–509, 1997.

30. Kallinowski, F. *et al.*, Glucose uptake, lactate release, ketone body turnover, metabolic micromilieu, and pH distributions in human breast cancer xenografts in nude rats. *Cancer Res.*, **48**(24 Pt 1), pp. 7264–7272, 1988.

31. Clavo, A. C., Brown, R. S. and Wahl, R. L., Fluorodeoxyglucose uptake in human cancer cell lines is increased by hypoxia. *J Nucl Med.*, **36**(9), pp. 1625–1632, 1995.

32. Airley, R. *et al.*, Glucose transporter glut-1 expression correlates with tumor hypoxia and predicts metastasis-free survival in advanced carcinoma of the cervix. *Clin. Cancer Res.*, **7**(4), pp. 928–934, 2001.

33. Choi, N. *et al.*, Predictive factors in radiotherapy for non-small cell lung cancer: present status. *Lung Cancer*, **31**(1), pp. 43–56, 2001.

34. Jonathan, R. A. *et al.*, The prognostic value of endogenous hypoxia-related markers for head and neck squamous cell carcinomas treated with ARCON. *Radiother. Oncol.*, **79**(3), pp. 288–297, 2006.

35. Iyer, N. V. *et al.*, Cellular and developmental control of O2 homeostasis by hypoxia-inducible factor 1 alpha. *Genes Dev.*, **12**(2), pp. 149–162, 1998.

36. Denko, N. *et al.*, Epigenetic regulation of gene expression in cervical cancer cells by the tumor microenvironment. *Clin. Cancer Res.*, **6**(2), pp. 480–487, 2000.

37. Denko, N. C. *et al.*, Investigating hypoxic tumor physiology through gene expression patterns. *Oncogene*, **22**(37), pp. 5907–5914, 2003.

38. Wykoff, C. C. *et al.*, Identification of novel hypoxia dependent and independent target genes of the von Hippel-Lindau (VHL) tumour suppressor by mRNA differential expression profiling. *Oncogene*, **19**(54), pp. 6297–6305, 2000.

39. Patra, K. C. *et al.*, Hexokinase 2 is required for tumor initiation and maintenance and its systemic deletion is therapeutic in mouse models of cancer. *Cancer Cell*, **24**(2), pp. 213–228, 2013.

40. Li, B. *et al.*, Fructose-1,6-bisphosphatase opposes renal carcinoma progression. *Nature*, **513**(7517), pp. 251–255, 2014.

41. Christofk, H. R. *et al.*, The M2 splice isoform of pyruvate kinase is important for cancer metabolism and tumour growth. *Nature*, **452**(7184), pp. 230–233, 2008.

42. Ritterson Lew, C., and Tolan, D. R., Targeting of several glycolytic enzymes using RNA interference reveals aldolase affects cancer cell proliferation through a non-glycolytic mechanism. *J. Biol. Chem.*, **287**(51), pp. 42554–42563, 2012.

43. Lay, A. J. *et al.*, Phosphoglycerate kinase acts in tumour angiogenesis as a disulphide reductase. *Nature*, **408**(6814), pp. 869–873, 2000.

44. Chen, Y. *et al.*, Oxygen consumption can regulate the growth of tumors, a new perspective on the Warburg effect. *PLoS One*, **4**(9), p. e7033, 2009.

45. Firth, J. D., Ebert, B. L., and Ratcliffe, P. J., Hypoxic regulation of lactate dehydrogenase A. Interaction between hypoxia-inducible factor 1 and cAMP response elements. *J. Biol. Chem.*, **270**(36), pp. 21021–21027, 1995.

46. Perez de Heredia, F., Wood, I. S., and Trayhurn, P., Hypoxia stimulates lactate release and modulates monocarboxylate transporter (MCT1, MCT2, and MCT4) expression in human adipocytes. *Pflugers Arch.*, **459**(3), pp. 509–518, 2010.

47. Fantin, V. R., St-Pierre, J., and Leder, P., Attenuation of LDH-A expression uncovers a link between glycolysis, mitochondrial physiology, and tumor maintenance. *Cancer Cell*, **9**(6), pp. 425–434, 2006.

48. Lee, D. C. *et al.*, A lactate-induced response to hypoxia. *Cell*, **161**(3), pp. 595–609, 2015.

49. Benej, M., Pastorekova, S., and Pastorek, J., Carbonic anhydrase IX: regulation and role in cancer. *Subcell Biochem.*, **75**, pp. 199–219, 2014.

50. Giatromanolaki, A. *et al.*, Expression of hypoxia-inducible carbonic anhydrase-9 relates to angiogenic pathways and independently to poor outcome in non-small cell lung cancer. *Cancer Res.*, **61**(21), pp. 7992–7998, 2001.

51. Kim, J. W. *et al.*, HIF-1-mediated expression of pyruvate dehydrogenase kinase: a metabolic switch required for cellular adaptation to hypoxia. *Cell Metab.*, **3**(3), pp. 177–185, 2006.

52. Papandreou, I. *et al.*, HIF-1 mediates adaptation to hypoxia by actively downregulating mitochondrial oxygen consumption. *Cell Metab.*, **3**(3), pp. 187–197, 2006.

53. Lu, C. W. *et al.*, Induction of pyruvate dehydrogenase kinase-3 by hypoxia-inducible factor-1 promotes metabolic switch and drug resistance. *J. Biol. Chem.*, **283**(42), pp. 28106–28114, 2008.

54. Korotchkina, L. G., and Patel, M. S., Mutagenesis studies of the phosphorylation sites of recombinant human pyruvate dehydrogenase. Site-specific regulation. *J. Biol. Chem.*, **270**(24), pp. 14297–14304, 1995.

55. Patel, M. S. *et al.*, The pyruvate dehydrogenase complexes: structure-based function and regulation. *J. Biol. Chem.*, **289**(24), pp. 16615–16623, 2014.

56. Korotchkina, L. G., and Patel, M. S., Site specificity of four pyruvate dehydrogenase kinase isoenzymes toward the three phosphorylation sites of human pyruvate dehydrogenase. *J. Biol. Chem.*, **276**(40), pp. 37223– 37229, 2001.

57. McFate, T. *et al.*, Pyruvate dehydrogenase complex activity controls metabolic and malignant phenotype in cancer cells. *J. Biol. Chem.*, **283**(33), pp. 22700–22708, 2008.

58. Hitosugi, T. *et al.*, Tyrosine phosphorylation of mitochondrial pyruvate dehydrogenase kinase 1 is important for cancer metabolism. *Mol. Cell*, **44**(6), pp. 864–877, 2011.

59. Fan, J. *et al.*, Tyr-301 phosphorylation inhibits pyruvate dehydrogenase by blocking substrate binding and promotes the Warburg effect. *J. Biol. Chem.*, **289**(38), pp. 26533–26541, 2014.

60. Fukuda, R. *et al.*, HIF-1 regulates cytochrome oxidase subunits to optimize efficiency of respiration in hypoxic cell. *Cell*, **129**(1), pp. 111–122, 2007.

61. David, P. S., and Poyton, R. O., Effects of a transition from normoxia to anoxia on yeast cytochrome c oxidase and the mitochondrial respiratory chain: implications for hypoxic gene induction. *Biochim. Biophys. Acta.*, **1709**(2), pp. 169–180, 2005.

62. Tello, D. *et al.*, Induction of the mitochondrial NDUFA4L2 protein by HIF-1alpha decreases oxygen consumption by inhibiting Complex I activity. *Cell Metab.*, **14**(6), pp. 768–779, 2011.

63. Bellot, G. *et al.*, Hypoxia-induced autophagy is mediated through hypoxia-inducible factor induction of BNIP3 and BNIP3L via their BH3 domains. *Mol. Cell Biol.*, **29**(10), pp. 2570–2581, 2009.

64. Zhang, H. *et al.*, Mitochondrial autophagy is an HIF-1-dependent adaptive metabolic response to hypoxia. *J. Biol. Chem.*, **283**(16), pp. 10892–10903, 2008.

65. Tian, W. *et al.*, Phosphorylation of ULK1 by AMPK regulates translocation of ULK1 to mitochondria and mitophagy. *FEBS Lett.*, **589**(15), pp. 1847–1854, 2015.

66. Papandreou, I. *et al.*, Hypoxia signals autophagy in tumor cells via AMPK activity, independent of HIF-1, BNIP3, and BNIP3L. *Cell Death Differ*, **15**(10), pp. 1572–1581, 2008.

67. Iresjo, B. M. *et al.*, Appearance of individual amino acid concentrations in arterial blood during steady-state infusions of different amino acid formulations to ICU patients in support of whole-body protein metabolism. *JPEN J Parenter Enteral Nutr.*, **30**(4), pp. 277–285, 2006.

68. Lee, J. C. *et al.*, Plasma amino acid levels in patients with colorectal cancers and liver cirrhosis with hepatocellular carcinoma. *Hepatogastroenterology*, **50**(53), pp. 1269–1273, 2003.

69. DeBerardinis, R. J. *et al.*, Beyond aerobic glycolysis: transformed cells can engage in glutamine metabolism that exceeds the requirement for protein and nucleotide synthesis. *Proc. Natl. Acad. Sci. USA.*, **104**(49), pp. 19345–19350, 2007.

70. Wise, D. R. *et al.*, Hypoxia promotes isocitrate dehydrogenase-dependent carboxylation of alpha-ketoglutarate to citrate to support cell growth and viability. *Proc. Natl. Acad. Sci. USA.*, **108**(49), pp. 19611–19616, 2011.

71. Wise, D. R. *et al.*, Myc regulates a transcriptional program that stimulates mitochondrial glutaminolysis and leads to glutamine addiction. *Proc. Natl. Acad. Sci. USA.*, **105**(48), pp. 18782–18787, 2008.

72. Son, J. *et al.*, Glutamine supports pancreatic cancer growth through a KRAS-regulated metabolic pathway. *Nature*, **496**(7443), pp. 101–5, 2013.

73. Holleran, A. L. *et al.*, Glutamine metabolism in AS-30D hepatoma cells. Evidence for its conversion into lipids via reductive carboxylation. *Mol. Cell Biochem.*, **152**(2), pp. 95–101, 1995.

74. Metallo, C. M. *et al.*, Reductive glutamine metabolism by IDH1 mediates lipogenesis under hypoxia. *Nature*, **481**(7381), pp. 380–384, 2012.

75. Mullen, A. R. *et al.*, Reductive carboxylation supports growth in tumour cells with defective mitochondria. *Nature*, **481**(7381), pp. 385–388, 2012.

76. Sun, R. C., and Denko, N. C., Hypoxic regulation of glutamine metabolism through HIF1 and SIAH2 supports lipid synthesis that is necessary for tumor growth. *Cell Metab.*, **19**(2), pp. 285–292, 2014.

77. Brugarolas, J., Molecular genetics of clear-cell renal cell carcinoma. *J. Clin. Oncol.*, **32**(18), pp. 1968–1976, 2014.

78. Favaro, E. *et al.*, Glucose utilization via glycogen phosphorylase sustains proliferation and prevents premature senescence in cancer cells. *Cell. Metab.*, **16**(6), pp. 751–764, 2012.

79. Fu, L. *et al.*, Activation of HIF2alpha in kidney proximal tubule cells causes abnormal glycogen deposition but not tumorigenesis. *Cancer Res.*, **73**(9), pp. 2916–2925, 2013.

80. Hughes, A. L., Todd, B. L., and Espenshade, P. J., SREBP pathway responds to sterols and functions as an oxygen sensor in fission yeast. *Cell*, **120**(6), pp. 831–842, 2005.

81. Ackerman, D., and Simon, M. C., Hypoxia, lipids, and cancer: surviving the harsh tumor microenvironment. *Trends Cell. Biol.*, **24**(8), pp. 472–478, 2014.

82. Young, R. M. *et al.*, Dysregulated mTORC1 renders cells critically dependent on desaturated lipids for survival under tumor-like stress. *Genes Dev.*, **27**(10), pp. 1115–1131, 2013.

83. Qiu, B. *et al.*, HIF2alpha-dependent lipid storage promotes endoplasmic reticulum homeostasis in clear-cell renal cell carcinoma. *Cancer Discov.*, **5**(6), pp. 652–667, 2015.

84. Kamphorst, J. J. *et al.*, Hypoxic and Ras-transformed cells support growth by scavenging unsaturated fatty acids from lysophospholipids. *Proc. Natl. Acad. Sci. USA.*, **110**(22), pp. 8882–8887, 2013.

85. Kamphorst, J. J. *et al.*, Quantitative analysis of acetyl-CoA production in hypoxic cancer cells reveals substantial contribution from acetate. *Cancer Metab.*, **2**, p. 23, 2014.

86. Schug, Z. T. *et al.*, Acetyl-CoA synthetase 2 promotes acetate utilization and maintains cancer cell growth under metabolic stress. *Cancer Cell*, **27**(1), pp. 57–71, 2015.

87. Zaugg, K. *et al.*, Carnitine palmitoyltransferase 1C promotes cell survival and tumor growth under conditions of metabolic stress. *Genes Dev.*, **25**(10), pp. 1041–1051, 2011.

88. Chaban, V. V., and Khandelia, H., Distribution of neutral lipids in the lipid droplet core. *J. Phys. Chem. B.*, **118**(38), pp. 11145–11151, 2014.

89. Roy, D. *et al.*, Loss of HSulf-1 promotes altered lipid metabolism in ovarian cancer. *Cancer Metab.*, **2**, p. 13, 2014.

90. Bensaad, K. *et al.*, Fatty acid uptake and lipid storage induced by HIF-1alpha contribute to cell growth and survival after hypoxia-reoxygenation. *Cell Rep.*, **9**(1), pp. 349–365, 2014.

91. Gimm, T. *et al.*, Hypoxia-inducible protein 2 is a novel lipid droplet protein and a specific target gene of hypoxia-inducible factor-1. *FASEB J.*, **24**(11), pp. 4443–4458, 2010.

92. McCarthy, N. Hypoxia: micro changes. *Nat. Rev. Cancer*, **14**(6), pp. 382–383, 2014.

93. el Azzouzi, H. *et al.*, The hypoxia-inducible microRNA cluster miR-199a approximately 214 targets myocardial PPARdelta and impairs mitochondrial fatty acid oxidation. *Cell Metab.*, **18**(3), pp. 341–354, 2013.

94. Huang, X. *et al.*, Hypoxia-inducible mir-210 regulates normoxic gene expression involved in tumor initiation. *Mol. Cell*, **35**(6), pp. 856–867, 2009.

95. Chan, S. Y. *et al.*, MicroRNA-210 controls mitochondrial metabolism during hypoxia by repressing the iron-sulfur cluster assembly proteins ISCU1/2. *Cell Metab.*, **10**(4), pp. 273–284, 2009.

96. Yao, M. *et al.*, Dicer mediating the expression of miR-143 and miR-155 regulates hexokinase II associated cellular response to hypoxia. *Am. J. Physiol. Lung. Cell. Mol. Physiol.*, **307**(11), pp. L829–L837, 2014.

97. Ho, J. J. *et al.*, Functional importance of Dicer protein in the adaptive cellular response to hypoxia. *J. Biol. Chem.*, **287**(34), pp. 29003–29020, 2012.

98. Jiang, H., Guo, R., and Powell-Coffman, J. A., The Caenorhabditis elegans hif-1 gene encodes a bHLH-PAS protein that is required for adaptation to hypoxia. *Proc. Natl. Acad. Sci. USA.*, **98**(14), pp. 7916–7921, 2001.

# Chapter 7

# Regulation of DNA Repair by Hypoxia

Yuhong Lu* and Peter M. Glazer*[,†,‡]

*Department of Therapeutic Radiology, Yale School of Medicine,
New Haven, CT 06520, USA
†Department of Genetics, Yale School of Medicine,
New Haven, CT 06520, USA
‡peter.glazer@yale.edu

## 1. Introduction

Hypoxia is a key feature in solid tumors, constituting a characteristic microenvironment for cancer cells along with other factors, such as low pH and nutrient deprivation.[1,2] As a hallmark feature, hypoxia applies a selective pressure for cancer cells. Hypoxic cancer cells use genetic and adaptive changes to survive and proliferate under this stress condition, which in turn forces tumor cells to acquire aggressive phenotypes that allow them to invade and metastasize.[3,4] As a result, hypoxia generally correlates with features of aggressive tumors and is also identified as a strong and independent adverse prognostic factor for patient outcomes, such as in head and neck cancer, cervical cancer, and soft tissue sarcomas.[5–7] The poorer outcome of patients with hypoxic tumors compared to those with non-hypoxic tumors is associated with increased risk of metastasis and resistance to conventional cancer therapy.[5]

Tumor progression has been correlated with genetic instability, which is one of the key cellular events induced by hypoxia. This is because hypoxia is associated with increased levels of DNA damage, enhanced rate of mutagenesis, and functional impairment in DNA repair pathways.[8] Hypoxia has been shown to lead to both large-scale chromosomal aberrations and small-scale DNA mutations.[9–11] The current evidence strongly supports that hypoxia can drive cancer progression through its impact on genetic instability.

Epigenetic modifications are a type of DNA-independent regulations of gene expression, including histone modification, DNA methylation, nucleosome remodeling and RNA-mediated targeting.[12] Under the hypoxic stress, cells, including tumor cells, use various mechanisms to adapt to this unfavorable microenvironment, one of which is epigenetic modification. Hypoxic tumor cells display distinctive epigenetic profiles and chromatin alterations, including histone acetylation or deacetylation and histone methylation or demethylation, etc.[13,14]

## 2. Hypoxia Induces Genetic Instability

## 2.1. Increased DNA damage and mutations under hypoxia

Hypoxia has been associated with a variety of DNA lesions. Hypoxia and subsequent reoxygenation can cause numerous types of base damages. The most common alterations observed in purines (G, guanine and A, adenine) and pyrimidines (C, cytosine and T, thymine) are formation of 8-oxoguanine (8-oxoG) and thymine glycols, respectively.[15] The former alteration leads to GC to TA transversions.[16] Hypoxia and reoxygenation cycles also can induce single- and double-stranded DNA breaks although hypoxia *per se* does not induce DNA strand breaks as detected by the comet assay.[17] However, reoxygenation, as opposed to hypoxia, induces a significant level of DNA damage and the level of strand breaks observed in a severe hypoxia-reoxygenation cycle was similar to 4–5 Gray (Gy) exposure of ionizing radiation (IR).[18] This cause of DNA damage is especially relevant to tumor biology, as hypoxia often occurs transiently and heterogeneously within tumor microenvironment, resulting in frequent cycles of hypoxia and reoxygenation.

Hypoxia-reoxygenation cycles also induce aberrant DNA synthesis, resulting in DNA over-replication and gene amplification. Hypoxia can cause illegitimate rounds of DNA replication (termed "replicon misfiring") after the primary round of DNA synthesis is interrupted, resulting in DNA over-replication.[19] Many investigators have reported DNA over-replication after exposure to hypoxia,[20,21] which has been linked to tumor metastasis.[10] There is also evidence that hypoxia affects cell cycle by inducing cell cycle arrest. Severe hypoxia (usually less than 0.02% Oxygen) induces an S-phase arrest that is rapidly reversible upon reoxygenation,[17,22] which is in part associated with degradation of cyclin A.[22] In addition, hypoxia also induces a G1-arrest and this type of cell cycle arrest appears to occur predominantly in p53-null cells.[23,24] Subsequent studies suggest that the G1-arrest may involve induction of the cyclin-dependent kinase p21 and p27 in response to hypoxia.[25,26]

Gene amplification is associated with the overexpression of numerous oncogenes and is tightly linked to tumor progression.[27] Hypoxia potentially induces gene amplification through several mechanisms. DNA over-replication during the reoxygenation phase was observed to promote gene amplification.[10,28] For example, hypoxia induces gene amplification of the multiple drug-resistance gene, p-glycoprotein, which underlines the mechanism of adriamycin and doxorubicin resistance in several tumor cell lines.[21,29] Hypoxia also is a potent activator of fragile sites,[28,30] regions in chromosomes that are particularly susceptible to breaks, and these loci have been implicated in the formation of many types of chromosome rearrangement and oncogene amplification.[31,32] The activation of fragile sites has been shown to trigger breakage-fusion-bridge (BFB) cycles, leading to the formation of double minutes (DMs) and homogenously staining regions (HSRs). The finding that hypoxia is a potent inducer of fragile sites provides one of mechanisms of hypoxia-induced gene amplification.

In the early work, we reported that tumor cells grown as xenograft tumors have higher mutation frequencies compared to the same tumor cells grown in culture.[33,34] Several studies by others also provided evidence that cells in solid tumors show increased levels of genomic rearrangements and higher levels of point mutations and small deletions compared with cells grown in cell culture.[35,36] Wilkinson and colleagues have shown that murine fibrosarcoma cells grown as tumors in nude mice have a three-fold increase in mutation frequency of the hypoxanthine phosphoribosyltransferase (*hprt*) gene compared to the same cells grown in culture for same period of time when they were later incubated in culture in the presence of 6-thioguanine to select for *hrpt* mutants.[37] *In vitro*, cells exposed to hypoxic stress also showed similar genomic rearrangements, such as gene amplification, DNA over-replication, and DNA breaks, which is associated with elevated mutation frequency.[10,11,20,33,36] These studies provide further evidences that conditions within tumor microenvironment can induce significant gene mutations.

## 2.2. Impaired DNA repair under hypoxia

In addition to DNA damages induced by hypoxia and reoxygenation, hypoxia can also impact on multiple DNA repair pathways, depending upon the type and severity of hypoxia. Acute hypoxia rapidly stimulates changes in DNA repair genes through post-translational modifications (PTMs); however, prolonged, chronic hypoxia can suppress DNA repair pathways, either by decreased expression or functional inactivation of DNA repair genes.

PTMs, such as phosphorylation, ubiquitination, acetylation, and hydroxylation, allow rapid control of protein functionality in response to cellular signals and stressors. Emerging evidence suggests that severe hypoxia rapidly induces a wide spectrum of PTMs of proteins involved in the response to DNA damage and cell stress.[18,38] Although hypoxia, in the absence of reoxygenation, does not induce direct DNA damage, it does induce replication stress. With 6 hours of severe hypoxic stress, replication initiation and elongation stall, giving rise to accumulation of single-stranded DNA and replication protein A (RPA) foci.[39,40] In response to hypoxia-induced replication stress, the ataxia telangiectasia and Rad3-related (ATR) check point kinase is activated and required for phosphorylation of downstream targets, including Checkpoint Kinase 1 (CHK1), histone 2AX (H2AX), RAD17, and Nijmegen breakage syndrome 1

(NBS1).[17,18,40] In addition, ATR is also required for hypoxia-induced mono-ubiquitination of Fanconi anemia group D2 (FANCD2) and Fanconi anemia group I (FANCI).[41] The hypoxia-induced PTMs are critical; for stabilizing replication forks, as loss of ATR activity leads to DNA damage during hypoxia.[40,41] Similar to ATR, the ataxia telangiectasia mutated (ATM) check-point kinase is also activated by hypoxia, although there are no double-strand breaks (DSBs) detected during hypoxia.[42–44] Hypoxia-induced ATM activation is required for phosphorylation of downstream targets, including Checkpoint Kinase 2 (CHK2), p53 binding protein 1 (53BP1) and DNA-dependent protein kinase, catalytic subunit (DNA-PKcs). Recent evidence indicates that hypoxia-induced replication stress together with increased histone H3 lysine 9 trimethylation (H3K9me3) lead to ATM activation.[45] Moreover, hypoxia-induced ATM activation is required for promoting replication progression as inhibition of ATM leads to a decreased rate of DNA replication and an accumulation of DNA damage in S phase under hypoxic condition.[45] These results suggest that hypoxia-induced ATM signaling may serve multiple distinct functions. Upon reoxygenation after hypoxia, production of reactive oxygen species directly induces oxidative DNA damage, which, in turn, activates ATM-CHK2 pathway in the classical manner.[18,42] Both ATM and ATR pathways appear to protect the cells from both hypoxia-induced replication stress and reoxygenation-induced DNA damage.

Transcriptional regulation of gene expression enables cells to exert more sustained changes in protein function. Prolonged hypoxic exposure to cells induces a chronic response, in which genes from selected DNA repair pathway are coordinately suppressed. Hypoxia has been shown to lead to transcriptional downregulation of mismatch repair (MMR) genes, *MLH1*, *MSH2*, and *MSH6 in vitro* and *in vivo*. These changes are associated with significantly increased genetic instability in cells.[46–48] Under severe hypoxic conditions, *MLH1* and *MSH2* are downregulated at both protein and mRNA levels. Mechanistically, hypoxia induces substantial downregulation of Myc levels in many different cell lines.[49] The decreased Myc expression by hypoxia leads to a dynamic shift in occupancy at the E-box motifs in the proximal promoter regions of *MLH1* and *MSH2* from Myc/Max transcriptional activation to Mad1/Max and Mnt/Max transcriptional repression.[48]

Cellular homologous recombination (HR) capacity is diminished 3–8 fold in hypoxic cells as measured by recombination of a shuttle vector plasmid with donor DNA or by intrachromosomal DSB repair assays.[50–53] In a microarray-based study of gene expression changes in response to hypoxia, we found that hypoxia specifically down-regulates the expression of two key homology-dependent repair (HR) genes, *BRCA1* and *RAD51*.[50,51] Hypoxia-mediated RAD51 down-regulation *in vivo* was also confirmed in experimental tumors in mice.[50] The mechanism underlying this down-regulation appears to be coordinated transcriptional repression of *BRCA1*, and *RAD51* by the E2F transcription factor network at their two adjacent E2F sites.[50,51] Quantitative chromatin immuneprecipitation (qChIP) assays have revealed that this repression is mediated, at least in part, by hypoxia-induced dephosphorylation and nuclear accumulation of p130, a Rb-related pocket protein, leading to the formation of the repressive E2F4/p130 complex and its increased binding to the *BRCA1* and *RAD51* promoters. Our recent study has found that down-regulation of *FANCD2* by hypoxia also occurs through a similar mechanism.[41]

# 3. Global Regulation of Epigenetic Pathways by Hypoxia

Epigenetic changes, including histone modifications and DNA methylation, have been shown to play an important role of regulating gene expression and have a crucial function in tumor progression.[54] Both severe and moderate hypoxia induce global epigenetic alternations and generate novel chromatin modification signatures.[14,55,56] Hypoxia-induced epigenetic changes are mainly through histone modification and/or DNA methylation mediated by multiple regulatory proteins.[57]

## 3.1. Hypoxia-induced histone modifications

Hypoxic exposure has been shown to induce global epigenetic modification changes.[14,55,58–60] The most well characterized global histone modifications induced by hypoxia include di and trimethylation of histone

3 lysine 9 (H3K9).[14,55,59] At the same time, H3K9 acetylation level is globally decreased under hypoxic condition.[14,55,59] Both increases in H3K9 methylation and decreases in H3K9 acetylation are associated with transcriptional repression. Hypoxia also globally induces H3 lysine 4 (H3K4) di and trimethylation, both of which are usually associated with transcriptional activation.[58] Other global hypoxia-induced histone alterations are also found, including increased H3K14 acetylation, H3 lysine 79 (H3K79) dimethylation, and H4 arginine 3 (H4R3) dimethylation, which are markers of transcriptional activation, as well as decreased H4 acetylation, increased H3K36 trimethylation, and H3K27 di and trimethylation, which are markers of transcriptional repression.[14,55,56]

## 3.2. Hypoxia-dependent regulation of genes involved in histone modifications

Histone modification changes are regulated by the modifiers that add or remove the acetyl or methyl groups at N-terminal tails of histones.[61,62] Hypoxia-induced changes in histone modifications may result from changes in expression and activity of theses histone modifiers. The Jumonji C (JmjC)-domain containing histone demethylases (JHDM) belong to a large family of lysine demethylases. Several members of JHDM have been shown to be transcriptionally induced by hypoxia, including JMJD1A, JMJD2B, and JMJD2C.[58,63–65] Since the JHDM family members require oxygen for demethylation, their enzymatic activity is likely to be compromised under hypoxia. It has been proposed that JHDM induction by hypoxia tends to restore histone methylation homeostasis when oxygen level is low.[59] On other hand, G9a, a histone methyltransferase, is also upregulated by hypoxia.[55] Available evidence suggests that an increase of H3K9me2 is partially regulated by hypoxia-dependent induction of the G9a methyltransferase.[55] Additionally, the regulation of gene expression by hypoxia through covalent modification of histones is also supported by evidence that histone deacetylase (HDAC) expression and activity have been shown to be upregulated in hypoxia and to play a role in activation of many HIF-1 responsive genes.[66]

## 3.3.  DNA methylation regulated by hypoxia

DNA is methylated post-synthetically on cytosine residues predominantly in the sequence CpG, which generally leads to inactivation of gene expression.[67,68] In addition to histone modifications, hypoxia also alters DNA methylation. Generally, acute hypoxia leads to reduction of DNA methylation whereas prolonged exposure to moderate hypoxia increases DNA methylation.[16,69] The hypoxia induced DNA demethylation has been reported in human colorectal and melanoma cell lines.[70] Specifically, tumor-associated CpG demethylation results in increased HIF-1 binding to the hypoxia-responsive elements (HREs) and augments HIF-1-mediated effects on tumor progression in HCT116 colon cancer cell line.[70,71] However, under chronic hypoxic exposure, global DNA hypermethylation was observed in the PwR-1E benign prostate epithelial cell. In addition, treatment with 5-aza-dC results in an overall reduction in DNA methylation in hypoxic the PwR-1E cell line,[69] further supports hypoxia-induced DNA hypermethylation phenotype.

DNA cytosine methylation and various histone modifications can interact with each other to cause gene repression. It has been reported that the histone methyltransferase G9a complex can recruit DNMT3A and DNMT3B to mediate *de novo* DNA methylation at the promoter of the Oct4 gene.[72] Hypoxia also increase DNMT3B activity, which results in increases in DNA methylation.[69] Hypoxia also leads to the down-regulation of DNA methyltrasferases including DNMT1, DNMT3a, and DNMT3b, which contributes to DNA hypomethylaiton under hypoxia.[60,69] However, more epigenetic mechanisms mediating changes of DNA methylation status under hypoxia still remain to be explored.

## 4.  Hypoxia Drives Silencing of Specific DNA Repair Genes Through Epigenetic Regulation

In addition to global histone modification changes under hypoxia, hypoxia also induces promoter-specific epigenetic regulation. The promoters of the vascular endothelial growth factor (*VEGF*) and early growth response protein 1 (*EGR1*), both of which are HIF target genes, there is a marked increase in H3K9 acetylation and H3K4 trimethylation and a decrease in

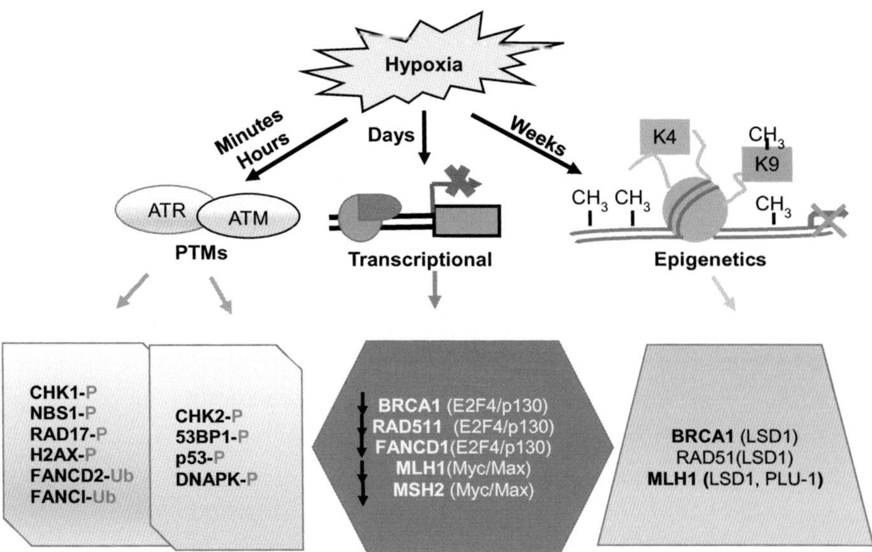


Fig. 1. Mechanisms of regulation of DNA repair pathways by hypoxia under different time course. Acute severe hypoxia activates DNA damage signaling pathways by PTMs. Chronic hypoxia leads to transcriptional downreglation of DNA repair capacity. Prolonged moderate hypoxia induces stable silencing specific DNA repair genes through epigenetic regulation.

H3K27 trimethylation.[14] The similar epigenetic changes have also been observed at the promoters of hypoxia-inducible genes erythropoietin (*EPO*), heme oxygenase (decycling) 1 (*HMOX1*) and decay-accelerating factor (*DAF*).[14,58] Our recent work has shown that hypoxia induces histone modifications at the *BRCA1* and *MLH1* promoters, which drives the silencing of these genes (see Fig. 1).[73,74]

## 4.1. Hypoxia-induced epigenetic silencing of the *BRCA1* promoter

Clinical evidence has shown that transcriptionally silenced *BRCA1* alleles are found in sporadic cancers, which is associated not only with promoter DNA hypermethylation,[75–77] but also with histone modifications in the promoter region.[78] By using qChIP to probe histone changes at *BRCA1* promoter during hypoxia, we found hypoxia causes substantial decreases in the levels of H3K4 methylation at the *BRCA1* promoter.[73] Other histone modifications induced by hypoxia at *BRCA1* promoter include significant increases in H3K9me3 levels and decreases in H3K9 acetylation levels. In contrast, H3K27 methylation levels are not significantly changed,[73] suggesting that hypoxia regulates specific pathways of histone modifications. Similar histone modification changes by hypoxia is also found at *RAD51* promoter.

Using a specifically designed reporter gene assay to identify cells in which the *BRCA1* promoter had been silenced, we have found that prolonged exposure to moderate hypoxia over the course of several weeks can promote the emergence of subclones in which *BRCA1* promoter has undergone long-term silencing.[73] The *BRCA1* silencing can persist for weeks even when cells are no longer cultured in hypoxic conditions.[73] In these silenced clones, the *BRCA1* promoter is marked by H3K4 demethylation and H3K9 deacetylation.[73] Consistent with histone modifications at *BRCA1* promoter in silenced clones, treatment of the silenced clones with the HDAC inhibitor, trichostatin A (TSA), reactivates the *BRCA1* promoter, suggesting that the repressive histone changes by hypoxia were partially reversed. H3K9 methylation has been recognized as a signal for DNA methylation and H3K4 demthylation is believed to be required for *de novo* DNA methylation.[79] Since hypoxia can induce both H3K9 methylation and H3K4 demethylation at *BRCA1* promoter, this points to a pathway of gene silencing initially driven by histone modifications, and also could provide the foundation for subsequent DNA methylation (see Fig. 2).

## 4.2. Hypoxia-induced epigenetic silencing of the promoters of mismatch repair genes

Like HR genes, several MMR genes, including *MLH1* and *MSH2*, are also downregulated by hypoxia. Interestingly, besides regulation by a shift in promoter occupancy from the activating Myc/Max to the repressive Mad1/Max and Mnt/Max complexes, downregulation of *MLH1* and *MSH2* by hypoxia also involves histone modifications at their promoters. The initial evidence has shown that the pathways mediating their

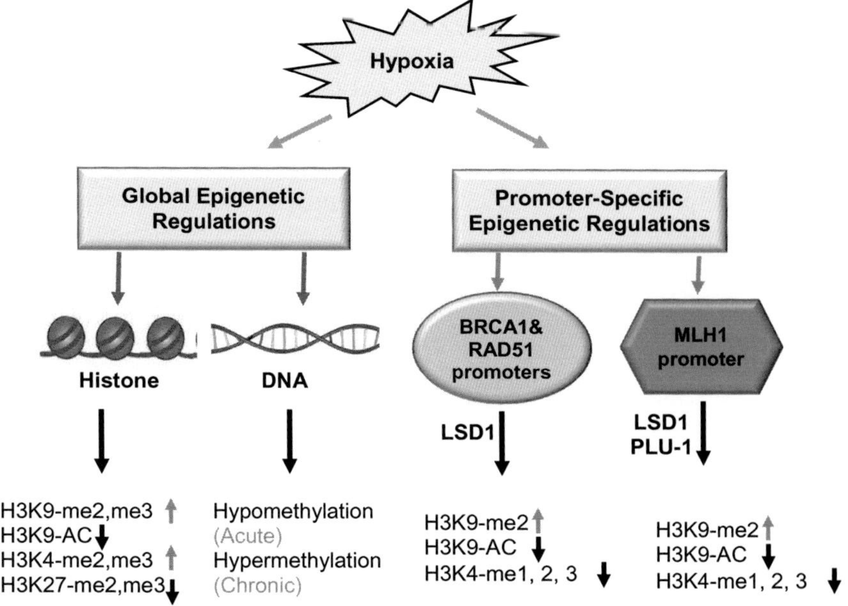



Fig. 2. Regulation of epigenetic pathways by hypoxia. Hypoxia induces global epigenetic modification changes that are associated with either transcriptional repression or activation. Also, hypoxia induces promoter-specific epigenetic regulation at DNA repair gene promoters that is associated gene silencing.

downregulation by transcription factors in hypoxia could be blocked by the HDAC inhibitor, TSA,[46,80,81] suggesting epigenetic regulation might be involved in this process.

Again by qChIP assay, the main findings of histone modification changes at *MLH1* promoter under hypoxic condition are similar to what we found at *BRCA1* and *RAD51* promoters; decreased H3K4 methylation and H3K9 acetylation at *MLH1* promoter, accompanied by increased H3K9 trimethylation.[74] We have also found that both the MLH1 protein levels and mRNA levels are reduced in conjunction with the changes in chromatin marks at the promoter in response to hypoxia.[74]

Using engineered assay system to select cells in which the *MLH1* promoter had undergone silencing, we found moderate hypoxia can promote *MLH1* promoter silencing in this system, and it is very clear that as the duration of hypoxic exposure increased, so did the frequency of *MLH1* promoter silenced colonies. These results provide evidence that hypoxia can enforce *MLH1* promoter silencing and that the silencing persists even after the cells are no longer in hypoxic conditions. In addition, we also found that about 25–30% of the hypoxia-induced *MLH1* promoters in the silenced cells were reactivated after treatment with the DNA methyltransferase inhibitor, 5-aza-2′-deoxycytidine (5-aza-dC),[74] suggesting that hypoxia-induced *MLH1* promoter silencing is partially associated with DNA methylation. Hence, we provide the evidence directly linking hypoxia with epigenetic regulation and durable long-term silencing of *MLH1*.

## 4.3. LSD1 mediates in H3K4 demethylation at the *BRCA1* promoter induced by hypoxia

To identify the histone demethylases that are involved in hypoxia-induced H3K4 demethylation at the *BRCA1* and *RAD51* promoters, we tested several H3K4 demethylases, including JARID1A/RBP2, JARKD1B/PLU-1, and LSD1/KDM1A. PLU-1 is the only one among the three whose expression is upregulated to responses to hypoxia, which makes it a good candidate for regulation of H3K4 demethylation at *BRCA1* and *RAD51* promoters. However, we found that knockdown of PLU-1 in MCF-7 cells did not prevent hypoxia-mediated suppression of *BRCA1* and *RAD51* at protein levels and at mRNA levels.[73] Similar negative results were seen in cells with shRNA-mediated knockdown of *RBP2/JARID1A*.[73]

However, we found knockdown of LSD1 clearly prevented the hypoxia-induced reduction in H3K4 methylation at both the *BRCA1* and *RAD51* promoters in MCF-7 cells.[73] Interestingly, LSD1 knockdown also blocked the reduction in H3K9 acetylation that otherwise occurs at the *BRCA1* and *RAD51* promoters in response to hypoxia, consistent with cross-talk between these modifications.[73] We also examined the changes in *BRCA1* and *RAD51* mRNA levels in response to hypoxia with or without LSD1 knockdown by using same cell lines. We found LSD1 knockdown blocked most of the reduction in mRNA levels for *BRCA1 and RAD51*, consistent with the key role for H3K4 methylation in promoter activation.[73] These results identify LSD1 as the key histone demethylase that mediates epigenetic regulation of *BRCA1* in response to hypoxia.

## 4.4. LSD1 and PLU1 are required for hypoxia induced histone modifications at the *MLH1* promoter

In the case of *MLH1*, we found that knockdown of LSD1 in SW480, a colon cancer cell line, only partially attenuated hypoxia-induced decreases in H3K4 methylation at *MLH1* promoter. Based on the finding that PLU-1 is upregulated by hypoxia, we next re-focused on the role of PLU-1 in H3K4 demethylation by hypoxia at *MLH1* promoter. Again we found that knockdown of PLU-1 in SW480 also partially attenuates hypoxia-induced H3K4 demethylation at *MLH1* promoter, with a level of attenuation similar to that knockdown of LSD1 in the SW480 cell line. However, when we simultaneously knocked down both LSD1 and PLU-1, we found that the dual knockdown in SW480 cells yielded greater inhibition of hypoxia-induced H3K4 demethylation than in the single knockdown of either of them.[74] These results indicate that LSD1 and PLU-1 have non-redundant functions (consistent with their slightly different substrate specificity for demethylation, as LSD1 cannot demethylate trimethylated H3K4)[82] and that both are involved in hypoxia-induced H3K4 demethylation at *MLH1* promoter. These results differ from the work implicating LSD1, by itself, in hypoxia-induced H3K4 demthylation at *BRCA1* promoters,[74] as PLU-1 does not play a significant role at these promoters.

Consistent with the histone modifications at *MLH1* promoter, we found that knockdown of either LSD1 or PLU-1 alone did not have statistically significant effects on the hypoxia-induced reduction of *MLH1* mRNA. However, double knockdown of LSD1 and PLU-1 did substantially prevent the downregulation of *MLH1* by hypoxia at both mRNA and protein levels.

## 5. Concluding Remarks and Future Perspectives

Tumor hypoxia is a dynamic process. As discussed above, the impact of hypoxia on both the genome and epigenome of malignant cells can be profound, which thus highlights hypoxia as a major factor in generating tumor heterogeneity and in cancer progression. These findings are now beginning to be applied towards clinical therapies. For example, targeting the DNA damage signaling pathways has been shown to sensitize cells to hypoxia-induced apoptosis; DNA damaging agents or poly ADP ribose polymerase (PARP) inhibitors may sensitize hypoxic tumor cells because of transcriptional downregulation of DNA repair genes by hypoxia.[83–85] As knowledge of the cancer epigenome accumulates, there is increasing interest in the development of epigenetic therapy for cancer treatment. The DNA methyltransferase inhibitors, azacitidine and decitabine, and the HDAC inhibitor, vorinostat, are already in clinic use. The epigenetic regulation by hypoxia and the consequent silencing of specific genes provides a further rationale to support the use of epigenetic therapy for cancer treatment because of the ubiquitous hypoxic microenvironment in solid tumors. Our work so far has demonstrated the role of LSD1 and to some extent PLU-1 in *BRCA1* and *MLH1* silencing, and so targeting LSD1 and PLU-1 may represent promising approaches that could be used alone or in combination with other such agents.

In the particular case of *MLH1*, prevention of silencing or reactivation of a silenced allele would not only serve to suppress genetic instability but also to restore the proapoptotic role of *MLH1* in the DNA-damage response, because cells deficient in *MLH1* show a damage-tolerant phenotype, and are resistant to cisplatin and temozolomide.[86,87] Hence, a pharmacologic strategy to inhibit or reverse *MLH1* silencing would be a valuable approach to render hypoxic cancer cells more sensitive to conventional chemotherapy.

## Acknowledgment

This work was supported by a Grant from the NIH (R01ES005775) to PMG.

## References

1. Hanahan, D., and Robert A., Weinberg, hallmarks of cancer: the next generation. *Cell*, **144**(5), pp. 646–674, 2011.
2. Vaupel, P., Tumor microenvironmental physiology and its implications for radiation oncology. *Semin. Radiat. Oncol.*, **14**(3), pp. 198–206, 2004.
3. Chang, J., and Erler, J., Hypoxia-mediated metastasis, in *Tumor Microenvironment and Cellular Stress: Signaling, Metabolism, Imaging, and*

*Therapeutic Targets*, Koumenis, C., Hammond, E., and Giaccia, A., eds. Springer New York: New York, NY. pp. 55–81, 2014.

4. Vaupel, P., and Mayer, A., Hypoxia in tumors: Pathogenesis-related classification, characterization of hypoxia subtypes, and associated biological and clinical implications, in *Oxygen Transport to Tissue XXXVI*, Swartz, H. M., Harrison, D. K., and Bruley, D. F., eds. Springer New York. pp. 19–24, 2014.

5. Vaupel, P., and Mayer, A., Hypoxia in cancer: significance and impact on clinical outcome. *Cancer and Metastasis Rev.*, **26**(2), pp. 225–239, 2007.

6. Jubb, A. M., Buffa, F. M., and Harris, A. L., Assessment of tumour hypoxia for prediction of response to therapy and cancer prognosis. *J. Cell. Mol. Med.*, **14**(1–2), pp. 18–29, 2010.

7. Vaupel, P., The Role of Hypoxia-Induced Factors in Tumor Progression. *Oncologist*, **9**(suppl 5), pp. 10–17, 2004.

8. Scanlon, S. E., and Glazer, P. M., Multifaceted control of DNA repair pathways by the hypoxic tumor microenvironment. *DNA Repair*, **32**, pp. 180–189, 2015.

9. Bindra, R. S., and Glazer, P. M., Genetic instability and the tumor microenvironment: towards the concept of microenvironment-induced mutagenesis. *Mutat. Res.-Fund. Mol. M.*, **569**(1–2), pp. 75–85, 2005.

10. Young, S. D., Marshall, R. S., and Hill, R. P., Hypoxia induces DNA over-replication and enhances metastatic potential of murine tumor cells. *P. Natl. Acad. Sci.USA.*, **85**(24), pp. 9533–9537, 1988.

11. Coquelle, A. *et al.*, A New Role for Hypoxia in Tumor Progression. *Mol. Cell*, **2**(2), pp. 259–265, 1998.

12. Dawson, Mark A., and Kouzarides, T., Cancer Epigenetics: From Mechanism to Therapy. *Cell*, **150**(1), pp. 12–27, 2012.

13. Tsai, Y.-P., and Wu, K.-J., Epigenetic regulation of hypoxia-responsive gene expression: Focusing on chromatin and DNA modifications. *Int. J. Cancer*, **134**(2), pp. 249–256, 2014.

14. Johnson, A. B., Denko, N., and Barton, M. C., Hypoxia induces a novel signature of chromatin modifications and global repression of transcription. *Mutat. Res.-Fund. Mol. M.*, **640**(1–2), pp. 174–179, 2008.

15. Lindahl, T., Instability and decay of the primary structure of DNA. *Nature*, **362**(6422), pp. 709–715, 1993.

16. Slupphaug, G., Kavli, B., and Krokan, H. E., The interacting pathways for prevention and repair of oxidative DNA damage. *Mutat. Res.-Fund. Mol. M.*, **531**(1–2), pp. 231–251, 2003.

17. Hammond, E. M. *et al.*, Hypoxia Links ATR and p53 through Replication Arrest. *Mol. Cell. Biol.*, **22**(6), pp. 1834–1843, 2002.

18. Hammond, E. M., Dorie, M. J., and Giaccia, A. J., ATR/ATM Targets Are Phosphorylated by ATR in Response to Hypoxia and ATM in Response to Reoxygenation. *J. Biol. Chem.*, **278**(14), pp. 12207–12213, 2003.

19. Varshavsky, A., On the possibility of metabolic control of replicon "misfiring": relationship to emergence of malignant phenotypes in mammalian cell lineages. *P. Natl. Acad. Sci. USA.*, **78**(6), pp. 3673–3677, 1981.

20. Rice, G. C., Hoy, C., and Schimke, R. T., Transient hypoxia enhances the frequency of dihydrofolate reductase gene amplification in Chinese hamster ovary cells. *P. Natl. Acad. Sci. USA.*, **83**(16), pp. 5978–5982, 1986.

21. Rice, G. C., Ling, V., and Schimke, R. T., Frequencies of independent and simultaneous selection of Chinese hamster cells for methotrexate and doxorubicin (adriamycin) resistance. *P. Natl. Acad. Sci. USA.*, **84**(24), pp. 9261–9264, 1987.

22. Seim, J. *et al.*, Hypoxia-induced irreversible S-phase arrest involves down-regulation of cyclin A. *Cell Proliferat.*, **36**(6), pp. 321–332, 2003.

23. Goda, N., Dozier, S. J., and Johnson, R. S., HIF-1 in cell cycle regulation, apoptosis, and tumor progression. *Antioxid Redox Signal*, **5**(4), pp. 467–73, 2003.

24. Graeber, T. G. *et al.*, Hypoxia induces accumulation of p53 protein, but activation of a G1-phase checkpoint by low-oxygen conditions is independent of p53 status. *Mol. Cell. Biol.*, **14**(9), pp. 6264–6277, 1994.

25. Green, S. L., Freiberg, R. A., and Giaccia, A. J., p21Cip1 and p27Kip1Regulate Cell Cycle Reentry after Hypoxic Stress but Are Not Necessary for Hypoxia-Induced Arrest. *Mol. Cell. Biol.*, **21**(4), pp. 1196–1206, 2001.

26. Gardner, L. B. *et al.*, Hypoxia Inhibits G1/S Transition through Regulation of p27 Expression. *J. Biol. Chem.*, **276**(11), pp. 7919–7926, 2001.

27. Brison, O., Gene amplification and tumor progression. *Biochimica et Biophysica Acta (BBA) — Rev. Cancer*, **1155**(1), pp. 25–41, 1993.

28. Coquelle, A. *et al.*, Expression of Fragile Sites Triggers Intrachromosomal Mammalian Gene Amplification and Sets Boundaries to Early Amplicons. *Cell*, **89**(2), pp. 215–225, 1997.

29. Luk, C. K. *et al.*, Effect of Transient Hypoxia on Sensitivity to Doxorubicin in Human and Murine Cell Lines. *J. Natl. Cancer Inst.*, **82**(8), pp. 684–692, 1990.

30. Coquelle, A. *et al.*, Induction of multiple double-strand breaks within an hsr by meganucleaseI-SceI expression or fragile site activation leads to formation of double minutes and other chromosomal rearrangements. *Oncogene*, **21**(50), pp. 7671–7679, 2002.

31. Hellman, A. *et al.*, A role for common fragile site induction in amplification of human oncogenes. *Cancer Cell*, **1**(1), pp. 89–97.

32. Smith, D.I., Huang, H., and Wang, L., Common fragile sites and cancer (review). *Int. J. Oncol*, **12**(1), pp. 187–96, 1998.

33. Reynolds, T. Y., Rockwell, S., and Glazer, P. M., Genetic Instability Induced by the Tumor Microenvironment. *Cancer Res.*, **56**(24), pp. 5754–5757, 1996.

34. Yuan, J. *et al.*, Diminished DNA Repair and Elevated Mutagenesis in Mammalian Cells Exposed to Hypoxia and Low pH. *Cancer Res.*, **60**(16), pp. 4372–4376, 2000.

35. Paquette, B., and Little, J. B., *In Vivo* Enhancement of Genomic Instability in Minisatellite Sequences of Mouse C3H/10T½ Cells Transformed *in vitro* by X-Rays. *Cancer Res.*, **54**(12), pp. 3173–3178, 1994.

36. Papp-Szabó, E., Josephy, P. D. and Coomber, B. L. Microenvironmental influences on mutagenesis in mammary epithelial cells. *Int. J. Cancer*, **116**(5), pp. 679–685, 2005.

37. Wilkinson, D. *et al.*, Hprt mutants in a transplantable murine tumour arise more frequently in vivo than *in vitro*. *Br. J. Cancer*, **72**(5), pp. 1234–1240, 1995.

38. Hammond, E. M., Green, S. L., and Giaccia, A. J., Comparison of hypoxia-induced replication arrest with hydroxyurea and aphidicolin-induced arrest. *Mutat. Res.-Fund. Mol. M.*, **532**(1–2), pp. 205–213, 2003.

39. Pires, I. M. *et al.*, Effects of Acute versus Chronic Hypoxia on DNA Damage Responses and Genomic Instability. *Cancer Res.*, **70**(3), pp. 925–935, 2010.

40. Hammond, E. M., and Giaccia, A. J., The role of ATM and ATR in the cellular response to hypoxia and re-oxygenation. DNA Repair, **3**(8–9), pp. 1117–1122, 2004.

41. Scanlon, S. E., and Glazer, P. M., Hypoxic Stress Facilitates Acute Activation and Chronic Downregulation of Fanconi Anemia Proteins. *Mol. Cancer Res.*, **12**(7), pp. 1016–1028, 2014.

42. Bencokova, Z. *et al.*, ATM Activation and Signaling under Hypoxic Conditions. *Mol. Cell. Biol.*, **29**(2), pp. 526–537, 2009.

43. Freiberg, R. A. *et al.*, DNA Damage during Reoxygenation Elicits a Chk2-Dependent Checkpoint Response. *Mol. Cell. Biol.*, **26**(5), pp. 1598–1609, 2006.

44. Freiberg, R. A. *et al.*, Checking in on hypoxia/reoxygenation. *Cell Cycle*, **5**(12), pp. 1304–1307, 2006.

45. Olcina, Monica M. *et al.* Replication Stress and Chromatin Context Link ATM Activation to a Role in DNA Replication. *Mol. Cell*, **52**(5), pp. 758–766, 2013.

46. Mihaylova, V. T. *et al.*, Decreased expression of the DNA mismatch repair gene Mlh1 under hypoxic stress in mammalian cells. *Mol. Cell. Biol.*, **23**(9), pp. 3265–3273, 2003.

47. Koshiji, M. *et al.*, HIF-1α induces genetic instability by transcriptionally downregulating MutSα expression. *Mol. Cell.*, **17**(6), pp. 793–803.

48. Bindra, R., Crosby, M., and Glazer, P., Regulation of DNA repair in hypoxic cancer cells. *Cancer Metastasis Rev.*, **26**(2), pp. 249–260, 2007.

49. Bindra, R. S., and Glazer, P. M., Co-repression of mismatch repair gene expression by hypoxia in cancer cells: Role of the Myc/Max network. *Cancer Lett.*, **252**(1), pp. 93–103, 2007.

50. Bindra, R. S. *et al.*, Down-regulation of Rad51 and decreased homologous recombination in hypoxic cancer cells. *Mol. Cell. Biol.*, **24**(19), pp. 8504–8518, 2004.

51. Bindra, R. S. *et al.*, Hypoxia-Induced Down-regulation of BRCA1 Expression by E2Fs. *Cancer Res.*, **65**(24), pp. 11597–11604, 2005.

52. Bindra, R. S. *et al.*, Alterations in DNA repair gene expression under hypoxia: elucidating the mechanisms of hypoxia-induced genetic instability. *Ann. NY. Acad. Sci.*, **1059**(1), pp. 184–195, 2005.

53. Chan, N. *et al.*, Chronic hypoxia decreases synthesis of homologous recombination proteins to offset chemoresistance and radioresistance. *Cancer Res.*, **68**(2), pp. 605–614, 2008.

54. Baxter, E. *et al.*, Epigenetic regulation in cancer progression. *Cell Biosci.*, **4**(1), pp. 1–11, 2014.

55. Chen, H. *et al.*, Hypoxic stress Induces dimethylated histone H3 lysine 9 through histone methyltransferase G9a in mammalian cells. *Cancer Res.*, **66**(18), pp. 9009–9016, 2006.

56. Tausendschön, M., Dehne, N., and Brüne, B., Hypoxia causes epigenetic gene regulation in macrophages by attenuating Jumonji histone demethylase activity. *Cytokine*, **53**(2), pp. 256–262, 2011.

57. Ramachandran, S. *et al.*, Epigenetic therapy for solid tumors: highlighting the impact of tumor hypoxia. *Genes*, **6**(4), p. 935, 2015.

58. Zhou, X. *et al.*, Hypoxia induces trimethylated H3 lysine 4 by inhibition of JARID1A demethylase. *Cancer Res.*, **70**(10), pp. 4214–4221, 2010.

59. Xia, X. *et al.*, Integrative analysis of HIF binding and transactivation reveals its role in maintaining histone methylation homeostasis. *P. Natl. Acad. Sci.*, **106**(11), pp. 4260–4265, 2009.

60. Watson, J. A. *et al.,* Epigenetics, the epicenter of the hypoxic response. *Epigenetics*, **5**(4), pp. 293–296, 2010.

61. Santos-Rosa, H., and Caldas, C., Chromatin modifier enzymes, the histone code and cancer. *Eur. J. Cancer*, **41**(16), pp. 2381–2402, 2005.

62. Verger, A., and Crossley, M., DNA damage repair and transcription. *Cell. Mol. Life Sci.* (CMLS), **61**(17), pp. 2154–2162, 2004.

63. Krieg, A. J. *et al.,* Regulation of the histone demethylase JMJD1A by hypoxia-inducible factor $1\alpha$ enhances hypoxic gene expression and tumor growth. *Mol. Cell. Biol.*, **30**(1), pp. 344–353, 2010.

64. Beyer, S. *et al.,* The histone Demethylases JMJD1A and JMJD2B are transcriptional targets of hypoxia-inducible factor HIF. *J. Biol. Chem.*, **283**(52), pp. 36542–36552, 2008.

65. Pollard, P. J. *et al.,* Regulation of Jumonji-domain-containing histone demethylases by hypoxia-inducible factor (HIF)-1alpha. *Biochem J.*, **416**(3), pp. 387–394, 2008.

66. Kim, M.S. *et al.,* Histone deacetylases induce angiogenesis by negative regulation of tumor suppressor genes. *Nat. Med.*, **7**(4), pp. 437–443, 2001.

67. Jaenisch, R., and Bird, A., Epigenetic regulation of gene expression: how the genome integrates intrinsic and environmental signals. *Nat. Genet.*, 2003.

68. Recillas-Targa, F., DNA Methylation, Chromatin Boundaries, and Mechanisms of Genomic Imprinting. *Arch. Med. Res.*, **33**(5), pp. 428–438, 2002.

69. Watson, J. A. *et al.,* Generation of an epigenetic signature by chronic hypoxia in prostate cells. *Human Mol. Genet.*, **18**(19), pp. 3594–3604, 2009.

70. Shahrzad, S. *et al.,* Induction of DNA hypomethylation by tumor hypoxia. *Epigenetics*, **2**(2), pp. 119–125, 2007.

71. Koslowski, M. *et al.,* Tumor-associated CpG demethylation augments hypoxia-induced effects by positive autoregulation of HIF-1[alpha]. *Oncogene*, **30**(7), pp. 876–882, 2011.

72. Bernstein, B. E. *et al.,* A Bivalent Chromatin Structure Marks Key Developmental Genes in Embryonic Stem Cells. *Cell*, **125**(2), pp. 315–326, 2006.

73. Lu, Y. *et al.,* Hypoxia-Induced Epigenetic Regulation and Silencing of the BRCA1 Promoter. *Mol. Cell. Biol.*, **31**(16), pp. 3339–3350, 2011.

74. Lu, Y. *et al.,* Silencing of the DNA Mismatch Repair Gene <em>MLH1 </em> Induced by Hypoxic Stress in a Pathway Dependent on the Histone Demethylase LSD1. *Cell Rep.*, **8**(2), pp. 501–513, 2014.

75. Esteller, M. *et al.,* A Gene Hypermethylation Profile of Human Cancer. *Cancer Res.*, **61**(8), pp. 3225–3229, 2001.

76.	Mirza, S. *et al.,* Promoter hypermethylation of TMS1, BRCA1, ER$\alpha$ and PRB in serum and tumor DNA of invasive ductal breast carcinoma patients. *Life Sci.,* **81**(4), pp. 280–287, 2007.

77.	Vasilatos, S. N. *et al.,* CpG Island Tumor Suppressor Promoter Methylation in Non-BRCA-Associated Early Mammary Carcinogenesis. *Cancer Epidem. Biomar.,* **18**(3), pp. 901–914, 2009.

78.	Jin, W. *et al.,* UHRF1 is associated with epigenetic silencing of BRCA1 in sporadic breast cancer. *Breast Cancer Res. Tr.,* **123**(2), pp. 359–373, 2010.

79.	Ooi, S. K. T. *et al.,* DNMT3L connects unmethylated lysine 4 of histone H3 to *de novo* methylation of DNA. *Nature,* **448**(7154), pp. 714–717, 2007.

80.	Rodríguez-Jiménez, F. J. *et al.,* Hypoxia Causes Downregulation of Mismatch Repair System and Genomic Instability in Stem Cells. *Stem Cells,* **26**(8), pp. 2052–2062, 2008.

81.	Nakamura, H. *et al.,* Human mismatch repair gene, MLH1, is transcriptionally repressed by the hypoxia-inducible transcription factors, DEC1 and DEC2. *Oncogene,* **27**(30), pp. 4200–4209, 2008.

82.	Li, Q. *et al.,* Binding of the JmjC Demethylase JARID1B to LSD1/NuRD Suppresses Angiogenesis and Metastasis in Breast Cancer Cells by Repressing Chemokine CCL14. *Cancer Res.,* **71**(21), pp. 6899–6908, 2011.

83.	Lee, J.-m., Ledermann, J. A., and Kohn, E. C., PARP Inhibitors for BRCA1/2 mutation-associated and BRCA-like malignancies. *Annals of Oncology,* **25**(1), pp. 32–40, 2014.

84.	Helleday, T., Putting poly (ADP-ribose) polymerase and other DNA repair inhibitors into clinical practice. *Curr. Opin. Oncol.,* **25**(6), pp. 609–614, 2013.

85.	Carvalho, J. F., and Kanaar, R., Targeting homologous recombination-mediated DNA repair in cancer. *Expert Opin Ther Targets,* **18**(4), pp. 427–458, 2014.

86.	Aebi, S. *et al.,* Loss of DNA mismatch repair in acquired resistance to cisplatin. *Cancer Res.,* **56**(13), pp. 3087–3090, 1996.

87.	Brown, R. *et al.,* hMLH1 expression and cellular responses of ovarian tumour cells to treatment with cytotoxic anticancer agents. *Oncogene,* **15**(1), pp. 45–52, 1997.

# Chapter 8

# Regulation of the Hypoxic Response by Non-coding RNAs

Xin Huang*

*Magee-Womens Research Institute, Department of Obstetrics, Gynecology and Reproductive Sciences, University of Pittsburgh, School of Medicine, Pittsburgh, PA, USA
Women's Cancer Research Center, University of Pittsburgh, Cancer Institute, Pittsburgh, PA, USA
*huangx2@upmc.edu*

Hypoxia is a hallmark of solid tumors and is correlated with a poor clinical outcome in cancer patients, independent of tumor size, stage, histology, grade, and nodal status. Due to its clinical significance, much effort has been invested in understanding the mechanism of gene regulation in the hypoxic tumor microenvironment. Recent advances have suggested that, in addition to protein-coding genes, non-coding RNAs (ncRNAs) may play important roles in the adaptive response to low oxygen in tumors. These ncRNAs include long non-coding RNAs (lincRNAs), microR-NAs, transfer RNAs, natural anti-sense RNAs, and transcripts from ultraconserved genomic regions. To date, the best characterized hypoxia-responsive ncRNA is microRNA-210 (miR-210). miR-210 is a robust target of hypoxia-inducible factor 1 (HIF1) with diverse functions that regulate almost every aspect of cellular hypoxic response. More ncRNAs in the hypoxia pathway are expected to be discovered because of rapid advancement and quick adaptation of new sequencing technologies. Regulation of these ncRNAs may affect tumor development in numerous ways. Thus, a better understanding of the function of these ncRNAs may lead to novel cancer diagnostic biomarkers and therapeutics.

## 1. Introduction

Hypoxia, the condition of insufficient oxygen supply to tissues, results from a reduction in oxygen availability, inadequate oxygen transport, or the inability of the tissues to utilize oxygen. In normal tissues, high altitude exposure, anemia, and drugs can induce hypoxia responsive pathways in the body. Cells react to hypoxia in part via a transcriptional program that is largely orchestrated by the core component of the hypoxia-sensing machinery, the hypoxia-inducible factors (HIFs).[1,2] HIFs are heterodimers consisting of an oxygen sensitive alpha subunit (HIF-$\alpha$) and a constitutively active beta subunit (HIF-1$\beta$, also called aryl hydrocarbon receptor nuclear translocator (ARNT)). Among the three homologous HIF-$\alpha$ genes, HIF-1$\alpha$, HIF-2$\alpha$, and HIF-3$\alpha$, the functions of HIF-1$\alpha$ and HIF-2$\alpha$ are best characterized. HIF-1$\alpha$ is ubiquitously expressed in essentially all tissue types, while HIF-2$\alpha$ expression is more tissue-specific.[3] Although our understanding of HIF-3$\alpha$ function lags behind, recent advance has started to reveal its function in gene regulation under hypoxic conditions.[4] Under normoxia, HIF-$\alpha$ is hydoxylated by prolyl-4-hydroxylases (PHDs), targeting it for proteasome destruction mediated by the von Hippel–Lindau (VHL) protein, an E3 ubiquitin ligase.[5,6] Under hypoxic conditions, the activity of PHDs decreases and HIF-$\alpha$ is stabilized and forms a dimer with HIF-1$\alpha$. The HIF-$\alpha$/HIF-1$\beta$ dimer is then translocated into the nucleus and binds specifically to the promoters of target genes involved in adaptation and protection against low oxygen conditions.[7]

Hypoxia is also a hallmark of solid tumors, where cancer cells preferably utilize glycolysis even when the oxygen supply is plentiful.[8] Compared to normal tissues where the distance between blood vessels is carefully regulated, the vasculature of solid tumors is comparatively disorganized, with many irregularities and abnormalities, and a wide variation in the distance between blood vessels.[9] The abnormalities in tumor vasculature and the exaggerated intercapillary spacing lead to hypoxic microenvironments that do not exist in normal tissues.[10] This unique tumor microenvironment inhibits access of traditional anti-cancer agents to hypoxic tumor cells.[11] Tumor cells in these hypoxic zones are also relatively quiescent, which renders them refractory to most cancer chemotherapies that typically target the rapidly proliferating cells.[12] This intratumor hypoxic state leads to upregulation of genes that confer resistance to chemotherapeutic drugs and radiotherapy, as well as genes that play a major role in initiating angiogenesis. In addition, tumor-associated hypoxia tends to select for cells that possess a profoundly malignant, metastatic phenotype,[13–15] which ultimately contributes to treatment relapse. As a consequence, tumor hypoxia has been associated with poor clinical outcome and is a negative prognostic indicator.[12] Thus, tumor hypoxia represents a compelling target for therapeutic intervention, and better understanding of hypoxia gene regulation will provide novel targets for cancer treatment.[16] Although it is well known that there are hundreds, if not thousands, of genes involved in adaptation to and protection against low oxygen conditions,[7] in this review, we will focus on the non-protein coding fraction of the transcriptome that are responsive to hypoxic conditions, many of which have only recently been discovered.

## 2. Non-coding RNAs — Not "Junk" Any More

Following the completion of the Human Genome Project, it was a surprise that the protein coding sequence only accounts for 1.1% of the entire human genome.[17] The rest was called genome "dark matter" or "junk DNA," without any coding capacity or obvious function. Since that time, it has been estimated that at least 80% of the human genome contains functional sequences, either transcribing ncRNAs or being involved in chromatin-associated regulatory function.[18] Given the pressure of natural selection that has shaped the human genome during evolution, it is unlikely that these non-coding transcripts are conserved in the human genome merely as "noises" to protein-coding gene transcription.

Over the last decade, largely owing to the rapid development of microarray and next generation sequencing technologies, the "dark matter" of the human genome has slowly been unveiled to encode tens of thousands of ncRNAs, including small nuclear RNAs (snRNAs), transfer RNAs (tRNAs), small interfering RNAs (siRNAs), piwi-associated RNAs (piRNAs), natural anti-sense RNAs (NATs), microRNAs (miRNAs), enhancer region RNAs (eRNAs), and long non-coding RNAs (lncRNAs). Despite their being incapable of being translated into proteins, many of them are known or suspected to regulate biological functions in almost any imaginable fashion. The transcription of miRNAs, lncRNAs, and NATs has been demonstrated to be regulated by HIFs under hypoxic conditions.[19] Thus, we will focus on these three classes of ncRNAs in this review. We will also briefly discuss the implication of recent findings regarding tRNA-derived RNA fragments (tRFs) that are processed under hypoxia. Figure 1 is a brief summary of the ncRNAs that have been discovered in the hypoxic pathway.

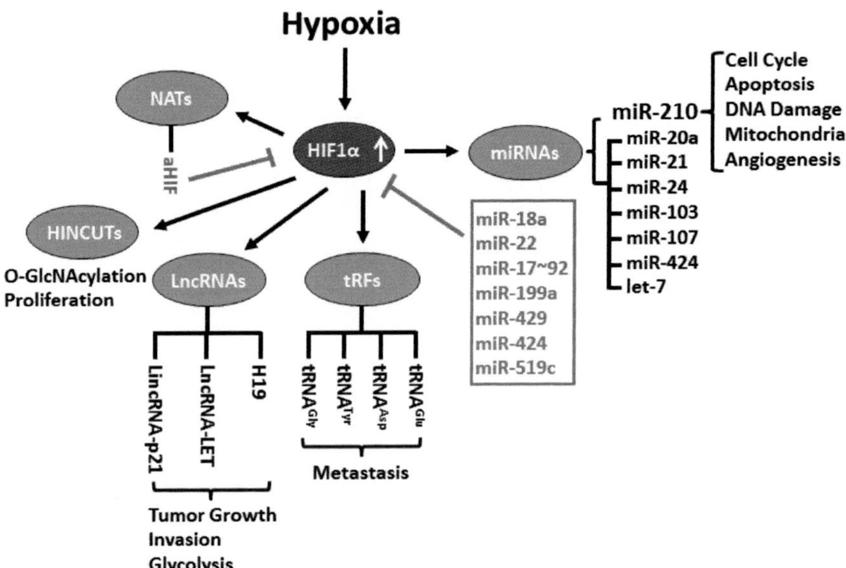


Fig. 1.   A summary of ncRNAs that have been discovered in the hypoxic pathway. The majority of ncRNAs is induced by HIF-1α. The ncRNAs that regulate HIF-1α were highlighted in grey.

# 3. Transfer RNA-Derived RNA Fragments (tRFs)

tRNAs play a central role in protein translation, acting as carriers of amino acids during peptide elongation. Although tRNAs are among the most abundant ncRNAs in the cell, only a small fraction of tRNAs are cleaved to produce tRFs, a class of single-stranded non-coding small RNAs, 18–25 nucleotides in length.[20] tRFs are abundant in cells and have been shown to be essential in cell proliferation and stress response.[21] tRNAs are cleaved by endoribonucleases, such as Dicer or Angiogenin to give rise to tRFs.[20,22] Interestingly, hypoxic stress can induce specific tRFs,[23] but their function remained largely unknown until a recent study that provided some mechanistic insight on hypoxia-induced tRFs as suppressors of breast cancer metastasis.[24] In this study, the authors found that a class of tRFs, derived from tRNA$^{Glu}$, tRNA$^{Asp}$, tRNA$^{Gly}$, and tRNA$^{Tyr}$, are induced, under hypoxic conditions, specifically in breast cancer cells with a low metastatic potential. These tRFs can suppress the stability of several onco-genic transcripts in breast cancer cells by displacing their 3′untranslated regions (UTRs) from the RNA-binding protein YBX1. Provocatively, the authors found that highly metastatic breast cancer cells attenuate the hypoxic induction of these tRFs and thus evade this tumor-suppressive mechanism. It is well known that a plethora of pro-metastatic genes, such as *LOX*, *CTGF*, and *VEGF*,[25–27] can be induced under hypoxia, which is a known factor contributing to a poor clinical outcome in cancer patients. The discovery of these hypoxia-inducible tRFs presents a new paradigm of hypoxia regulation of cancer cell metastasis. We believe this elegant study is merely the tip of the iceberg, that more hypoxia-induced tRFs will be discovered in the near future, and that their functions are likely to expand into additional aspects of cancer biology.

# 4. lncRNAs

"lncRNA" may be loosely defined as ncRNA molecules longer than 200 nucleotides.[28] *XIST*, a master regulator of X chromosome inactivation,[29] may be the best known lncRNA. *XIST* is transcribed from the X chromo-some and serves as a center to initiate and spread X inactivation in *cis*.[30] The discovery of the *HOTAIR* lncRNA demonstrated for the first time that lncRNA can function in *trans*.[31] It is generally believed that transacting lncRNAs function as a scaffold to facilitate the formation of ribonucleo-protein (RNP) complexes with numerous chromatin regulators and tran-scription factors to regulate target gene expression.[28] Despite the recent rapid progress of lncRNA study, the role of hypoxia in regulating lncRNA expression has just started to be appreciated. Given the large number of lncRNAs that have been discovered[32] and rapid technical advancement, the number of hypoxia-inducible lncRNAs is expected to increase signifi-cantly in the near future.

## 4.1. H19

H19 is best known as a maternally imprinted lncRNA.[33] H19 is robustly induced under hypoxic conditions, and its induction is abolished by HIF-1$\alpha$ knockdown.[34,35] Although H19 has been shown as a primary pre-cursor for miR-675,[36] miR-675 has not been reported as a hypoxia-inducible miRNA to date. Thus, it remains unclear whether miR-675 is a mediator of H19 function under hypoxia or is merely an RNA splicing byproduct in this context. H19 has been reported as a promoter of tumori-genesis in numerous cancers,[34,37,38] consistent with the general role of hypoxia in promoting tumor progression. However, the mechanism of hypoxia-induced H19 function remains largely unknown at present.

## 4.2. lincRNA-p21

Long intergenic non-coding RNAs (lincRNAs) are a subgroup of lncRNA that are transcribed from non-coding DNA sequences between protein-coding genes.[39] lincRNA-p21 was first identified as a p53-responsive ncRNA that represses p53-dependent transcription in mouse cells.[40] Interestingly, lincRNA-p21 selectively regulates the apoptotic pathway but not the cell cycle arrest pathway downstream of the p53 response. Recently, a bioinformatic search identified the presence of hypoxia-responsive elements in the promoter and exon 2 of the lincRNA-p21 gene in humans.[41] Expression of lincRNA-p21 can be induced by HIF-1$\alpha$, but not HIF-2$\alpha$, to regulate hypoxia-enhanced glycolysis. Mechanistically, hypoxia-induced lincRNA-p21 binds HIF-1$\alpha$ and VHL and disrupts the

VHL/HIF-1$\alpha$ interaction. Attenuated VHL-mediated HIF-1$\alpha$ ubiquitination leads to HIF-1$\alpha$ stabilization and, consequently, to enhanced glycolysis. Surprisingly, unlike its mouse counterpart, expression of human lincRNA-p21 is not regulated by p53 under hypoxia, and human lincRNA-p21 has no role in doxorubicin-induced apoptosis. We believe that this may be explained, at least partially, by the lack of conservation between human and mouse lincRNA-p21 that is commonly seen among lncRNAs.[42]

## 4.3. lncRNA-LET

lncRNA-light energy transfer (LET) is relatively less well studied, with only a handful of publications to date, all in the context of cancer. Expression of lncRNA-LET is frequently downregulated in hepatocellular and squamous-cell lung carcinomas and in gastric, cervical, and colorectal cancers.[43–45] lncRNA-LET expression is repressed under 1% oxygen through promoter histone deacetylation that is mediated by hypoxia-induced HDAC3 expression.[43] lncRNA-LET can bind NF90, a double-stranded RNA-binding protein, to decreases HIF-1$\alpha$ and cell division cycle 42 (CDC42) mRNA stability. The lncRNA-LET/NF90/HIF-1$\alpha$ axis and the lncRNA-LET/NF90/CDC42 axis may be partially responsible for cancer cell invasiveness under hypoxic and normoxic conditions, respectively. Thus, lncRNA-LET presents another example of the complexity of hypoxia gene regulation.

## 4.4. Hypoxia-induced non-coding ultraconserved transcripts (HINCUTs)

In the human genome, segments that are longer than 200 base pairs with 100% conservation between orthologous regions of the human, rat, and mouse genomes are called ultraconserved regions (UCRs).[46] It was found that UCRs encode ncRNAs that are dysregulated in human cancers,[47] suggesting a functional role for these ncRNAs in tumorigenesis. Recently, UCR-encoded ncRNAs have been found to be induced by hypoxia.[48] This class of lncRNAs, also termed "HINCUTs," may play important roles in mediating functions in the hypoxia response pathways. One of the

HINCUTS, HINCUT-1, has been demonstrated to regulate cell proliferation and optimal O-GlcNAcylation of proteins specifically under hypoxic conditions. However, the biological functions and mechanisms of action remain elusive for the majority of HINCUTs.

## 5.  NATs

NATs are a class of ncRNAs that are transcribed from the opposite strand of a coding gene and capable of regulating the expression of their sense gene pair or of several related genes.[49] Transcription of NATs is ubiquitous in the mammalian genome and NATs can regulate the gene transcribed from the sense strand.[50,51] Hypoxia regulation of NAT expression was first reported in 1999.[52] The NAT, aHIF was found to be specifically over-expressed in all non-papillary clear-cell renal cell carcinomas, a tumor type with mutations of the *VHL* gene and subsequent constitutive stabilization of HIF-1$\alpha$. The aHIF transcript has an 882-nucleotide overlap with the 3'UTR of HIF-1$\alpha$ and is robustly induced under hypoxic conditions, suggesting it as a potential HIF-1$\alpha$ target. It was later confirmed that the aHIF promoter does contain several functional hypoxia-responsive elements (HREs) and that both HIF-1$\alpha$ and HIF-2$\alpha$ can regulate the HREs.[53,54] Different kinetics of HIF-1$\alpha$ and HIF-2$\alpha$ accumulation, under prolonged hypoxia, have long been observed, with a quick stabilization of HIF-1$\alpha$ at the beginning of hypoxia but levels gradually decreasing after 10–12 hours, while HIF-2$\alpha$ levels stayed relatively constant once stabilized. The sequence complementarity between the 5'aHIF transcript and the 3'UTR of HIF-1$\alpha$ provides a plausible explanation for this phenomenon: that is, aHIF can specifically bind to HIF-1$\alpha$ transcript and thus destabilize HIF-1$\alpha$ mRNA under prolonged hypoxia. Despite the rapid development of sequencing technology and the recent explosion in knowledge on ncRNAs, there is currently only a nascent understanding of hypoxia regulation of NAT. We expect that much is to be learned in the near future.

## 6.  miRNAs

miRNAs are single-stranded non-coding small RNA molecules (~22 nucleotides in length). Genes encoding miRNAs are initially transcribed by RNA polymerase II as part of much longer primary transcripts (pri-miRNAs),[55,56] typically containing the cap structure and the poly(A) tails. In the second step, pri-miRNAs are processed by the nuclear RNase III Drosha, leading to ~70-nucleotide hairpin-shaped intermediates, termed precursor miRNAs (pre-miRNAs). Pre-miRNAs are subsequently exported out of the nucleus by exportin-5 and cleaved by the cytoplasmic RNase III Dicer into a *short* miRNA duplex. One strand of this short-lived duplex is degraded, while the other strand is retained as mature miRNA and incorporated into the RNA-induced silencing complex (RISC), an RNA-protein complex with proteins from the Argonaute family.[57] The mature miRNA guides the RISC to recognize its target mRNA based on sequence complementarity, most importantly between the "seed region" of mature miRNAs, nucleotides 2–8, and the 3′ UTRs of their target genes, which generally leads to translation inhibition and/or mRNA degradation.[58,59] Because usually a perfect sequence complementarity is only required between the "seed region" of a miRNA and the 3′ UTR of its target mRNA, theoretically, a single miRNA can regulate multiple mRNAs, often hundreds, and the 3′ UTR of an mRNA may contain several miRNA-recognition sequences in its 3′UTR. This relative lack of specificity poses significant challenges for identifying authentic miRNA targets and also dictates the way miRNAs regulate their target genes — by exerting relatively mild influences over a large number of targets.[60,61]

Although such cases are much fewer in number, miRNAs have also been found to bind to the 5′ UTRs or in the gene coding region of their target genes,[62,63] suggesting that miRNAs can bind to virtually any region in their target transcripts, greatly expanding the number of their potential targets and making precise prediction of miRNA targets a challenge. In addition to their canonical function of repressing target gene expression, miRNAs have also been identified to activate target gene transcription or enhance protein translation,[64–66] further complicating decipherment of the mechanisms of miRNA function. According to the most recent count (miRBase Release 21, retrieved from http://www.mirbase.org), 2,809 mature miRNAs have been identified in the human genome. Experimental evidence has demonstrated that miRNAs are regulators of almost every aspect of cellular function.[67] Given the large number of miRNAs discovered to date and the versatile functions they may have, we believe that essentially all genes, protein-coding genes or ncRNAs, are subject to miRNA regulation.

In this review, we are focusing on miRNA function in cancer biology. Evidence of aberrant miRNA expression has been presented in all cancers.[68,69] While the mechanisms behind specific miRNA expression profiles in different tumors remain largely obscure, recent advances in cancer genome sequencing have provided some clues; frequent mutations of DROSHA and DICER, key members of the miRNA biogenesis pathway, have been found in certain cancers.[70–72] Understanding of miRNA responses to microenvironment stresses and oncogenic alterations have also provided useful clues.[73,74] As one of the most important microenvironment factors during tumor initiation and development, tumor hypoxia has been found to influence miRNA expression, while miRNAs have also been found to regulate many aspects of cellular hypoxic response.[75–82] In the sections below, we will summarize current knowledge of miRNAs involvement in the hypoxic response pathway, discuss challenges we face in elucidating their functions, and speculate about opportunities for using miRNAs for cancer diagnosis and treatment.

## 6.1. miRNAs that regulate HIF-1$\alpha$

HIF-1$\alpha$ is the major transcriptional factor that regulates cellular response to a hypoxic microenvironment.[83] Thus, it is not surprising that miRNAs have been identified that modulate the hypoxic pathway both upstream and downstream of HIF-1$\alpha$. miR-18a, the miR-17–92 cluster, miR-22, miR-199a, miR-210, miR-429, and miR-519c have been demonstrated to repress HIF1$\alpha$ expression by directly binding to the 3′ UTR of HIF-1$\alpha$ in a variety of cells,[84–90] affecting functions that are known to be tightly linked to HIF-1$\alpha$, such as tumor metastasis, angiogenesis, and immune function. Interestingly, two of these miRNAs, miR-429, and miR-210, are also induced by HIF-1$\alpha$; thus, they form negative feedback loops that fine-tune the cellular hypoxic response regulated by HIF-1$\alpha$.[88,89]

Just like anything in nature, if there is a Ying, there must be a Yang: miRNAs that upregulate HIF-1$\alpha$ have also been identified. miR-424, a hypoxia-inducible miRNA in human endothelial cells, can target cullin 2 (CUL2), a scaffolding protein critical to the assembly of the ubiquitin ligase system, to stabilize HIF-1$\alpha$.[91] miR-494 was found to be induced to a maximal level in a human hepatic cell line when the cells were exposed to 1% oxygen for only four hours, suggesting miR-494 as an early responder to the hypoxia challenge.[92] Although the exact mechanism remains unclear, the authors suggested that miR-494 can upregulate HIF-1$\alpha$ gene transcription by activating the PI3K/AKT pathway. Compared to the rapid progress we have made in elucidating the function of miRNAs induced by HIF1$\alpha$, a lot more is yet to be learned about miRNAs that regulate the HIFs. Given the nature of miRNA regulation of their targets, we are unlikely to identify miRNAs that can function as on-and-off switches for HIFs, but these miRNAs may still play important roles in cell type or context-specific manners.

## 6.2. miRNAs induced under hypoxia

In the past several years, a plethora of hypoxia-induced miRNAs have been identified in a variety of cells with diverse genetic background, such as miR-20a, miR-21, miR-24, miR-103, miR-107, miR-210, miR-424, and let-7.[76,80,91,93–95] Many of these miRNAs are only reported in limited studies, indicating a tissue- or cell type-specific hypoxic response of miRNA expression. However, miR-210 stands out as the only miRNA consistently and robustly induced under hypoxic conditions in essentially all experimental systems, suggesting that miR-210 is the dominant responder, in the miRNA realm, to hypoxic stress. The following sections will focus on miR-210's role in cancer biology.

### 6.2.1. *miR-210, a marker for tumor hypoxia*

miR-210 has been identified as a HIF-1$\alpha$ target in a majority of experiments.[96] HIF-1$\alpha$ directly binds an HRE on the proximal miR-210 promoter.[80] This HRE site is highly conserved across species, indicating the importance of hypoxia in regulating miR-210 expression. This highly conserved HRE was confirmed to be the functional HRE that is responsible for the robust hypoxic induction of mouse miR-210 expression.[97] Our discovery that miR-210 expression is correlated with a gene expression signature of tumor hypoxia in primary head and neck tumors[80] further support the notion that miR-210 expression may reflect the *in vivo* hypoxic microenvironment of solid tumors.

miR-210 is upregulated in most solid tumors, and its levels correlate with a negative clinical outcome.[77,98–103] Strikingly, when these studies were pooled for a meta-analysis, elevated miR-210 was found to be a strong prognostic factor of poor patient survival for a variety of carcinomas.[104,105] These observations were supported by the finding that miR-210 belongs to a pan-cancer, coregulated oncogenic miRNA "superfamily," which cotargets critical tumor suppressors via a central GUGC core seed motif.[106] However, whether these close associations between miR-210 expression and poor survival in cancer patients actually reflect a pro-oncogenic role for miR-210 remains controversial. Because miR-210 is such a robust HIF-1$\alpha$ target, its overexpression in these tumors may merely reflect the *in vivo* state of tumor hypoxia, a well-established prognostic factor for poor patient outcomes[12] but irrelevant to any role it may play during tumorigenesis. In support of this argument, we have found that ectopic expression of miR-210 suppresses xenograft tumor initiation by downregulating *HOXA1* and other potential tumor promoting genes,[80] suggesting a tumor suppressor function of miR-210. Our study was further supported by findings that miR-210 could repress a host of genes that are critical for mitosis, such as *Cdc25B*, *Plk1*, *E2F3*, and *Ccnf*.[79,107] Thus, we should be cautious in inferring potential miR-210 function on the basis of its ubiquitous overexpression in human cancers before its role in tumorigenesis is better defined using spontaneous cancer models in animals with miR-210 knockout.

## 6.2.2. *miR-210 target identification*

Currently, the most frequently employed approach to identifying miRNA targets is through computational prediction, which is based on the complementarity of target gene 3′ UTR sequence to the "seed region" sequence of a miRNA.[108] Due to the short seed sequence required (only 6–7 nucleotides) for miRNA binding to the 3′ UTR of their targets, reliably predicting miRNA targets has always been a bioinformatics challenge. Any given miRNA may be predicted to regulate hundreds of target genes. When the search is extended to the 5′UTR, the coding region, or even "seedless" targets,[109,110] the number of potential miRNA targets is expected to be even higher. Thus, false positive prediction has become the major limitation for computational prediction. Furthermore, due to insufficient understanding of how miRNAs recruit and bind their targets, algorithms used for prediction sometimes generate drastically different lists of target genes, with little overlap.[60] Thus, predicted targets are usually used as a guide for experimental validation of biologically relevant miRNA target genes.

Theoretically, proteomic profiling is best suited for unbiased and comprehensive identification of miRNA targets. This approach has been successfully utilized in numerous studies.[111–113] However, the lack of sufficient sensitivity and the requirement of sophisticated and expensive equipment for proteomics have prevented broad application of this promising strategy.

A major mechanism that miRNAs utilize to downregulate their target genes is to degrade their mRNAs[114,115]; this can be reliably detected by microarray or whole transcriptome RNA sequencing (RNA-Seq). This strategy has been used successfully in identifying miR-210 targets.[116,117] However, this approach may miss authentic targets because miRNA can inhibit target gene protein translation without disturbing their mRNA expression.[61] To overcome this problem, Argonaute protein immunoprecipitation (miRNP-IP) has been used prior to microarray or RNA-Seq to identify targets that directly interact with miRNAs.[118] miRNP-IP has been successfully used to identify miR-210 targets.[80,119] To further improve the specificity of miRNP-IP, ultraviolet irradiation has been used to covalently crosslink RNA–Argonaute protein complexes, allowing them to be more stringently purified. This approach, termed crosslinking immunoprecipitation (CLIP), can be used to identify miRNA targets with a high confidence.[120,121] However, no published report has utilized this promising approach for miR-210 target identification yet.

With the lowering cost of RNA-Seq, the combination of more accurate computational algorithms and miRNP-IP/CLIP will provide more complete and accurate identification of physiologically relevant miR-210 targets. The function of some of these reported miR-210 target genes will be further discussed below.

### 6.2.3. *miR-210 regulates DNA damage response*

Cellular responses to DNA damage involve complex mechanisms that detect and repair genomic lesions. Severe hypoxia (< 0.1% Oxygen) is known to induce replication arrest, which subsequently can initiate a unique DNA damage response (DDR) that includes both ATR- and ATM-mediated signaling.[122] We have found that miR-210 is robustly induced under anoxic condition,[80] raising an interesting question as to whether miR-210 may be involved in the hypoxia-induced DDR. The discovery that miR-210 targets *RAD52*,[119,123] a key gene in the homologous recombination (HR)-mediated repair of double-strand breaks (DSBs), shed new light on the mechanism of compromised HR repair activity in hypoxic cells.[124] miR-210's role in repressing cellular DDR is further supported by a study in which expression of miR-210 leads to double-strand DNA breaks in cultured Fibroblasts.[209] Paradoxically, overexpressing miR-210 in lung cancer cells led to accelerated clearance of DSB foci following radiation,[125] suggesting that miR-210 expression promotes a more efficient DSB repair and thus contributes to radioresistance in cancer cells. Given the significance of DDR in cancer therapy, miR-210's role in DDR warrants further study.

### 6.2.4. *miR-210 regulation of apoptosis*

Apoptosis is essential for tissue homeostasis in multicellular organisms. HIF-1$\alpha$ plays a well-established role in regulating apoptotic pathways under hypoxia.[126] As the most consistently hypoxia-induced miRNA, miR-210 has been shown to regulate apoptosis. The majority of evidence supports an anti-apoptotic property of miR-210; expression of miR-210 can protect cells from apoptosis,[76,127–130] while downregulation of miR-210 leads to apoptosis.[76,78,131–134] Several targets have been identified to mediate miR-210's anti-apoptotic function in various experimental systems, such as *E2F3*,[131] *Ptp1b* (also named *PTPN1*),[129,135] caspase-8-associated protein-2 (*CASP8AP2*),[127,136] and mitochondrion-associated, 3 (*AIFM3*).[133] However, the majority of these targets has only been vigorously validated, making it difficult to generalize these findings.

Despite overall evidence suggesting an anti-apoptotic function for miR-210, a recent report suggested that miR-210 may have a pro-apoptotic function through targeting anti-apoptotic protein BCL2 to mediate hypoxia-induced apoptosis in neuroblastoma cells.[137] However, this result is disputed by another study, where overexpressing miR-210 suppressed apoptosis concurrent with increased BCL2 level.[138] The HIF-1$\alpha$/miR-210/*BCL2* axis has also been implicated in the autophagy.[139] In the study, HIF-1$\alpha$ induces miRNA-210, which in turn, enhances autophagy and reduces radiosensitivity by downregulating *BCL2* expression in colon cancer cells. When miR-210 expression is suppressed, *BCL2* expression is upregulated, leading to apoptosis of colon cancer cells after radiation treatment.

In summary, the vast majority of evidence supports an anti-apoptotic function for miR-210. However, the mechanism of the miR-210-mediated anti-apoptotic function remains elusive.

## 6.2.5. *miR-210 regulation of cell cycle*

It is well established that HIF-1$\alpha$ is essential for hypoxia-induced cell cycle arrest.[140] Now, accumulating evidence suggests that miR-210 may also play a role in this process. One of the best characterized miR-210 targets on cell cycle control is *E2F3*, a promoter of the G1/S transition.[141] *E2F3* has been reported to be a miR-210 target in ovarian cancer,[79] clear cell renal cell carcinoma,[142] ischemic wounds and keratinocytes,[143] and HEK293 cells.[119] In addition to *E2F3*, fibroblast growth factor receptor-like 1 (*FGFRL1*) was also identified as a miR-210 target involved in cell cycle control.[144] Decreased miR-210 expression in esophageal squamous cell carcinomas released *FGFRL1* from miR-210 repression, leading to accelerated cell cycle progression. In contrast, overexpressed miR-210 induces cell cycle arrest in G1/G0 and G2/M phases.[144] This work is further supported by a recent report showing that miR-210 overexpression or knockdown of *FGFRL1* suppressed cell proliferation by increasing head and neck cancer cells in G1/G0 phase while reducing cells in S and G2/M phases.[145] Furthermore, when cells ectopically expressing miR-210 were implanted into nude mice, tumor growth was significantly suppressed compared to vector controls. However, when *FGFRL1* is coexpressed, tumor growth inhibition can be partially alleviated, consistent with our early report.[80] Additional work has suggested that miR-210 may have a much broader effect on cell cycle regulation, as a group of mitosis-related genes, including *Plk1*, *Cdc25B*, Cyclin F, *Bub1B*, and *Fam83D*, have been identified as direct miR-210 targets.[107]

In contrast to its role in suppressing cell cycle progression by targeting *E2F3* and *FGFRL1*, miR-210 can also promote cell cycle progression by downregulating *MNT*.[81,116,146] *MNT* is a member of the *MYC/MAX/MAD* network with a basic-helix-loop-helix-zipper domain and represses *MYC* target genes by binding the E box DNA sequence (CANNTG) after forming heterodimers with MAX.[147,148] Because a major mechanism of HIF-1$\alpha$-induced cell cycle arrest is through antagonizing *c-MYC* function,[149] the miR-210/*MNT* axis unveils yet another layer of the complex mechanism for regulating cell cycle progression under hypoxic conditions.

Despite the aforementioned evidence supporting miR-210's role in regulating cell cycle progression, it remains debatable whether this is a major function of miR-210. In some studies,[80,150] no obvious differences in cell proliferation were detected when miR-210 was overexpressed, suggesting that miR-210's impact on cell proliferation may be cell type or context-dependent. Clearly, much more effort is needed to better address this question.

## 6.2.6. *miR-210 regulation of angiogenesis*

Hypoxia is one of the best characterized factors in the tumor microenvironment to promote angiogenesis.[9] Numerous pro-angiogenic factors are up-regulated in cells responding to a hypoxic microenvironment,[10] with vascular endothelial growth factor (VEGF) being the best example.[27,151] The identification of miR-210 has shed new light on the complexity of organisms' angiogenic response to hypoxia.

In two studies, ectopic miR-210 expression in normoxic human umbilical vein endothelial cells (HUVECs) was found to stimulate the formation of capillary-like structures as well as VEGF-induced cell migration, while inhibiting miR-210 antagonizes both tubulogenesis and VEGF-mediated endothelial chemotaxis,[78,152] supporting a causal role for miR-210 in promoting angiogenesis. The receptor tyrosine kinase ligand, Ephrin-A3 (*EFNA3*), was identified as a miR-210 target.[78] The authors further demonstrated that suppression of *EFNA3* by miR-210 is necessary for miR-210-mediated stimulation of tubulogenesis and chemotaxis. Although the function of *EFNA3* has not yet been clearly defined, members of the ephrin family are known to be important factors in the development of the cardiovascular system and in vascular remodeling.[153] Paradoxically, despite being one of the most consistent miR-210 target genes,[78,80,119,154,155] *EFNA3* expression is also highly induced in post-ischemic mouse hippocampus or under hypoxic conditions.[78,156,157] A recent study presented surprising, but convincing, evidence to indicate that the *EFNA3* mRNA is not responsive to hypoxia treatment, but the two lncRNAs encoded at the *EFNA3* locus are.[158] Thus, the previously observed induction of *EFNA3* mRNA under hypoxic conditions may actually reflect the increased expression of these lncRNAs. Because the EFNA3 protein was induced under hypoxia, it suggests that the *EFNA3* lncRNA may serve as a competing endogenous RNA to saturate miR-210 and consequently, relieve *EFNA3* mRNA from miR-210 inhibition for efficient translation. It is somewhat surprising that the cells developed such a complex mechanism to regulate EFNA3 protein output under hypoxia. Thus, we speculate that *EFNA3* may have a critical, yet unidentified, function in hypoxic cells.

*Ptp1b*, a protein tyrosine phosphatase, was identified as another miR-210 target that promotes angiogenesis and inhibits cellular apoptosis following mouse myocardial infarction.[135] PTP1B can negatively regulate the activation of a VEGF receptor, VEGFR2, via binding to the receptor or by stabilizing cell-cell adhesions through reducing tyrosine phosphorylation of vascular endothelial cadherin in endothelial cells.[159] Thus, by inhibiting *Ptp1b* and *Efna3*, both negative regulators of angiogenesis, miR-210 could promote angiogenesis. This mechanism is further supported by recent findings that overexpression of miR-210 in HUVECs can enhance *VEGF* and *VEGFR2* expression to augment angiogenesis despite no miR-210 targets being identified in the study.[160] In addition, recent studies also suggest a positive role for miR-210 in promoting angiogenesis by regulating the *VEGF* or Notch signaling pathways.[152,161,162]

In breast cancer patients, miR-210 expression was found to correlate closely with *VEGF* signaling.[163] However, given miR-210's close association with hypoxia, a positive correlation does not necessarily suggest a causal relationship between miR-210 and breast cancer angiogenesis. Angiogenesis is critical for tumor growth and metastasis. Although accumulated evidence suggests a role for miR-210 in promoting angiogenesis, the mechanism remains largely unclear.

## 6.2.7. *miR-210 regulates mitochondrial metabolism*

One of the most important changes cells have to make under hypoxic conditions is in how energy is generated. Under normoxia, cells generate ATP mainly through oxidative phosphorylation (OXPHOS). When the oxygen supply is limited, glycolysis, a much less efficient pathway in generating ATP, is utilized. HIF-1$\alpha$ is arguably the most important factor regulating glycolysis by upregulating essentially all the enzymes in the glycolytic pathway.[164] However, how HIF-1$\alpha$ downregulates mitochondrial OXPHOS is less clear. Accumulating evidence suggests that miR-210 is a new player during this metabolic shift by downregulating mitochondrial electron transport chain (ETC) activity. One of the major targets of miR-210 mediating this effect is the iron–sulfur (Fe–S) cluster scaffold proteins, ISCU1 and ISCU2.[119,165–171] ISCU is part of an ancient machinery that facilitates the assembly of Fe–S clusters that are then incorporated into enzymes that function in the tricarboxylic acid cycle, such as aconitase and the mitochondrial ETC complexes I, II, and III.[172]

Several additional mitochondrial ETC components have also been reported to be miR-210 targets, such as NADH dehydrogenase (ubiquinone) 1 alpha subcomplex 4 (*NDUFA4*),[79] succinate dehydrogenase complex, subunit D (*SDHD*),[117] and cytochrome c oxidase assembly homolog 10 (*COX10*).[166] NDUFA4 is a subunit of Complex IV, and its mutation has been found to cause human neurological disease.[173,174] SDHD is a subunit of Complex II and is also a tumor suppressor.[175,176] By targeting multiple components along the mitochondrial ETC, robust induction of miR-210 under hypoxia is an efficient mechanism to attenuate mitochondrial respiration.

In addition to the ETC components, another intriguing miR-210 target with mitochondria-related function is glycerol-3-phosphate dehydrogenase 1-like (*GPD1L*).[177,178] Although *GPD1L* function remains unclear, its homology to glycerol-3-phosphate dehydrogenase (*GPD*), the catalyst of the glycerol phosphate shuttle that transfers electrons from cytoplasmic NADH to the mitochondrial ETC,[179] suggests that GPD1L may possess a similar metabolic function. Interestingly, suppression of *GPD1L* by miR-210 contributes to inactivation of HIF prolyl hydroxylase activity, resulting in increased HIF-1$\alpha$ expression.[177] A separate study also demonstrated that a high miR-210 level contributes to the maintenance of stabilized HIF-1$\alpha$ during hypoxia,[117] suggesting that miR-210 and HIF-1$\alpha$ may form a feed-forward loop to enhance glycolysis. Collectively, these data support the notion that miR-210 may be a critical regulator of mitochondrial respiration in the HIF-1$\alpha$ pathway.

It is well-known that tumors rely on glycolysis even when a sufficient oxygen supply is available, a phenomenon termed "the Warburg effect",[180] in which HIF-1$\alpha$ plays an important role.[8] Given the potential feed-forward mechanism between HIF-1$\alpha$ and miR-210, we speculate that the frequent overexpression of miR-210 in human cancer may promote the Warburg effect in these tumors by helping to stabilize HIF-1$\alpha$. However, loss-of-function studies, especially these in spontaneous tumor models, are essential to provide an unequivocal answer to this attractive hypothesis.

## 6.2.8. *miR-210 as a potential cancer therapeutic target*

Increased expression of miR-210 is generally linked to adverse prognosis in pan-cancer meta-analysis,[103–105,181] suggesting that miR-210 may be exploited as a potential therapeutic target. Indeed, targeting miR-210 has been shown to sensitize tumor cells to radiation in a variety of cancers,[81,125,133,182] inhibit the migration and invasion of renal cell carcinoma cells,[183] and lead to enhanced cell death.[184] Thus, agents that target miR-210 may be especially detrimental to highly hypoxic tumor cells that are usually resistant to radiation and chemotherapy. It may be a more effective strategy to combine conventional cytotoxic agents that eliminate well-oxygenated, fast-growing tumor cells with agents that target miR-210 for cancer treatment.

## 6.2.9. *Circulating miR-210 as a promising biomarker for cancer diagnosis and prognosis*

The presence of nucleic acids in the circulation has been known in healthy and diseased people.[210] However, the discovery of circulating miRNAs in human blood in 2008 has caused great excitement for their potential use as biomarkers for early cancer detection, diagnosis, and prognosis and for monitoring cancer progression,[185–191] mostly due to their exceptional stability and abundance. Recently, it was found that miRNAs in exosomes secreted by cancer cells can mediate metastasis and promote tumorigenesis,[192,193] providing examples for explaining the function of large amounts of cell-free miRNAs in the human circulation. In addition, secreted miRNAs can also function as ligands to bind to receptors of the toll-like receptor family,[207] serving as a "hormone" in paracrine or endocrine signaling.

Interestingly, an elevated miR-210 level in the serum of patients with diffuse large $\beta$-cell lymphoma was among the first evidence supporting the presence of miRNAs in human circulation.[189] Recently, exosomes from mouse breast cancer 4T1 cells transfected with miR-210 were found to significantly enhance the migration and capillary formation of HUVECs,[208] indicating a functional role for secreted miR-210 in the circulation. In addition, secreted miR-210 in the conditioned medium from donor cells was found to be taken up by recipient cells and to regulate mitochondrial function in them by repressing ISCU,[194] further indicating the functional role of circulating miR-210. However, whether these findings could be generalized to support a broader function for circulating miR-210 in human cancers remains to be determined.

Significantly elevated circulating miR-210 levels have been found in many tumor types, including clear cell renal cell carcinoma (ccRCC),[195,196] pancreatic cancer,[197,198] breast cancer,[199,200] adrenocortical tumors,[201] melanoma,[202] and glioma.[203] Pancreatic cancer is known for the presence of highly hypoxic tumors,[204] while constitutive stabilization of HIF-1$\alpha$ is ubiquitous in ccRCC due to frequent mutations of *VHL*, a negative regulator of HIF-1$\alpha$. Detection of elevated circulating miR-210 in ccRCC and pancreatic cancer patients is particularly interesting because these studies raise the possibility of using circulating miR-210 as a surrogate biomarker for non-invasive detection of tumor hypoxia. In addition, a study has shown that plasma miR-210 is correlated with sensitivity to trastuzumab and tumor presence in breast cancer patients.[205] Although the biology behind this correlation remains to be elucidated, it nevertheless raises the exciting possibility of using circulating miR-210 for non-invasive monitoring of patient response to cancer therapy.

Circulating miRNA offers exciting opportunities for cancer biomarker discovery. Since its discovery in 2008, this field has been experiencing an exponential growth as part of the "liquid biopsy" movement. Given its robust induction under hypoxic conditions, we speculate that miR-210 may represent one of the best biomarkers for tumor hypoxia and other clinical characteristics closely related to hypoxia. However, stringent criteria in design, execution, and interpretation of experimental data need to be followed in such studies, especially when the biological significance of miR-210 as such a biomarker remains to be determined.

# 7.  Concluding Remarks

From the current literature discussed above, it is clear that ncRNAs are an important component of the cellular response to hypoxic stress, especially in the context of tumor hypoxia. Compared to the rich knowledge we have gained on protein-coding genes since the characterization of HIF-1$\alpha$ in 1995,[1] hypoxic regulation of ncRNAs is still a nascent field, with the exception of miRNAs. The rapid advancement of sequencing technology will only reveal many more new hypoxia-regulated ncRNAs that may play roles completely unexpected at present. Given that the majority of the human genome has been transcribed,[206] the major challenge will be the elucidation of their functions, miR-210 serving as a good example in this regard. Since its discovery in 2007,[76] hundreds of papers have been published with miR-210 as the study subject. However, miR-210's physiological function and the significance of its role in cancer development *in vivo* remain largely elusive. The emergence of new technologies, such as genome editing and nanopore sequencing, new animal models, and computational capacity to mine the vast clinical data for cancer patients, will provide unprecedented opportunities for us to tackle these difficult questions.

## Acknowledgments

This work was supported, in part, by an American Cancer Society Research Scholar Grant (RSG-12-188-01-RMC) and the Liz Tilberis Scholars Award from the Ovarian Cancer Research Fund (OCRF 258940).

## References

1. Wang, G. L. *et al.*, Hypoxia-inducible factor 1 is a basic-helix-loop-helix-PAS heterodimer regulated by cellular O2 tension. *P. Nat. Acad. Sci.*, **92**(12), pp. 5510–5514, 1995.
2. Wang, G. L., and Semenza, G. L., Purification and Characterization of Hypoxia-inducible Factor 1. *J. Biol. Chem.*, **270**(3), pp. 1230–1237, 1995.
3. Wiesener, M. S. *et al.*, Widespread hypoxia-inducible expression of HIF-2α in distinct cell populations of different organs. *FASEB J.*, **17**(2), pp. 271–273, 2003.
4. Zhang, P. *et al.*, Hypoxia-Inducible Factor 3 Is an Oxygen-Dependent Transcription Activator and Regulates a Distinct Transcriptional Response to Hypoxia. *Cell Reports*, **6**(6), pp. 1110–1121, 2014.
5. Jaakkola, P. *et al.*, Targeting of HIF-alpha to the von Hippel-Lindau Ubiquitylation Complex by O2-Regulated Prolyl Hydroxylation. *Science*, **292**(5516), pp. 468–472, 2001.
6. Ivan, M. *et al.*, HIFalpha Targeted for VHL-Mediated Destruction by Proline Hydroxylation: Implications for O2 Sensing. *Science*, **292**(5516), pp. 464–468, 2001.
7. Semenza, G. L., Hypoxia-Inducible Factors in Physiology and Medicine. *Cell*, **148**(3), pp. 399–408, 2012.
8. Kim, J.-W., and Dang, C. V., Cancer's molecular sweet tooth and the Warburg effect. *Cancer Res.*, **66**(18), pp. 8927–8930, 2006.
9. Brown, J. M., and Giaccia, A. J., The unique physiology of solid tumors: opportunities (and problems) for cancer therapy. *Cancer Res.*, **58**(7), pp. 1408–1416, 1998.
10. Carmeliet, P., and Jain, R. K., Angiogenesis in cancer and other diseases. *Nature*, **407**(6801), pp. 249–257, 2000.

11. Minchinton, A. I., and Tannock, I. F., Drug penetration in solid tumours. *Nat. Rev. Cancer.*, **6**(8), pp. 583–592, 2006.

12. Vaupel, P., and Mayer, A., Hypoxia in cancer: significance and impact on clinical outcome. *Cancer Metastasis Rev.*, **26**(2), pp. 225–239, 2007.

13. Le, Q.-T., Denko, N. C., and Giaccia, A. J., Hypoxic gene expression and metastasis. *Cancer Metastasis Rev.*, **23**(3–4), pp. 293–310, 2004.

14. Sullivan, R., and Graham, C., Hypoxia-driven selection of the metastatic phenotype. *Cancer Metastasis Rev.*, **26**(2), pp. 319–331, 2007.

15. Chan, D., and Giaccia, A., Hypoxia, gene expression, and metastasis. *Cancer Metastasis Rev.*, **26**(2), pp. 333–339, 2007.

16. Wilson, W. R., and Hay, M. P., Targeting hypoxia in cancer therapy. *Nat. Rev. Cancer.*, **11**(6), pp. 393–410, 2011.

17. Venter, J. C. *et al.*, The Sequence of the Human Genome. *Science*, **291**(5507), pp. 1304–1351, 2001.

18. Consortium, T. E. P., An integrated encyclopedia of DNA elements in the human genome. *Nature*, **489**(7414), pp. 57–74, 2012.

19. Choudhry, H. *et al.*, Extensive regulation of the non-coding transcriptome by hypoxia: role of HIF in releasing paused RNApol2. *EMBO Rep.*, **15**(1), pp. 70–76, 2014.

20. Thompson, D. M., and Parker, R., Stressing out over tRNA cleavage. *Cell*, **138**(2), pp. 215–219, 2009.

21. Lee, Y. S. *et al.*, A novel class of small RNAs: tRNA-derived RNA fragments (tRFs). *Gene Dev*, **23**(22), pp. 2639–2649, 2009.

22. Cole, C. *et al.*, Filtering of deep sequencing data reveals the existence of abundant Dicer-dependent small RNAs derived from tRNAs. *RNA*, **15**(12), pp. 2147–2160, 2009.

23. Mizuno, Y. *et al.*, miR-210 promotes osteoblastic differentiation through inhibition of AcvR1b. *FEBS Lett.*, **583**(13), pp. 2263–2268, 2009.

24. Goodarzi, H. *et al.*, Endogenous tRNA-derived fragments suppress breast cancer progression via YBX1 displacement. *Cell*, **161**(4), pp. 790–802, 2015.

25. Erler, J. T. *et al.*, Lysyl oxidase is essential for hypoxia-induced metastasis. *Nature*, **440**(7088), pp. 1222–1226, 2006.

26. Bennewith, K. L. *et al.*, The role of tumor cell-derived connective tissue growth factor (CTGF/CCN2) in pancreatic tumor growth. *Cancer Res.*, **69**(3), pp. 775–784, 2009.

27. Liu, Y. *et al.*, Hypoxia regulates vascular endothelial growth factor gene expression in endothelial cells: identification of a 5' enhancer. *Circ. Res.*, **77**(3), pp. 638–643, 1995.

28. Rinn, J. L., and Chang, H. Y., Genome Regulation by Long Noncoding RNAs. *Ann. Rev. Biochem.*, **81**, pp. 145–166, 2012.

29. Chow, J. C. *et al.*, Silencing of the mammalian X chromosome. *Ann. Rev. Genomics Hum Genet.*, **6**(1), pp. 69–92, 2005.

30. Herzing, L. B. K. *et al.*, Xist has properties of the X-chromosome inactivation centre. *Nature*, **386**(6622), pp. 272–275, 1997.

31. Rinn, J. L. *et al.*, Functional demarcation of active and silent chromatin domains in human HOX Loci by noncoding RNAs. *Cell*, **129**(7), pp. 1311–1323, 2007.

32. Derrien, T. *et al.*, The GENCODE v7 catalog of human long noncoding RNAs: Analysis of their gene structure, evolution, and expression. *Genome Res.*, **22**(9), pp. 1775–1789, 2012.

33. Gabory, A. *et al.*, The H19 gene: regulation and function of a non-coding RNA. *Cytogenet Genome Res.*, **113**(1–4), pp. 188–193, 2006.

34. Matouk, I. J. *et al.*, The H19 non-coding RNA is essential for human tumor growth. *PLoS ONE*, **2**(9), p. e845, 2007.

35. Matouk, I. J. *et al.*, The oncofetal H19 RNA connection: Hypoxia, p53 and cancer. *Mol. Cell Res., Biochimica et Biophysica Acta (BBA).* **1803**(4), pp. 443–451, 2010.

36. Cai, X., and Cullen, B. R., The imprinted H19 noncoding RNA is a primary microRNA precursor. *RNA*, **13**(3), pp. 313–316, 2007.

37. Berteaux, N. *et al.*, H19 mRNA-like noncoding RNA promotes breast cancer cell proliferation through positive control by E2F1. *J. Biol. Chem.*, **280**(33), pp. 29625–29636, 2005.

38. Lottin, S. *et al.*, Overexpression of an ectopic H19 gene enhances the tumorigenic properties of breast cancer cells. *Carcinogenesis*, **23**(11), pp. 1885–1895, 2002.

39. Ulitsky, I., and Bartel, D. P., LincRNAs: genomics, evolution, and mechanisms. *Cell*, **154**(1), pp. 26–46, 2013.

40. Huarte, M. *et al.*, A large intergenic noncoding RNA induced by p53 mediates global gene repression in the p53 response. *Cell*, **142**(3), pp. 409–419, 2010.

41. Yang, F. *et al.*, Reciprocal regulation of HIF-1α and LincRNA-p21 modulates the Warburg effect. *Mol. Cell*, **53**(1), pp. 88–100, 2014.

42. Pang, K. C., Frith, M. C., and Mattick, J. S., Rapid evolution of noncoding RNAs: lack of conservation does not mean lack of function. *Trends Gene.*, **22**(1), pp. 1–5, 2006.

43. Yang, F. *et al.*, Repression of the long noncoding RNA-LET by histone deacetylase 3 contributes to hypoxia-mediated metastasis. *Mol. Cell*, **49**(6), pp. 1083–1096, 2013.

44. Jiang, S., Wang, H.-L., and Yang, J., Low expression of long non-coding RNA LET inhibits carcinogenesis of cervical cancer. *Int. J. Clinical Experimental Pathology*, **8**(1), pp. 806–811, 2015.

45. Zhou, B. *et al.*, Down-regulation of long non-coding RNA LET is associated with poor prognosis in gastric cancer. *Int. J. Clinical Experimental Pathology*, **7**(12), pp. 8893–8898, 2014.

46. Bejerano, G. *et al.*, Ultraconserved elements in the human genome. *Science*, **304**(5675), pp. 1321–1325, 2004.

47. Calin, G. A. *et al.*, Ultraconserved regions encoding ncRNAs are altered in human leukemias and carcinomas. *Cancer Cell*, **12**(3), pp. 215–229, 2007.

48. Ferdin, J. *et al.*, HINCUTs in cancer: hypoxia-induced noncoding ultraconserved transcripts. *Cell Death Differ*, **20**(12), pp. 1675–1687, 2013.

49. Khorkova, O. *et al.*, Natural antisense transcripts. *Hum. Mol. Genet.*, **23**(R1), pp. R54–R63, 2014.

50. Katayama, S. *et al.*, Antisense transcription in the mammalian transcriptome. *Science*, **309**(5740), pp. 1564–1566, 2005.

51. Yelin, R. *et al.*, Widespread occurrence of antisense transcription in the human genome. *Nat. Biotech*, **21**(4), pp. 379–386, 2003.

52. Thrash-Bingham, C. A., and Tartof, K. D., aHIF: a natural antisense transcript overexpressed in human renal cancer and during hypoxia. *J. Nat. Cancer Inst.*, **91**(2), pp. 143–151, 1999.

53. Rossignol, F., Vaché, C., and Clottes, E., Natural antisense transcripts of hypoxia-inducible factor $1\alpha$ are detected in different normal and tumour human tissues. *Gene*, **299**(1–2), pp. 135–140, 2002.

54. Uchida, T. *et al.*, Prolonged hypoxia differentially regulates hypoxiainducible factor (HIF)-$1\alpha$ and HIF-$2\alpha$ expression in lung epithelial cells: implication of natural antisense HIF-$1\alpha$. *J. Biol. Chem.*, **279**(15), pp. 14871–14878, 2004.

55. Cai, X., Hagedorn, C. H., and Cullen, B. R., Human microRNAs are processed from capped, polyadenylated transcripts that can also function as mRNAs. *RNA*, **10**(12), pp. 1957–1966, 2004.

56. Lee, Y. *et al.*, MicroRNA genes are transcribed by RNA polymerase II. *The EMBO J.*, **23**(20), pp. 4051–4060, 2004.

57. Schwarz, D. S. *et al.*, Asymmetry in the assembly of the RNAi enzyme complex. *Cell*, **115**(2), pp. 199–208, 2003.

58. Djuranovic, S., Nahvi, A., and Green, R., A parsimonious model for gene regulation by miRNAs. *Science*, **331**(6017), pp. 550–553, 2011.

59. Djuranovic, S., Nahvi, A., and Green, R., miRNA-mediated gene silencing by translational repression followed by mRNA deadenylation and decay. *Science*, **336**(6078), pp. 237–240, 2012.

60. Baek, D. *et al.*, The impact of microRNAs on protein output. *Nature*, **455**(7209), pp. 64–71, 2008.
61. Selbach, M. *et al.*, Widespread changes in protein synthesis induced by microRNAs. *Nature*, **455**(7209), pp. 58–63, 2008.
62. Da Sacco, L., and Masotti, A., Recent insights and novel bioinformatics tools to understand the role of MicroRNAs binding to 5′ untranslated region. *Int. J. Mol. Sci.*, **14**(1), pp. 480–495, 2013.
63. Huang, S. *et al.*, MicroRNA-181a modulates gene expression of zinc finger family members by directly targeting their coding regions. *Nucleic Acids Res.*, **38**(20), pp. 7211–7218, 2010.
64. Mortensen, R. D. *et al.*, Posttranscriptional activation of gene expression in Xenopus laevis oocytes by microRNA-protein complexes (microRNPs). *P. Nat. Acad. Sci.*, **108**(20), pp. 8281–8286, 2011.
65. Place, R. F. *et al.*, MicroRNA-373 induces expression of genes with complementary promoter sequences. *P. Nat. Acad. Sci.*, **105**(5), pp. 1608–1613, 2008.
66. Vasudevan, S., Tong, Y., and Steitz, J. A., Switching from repression to activation: MicroRNAs can up-regulate translation. *Science*, **318**(5858), pp. 1931–1934, 2007.
67. Bushati, N., and Cohen, S. M., microRNA Functions. *Annual Review of Cell and Developmental Biology*, **23**(1), pp. 175–205, 2007.
68. Lu, J. *et al.*, MicroRNA expression profiles classify human cancers. *Nature*, **435**(7043), pp. 834–838, 2005.
69. Calin, G. A., and Croce, C. M., MicroRNA signatures in human cancers. *Nat. Rev. Cancer*, **6**(11), pp. 857–866, 2006.
70. Wegert, J. *et al.*, Mutations in the SIX1/2 pathway and the DROSHA/DGCR8 miRNA microprocessor complex underlie high-risk blastemal type Wilms tumors. *Cancer Cell*, **27**(2), pp. 298–311, 2015.
71. Foulkes, W. D., Priest, J. R., and Duchaine, T. F., DICER1: mutations, microRNAs and mechanisms. *Nat. Rev. Cancer.*, **14**(10), pp. 662–672, 2014.
72. Heravi-Moussavi, A. *et al.*, Recurrent somatic DICER1 mutations in nonepithelial ovarian cancers. *New Engl. J. Med.*, **366**(3), pp. 234–242, 2012.
73. Shen, J. *et al.*, EGFR modulates microRNA maturation in response to hypoxia through phosphorylation of AGO2. *Nature*, **497**(7449), pp. 383–387, 2013.
74. Qi, H. H. *et al.*, Prolyl 4-hydroxylation regulates Argonaute 2 stability. *Nature*, **455**(7211), pp. 421–424, 2008.

75. Donker, R. B. *et al.*, The expression of Argonaute2 and related microRNA biogenesis proteins in normal and hypoxic trophoblasts. *Mol. Hum. Reprod.*, **13**(4), pp. 273–279, 2007.

76. Kulshreshtha, R. *et al.*, A microRNA signature of hypoxia. *Mol. Cell. Biol.*, **27**(5), pp. 1859–1867, 2007.

77. Camps, C. *et al.*, hsa-miR-210 is induced by hypoxia and is an independent prognostic factor in breast cancer. *Clinical Cancer Res.* **14**(5), pp. 1340–1348, 2008.

78. Fasanaro, P. *et al.*, MicroRNA-210 modulates endothelial cell response to hypoxia and inhibits the receptor tyrosine kinase ligand ephrin-A3. *J. Biol. Chem.*, **283**(23), pp. 15878–15883, 2008.

79. Giannakakis, A. *et al.*, miR-210 links hypoxia with cell cycle regulation and is deleted in human epithelial ovarian cancer. *Cancer Biol. Ther.*, **7**(2), pp. 255–264, 2008.

80. Huang, X. *et al.*, Hypoxia-inducible mir-210 regulates normoxic gene expression involved in tumor initiation. *Molecular Cell*, **35**(6), pp. 856–867, 2009.

81. Yang, W. *et al.*, Knockdown of miR-210 decreases hypoxic glioma stem cells stemness and radioresistance. *Experimental Cell Res.*, **326**(1), pp. 22–35, 2014.

82. Suzuki, H. I. *et al.*, MicroRNA regulons in tumor microenvironment. *Oncogene*, **34**(24), pp. 3085–3094, 2015.

83. Semenza, G. L. Defining the role of hypoxia-inducible factor 1 in cancer biology and therapeutics. *Oncogene*, **29**(5), pp. 625–634, 2009.

84. Taguchi, A. *et al.*, Identification of hypoxia-inducible factor-1a as a novel target for miR-17-92 microRNA cluster. *Cancer Res.*, **68**(14), pp. 5540–5545, 2008.

85. Yamakuchi, M. *et al.*, MicroRNA-22 regulates hypoxia signaling in colon cancer cells. *PLoS ONE*, **6**(5), p. e20291, 2011.

86. Joshi, H. P. *et al.*, Dynamin 2 along with microRNA-199a reciprocally regulate hypoxia-inducible factors and ovarian cancer metastasis. *P. Nat. Acad. Sci.*, **111**(14), pp. 5331–5336, 2014.

87. Krutilina, R. *et al.*, MicroRNA-18a inhibits hypoxia-inducible factor $1\alpha$ activity and lung metastasis in basal breast cancers. *Breast Cancer Res.*, **16**(4), pp. 1–16, 2014.

88. Bartoszewska, S. *et al.*, The hypoxia-inducible miR-429 regulates hypoxia-inducible factor-$1\alpha$ expression in human endothelial cells through a negative feedback loop. *FASEB J.*, **29**(4), pp. 1467–1479, 2015.

89. Wang, H. *et al.*, Negative regulation of Hif1a expression and TH17 differentiation by the hypoxia-regulated microRNA miR-210. *Nat. Immunol.*, **15**(4), pp. 393–401, 2014.

90. Cha, S.-T. *et al.*, MicroRNA-519c suppresses hypoxia-inducible factor-1a expression and tumor angiogenesis. *Cancer Res.*, **70**(7), pp. 2675–2685, 2010.

91. Ghosh, G. *et al.*, Hypoxia-induced microRNA-424 expression in human endothelial cells regulates HIF-$\alpha$ isoforms and promotes angiogenesis. *J. Clinical Investigation*, **120**(11), pp. 4141–4154, 2010.

92. Sun, G. *et al.*, Over-expression of microRNA-494 up-regulates hypoxia-inducible factor-1 alpha expression via PI3K/Akt pathway and protects against hypoxia-induced apoptosis. *J. Biomedical Sci.*, **20**: p. 100, 2013.

93. Sarkar, J. *et al.*, MicroRNA-21 plays a role in hypoxia-mediated pulmonary artery smooth muscle cell proliferation and migration. *Am. J. Physiol.— Lung C.*, **299**(6), pp. L861–L871, 2010.

94. Lin, S.-C. *et al.*, Hypoxia-induced MicroRNA-20a expression increases ERK phosphorylation and angiogenic gene expression in endometriotic stromal cells. *J. Clinical Endocrinology Metabolism*, **97**(8), pp. E1515–E1523, 2012.

95. Chen, Z. *et al.*, Hypoxia-responsive miRNAs target argonaute 1 to promote angiogenesis. *J Clinical Investigation*, **123**(3), pp. 1057–1067, 2013.

96. Huang, X., Le, Q.-T., and Giaccia, A. J., MiR-210 — micromanager of the hypoxia pathway. *Trends Mole. Medicine*, **16**(5), pp. 230–237, 2010.

97. Cicchillitti, L. *et al.*, Hypoxia-inducible Factor 1-a induces miR-210 in normoxic differentiating myoblasts. *J. Biol. Chem.*, **287**(53), pp. 44761–44771, 2012.

98. Gee, H. E. *et al.*, hsa-miR-210 is a marker of tumor hypoxia and a prognostic factor in head and neck cancer. *Cancer*, **116**(9), pp. 2148–2158, 2010.

99. Rothe, F. *et al.*, Global MicroRNA Expression profiling identifies MiR-210 associated with tumor proliferation, invasion and poor clinical outcome in breast cancer. *PLoS ONE*, **6**(6), p. e20980, 2011.

100. Qu, A. *et al.*, Hypoxia-inducible MiR-210 is an independent prognostic factor and contributes to metastasis in colorectal Cancer. *PLoS ONE*, **9**(3), p. e90952, 2014.

101. Ge, Y.-Z. *et al.*, MicroRNA expression profiles predict clinical phenotypes and prognosis in chromophobe renal cell carcinoma. *Sci. Rep.*, **5**: p. 10328, 2015.

102. Samaan, S. *et al.*, miR-210 Is a Prognostic Marker in Clear Cell Renal Cell Carcinoma. *J. Mol. Diagn.*, **17**(2), pp. 136–144, 2015.

103. Hong, L. *et al.*, High expression of miR-210 predicts poor survival in patients with breast cancer: A meta-analysis. *Gene*, **507**(2), pp. 135–138, 2012.

104. Li, M. *et al.*, Prognostic role of MicroRNA-210 in various carcinomas: a systematic review and meta-analysis. *Dis. Markers*, **2014**, p. 106197, 2014.

105. Wang, J. *et al.*, Elevated expression of miR-210 predicts poor survival of cancer patients: a systematic review and meta-analysis. *PLoS ONE*, **9**(2), p. e89223, 2014.

106. Hamilton, M. P. *et al.*, Identification of a pan-cancer oncogenic microRNA superfamily anchored by a central core seed motif. *Nat. Commun.*, **4**, p. 2730, 2013.

107. He, J. *et al.*, MiR-210 disturbs mitotic progression through regulating a group of mitosis-related genes. *Nucleic Acids Res.*, **41**(1), pp. 498–508, 2013.

108. Bartel, D. P., MicroRNAs: target recognition and regulatory functions. *Cell*, **136**(2), pp. 215–233, 2009.

109. Lal, A. *et al.*, miR-24 inhibits cell proliferation by targeting E2F2, MYC, and other cell-cycle genes via binding to seedless 3' UTR MicroRNA recognition elements. *Mol. Cell*, **35**(5), pp. 610–625, 2009.

110. Fasanaro, P. *et al.*, ROD1 is a seedless target gene of hypoxia-induced miR-210. *PLoS ONE*, **7**(9), p. e44651, 2012.

111. Korpal, M. *et al.*, Direct targeting of Sec23a by miR-200s influences cancer cell secretome and promotes metastatic colonization. *Nat. Med.*, **17**(9), pp. 1101–1108, 2011.

112. Li, C. *et al.*, Quantitative proteomic strategies for the identification of microRNA targets. *Expert Rev. Proteomics*, **9**(5), pp. 549–559, 2012.

113. Bargaje, R. *et al.*, Identification of novel targets for miR-29a using miRNA proteomics. *PLoS ONE*, **7**(8), p. e43243, 2012.

114. Lim, L. P. *et al.*, Microarray analysis shows that some microRNAs downregulate large numbers of target mRNAs. *Nature*, **433**(7027), pp. 769–773, 2005.

115. Guo, H. *et al.*, Mammalian microRNAs predominantly act to decrease target mRNA levels. *Nature*, **466**(7308), pp. 835–840, 2010.

116. Zhang, Z., *et al.*, MicroRNA miR-210 modulates cellular response to hypoxia through the MYC antagonist MNT. *Cell Cycle*, **8**(17), pp. 2756–2768, 2009.

117. Puissegur, M. P. *et al.*, miR-210 is overexpressed in late stages of lung cancer and mediates mitochondrial alterations associated with modulation of HIF-1 activity. *Cell Death Differ.*, **18**(3), pp. 465–478, 2011.

118. Karginov, F. V. *et al.*, A biochemical approach to identifying microRNA targets. *Proc. Nat. Acad. Sci.*, **104**(49), pp. 19291–19296, 2007.

119. Fasanaro, P. *et al.*, An Integrated Approach for Experimental Target Identification of Hypoxia-induced miR-210. *J. Biol. Chem.*, **284**(50), pp. 35134–35143, 2009.

120. Chi, S. W. *et al.*, Argonaute HITS-CLIP decodes microRNA-mRNA interaction maps. *Nature*, **460**(7254), pp. 479–486, 2009.

121. Hafner, M. *et al.*, Transcriptome-wide identification of RNA-binding protein and microRNA target sites by PAR-CLIP. *Cell*, **141**(1), pp. 129–141, 2010.

122. Pires, I. M., Poole, R., and Hammond, E. M., *Chapter 10: Hypoxia and the DNA Damage Response, in Tumor Microenvironment*. John Wiley & Sons, Ltd., pp. 207–228, 2010.

123. Crosby, M. E., *et al.*, MicroRNA regulation of DNA repair gene expression in hypoxic stress. *Cancer Res.*, **69**(3), pp. 1221–1229, 2009.

124. Bindra, R., Crosby, M., and Glazer, P., Regulation of DNA repair in hypoxic cancer cells. *Cancer Metastasis Rev.*, **26**(2), pp. 249–260, 2007.

125. Grosso, S. *et al.*, MiR-210 promotes a hypoxic phenotype and increases radioresistance in human lung cancer cell lines. *Cell Death Dis.*, **4**, p. e544, 2013.

126. Carmeliet, P. *et al.*, Role of HIF-1$\alpha$ in hypoxia-mediated apoptosis, cell proliferation and tumour angiogenesis. *Nature*, **394**(6692), pp. 485–490, 1998.

127. Kim, H. W. *et al.*, Ischemic preconditioning augments survival of stem cells via miR-210 expression by targeting caspase-8-associated protein 2. *J. Biol. Chemistry.*, **284**(48), pp. 33161–33168, 2009.

128. Mutharasan, R. K. *et al.*, microRNA-210 is upregulated in hypoxic cardiomyocytes through Akt- and p53-dependent pathways and exerts cytoprotective effects. *Am. J. Physiol. Heart. C.*, **301**(4), pp. H1519–H1530, 2011.

129. Li, L. a. *et al.*, Hypoxia-induced miR-210 in epithelial ovarian cancer enhances cancer cell viability via promoting proliferation and inhibiting apoptosis. *Int. J. Oncology*, **44**(6), pp. 2111–2120, 2014.

130. Nie, Y. *et al.*, Identification of microRNAs involved in hypoxia- and serum deprivation-induced apoptosis in mesenchymal stem cells. *Int. J. Biol. Sci.*, **7**, p. 762–768, 2011.

131. Gou, D. *et al.*, miR-210 has an antiapoptotic effect in pulmonary artery smooth muscle cells during hypoxia. *Am. J. Physiol. — Lung C.*, **303**(8), pp. L682–L691, 2012.

132. Liu, Y. *et al.*, Synthetic miRNA-Mowers targeting miR-183-96-182 cluster or miR-210 inhibit growth and migration and induce apoptosis in bladder cancer cells. *PLoS ONE*, **7**(12), p. e52280, 2012.

133. Yang, W. *et al.*, Downregulation of miR-210 expression inhibits proliferation, induces apoptosis and enhances radiosensitivity in hypoxic human hepatoma cells in vitro. *Exp. Cell Res.*, **318**(8), pp. 944–954, 2012.

134. Qiu, J. *et al.*, MicroRNA-210 knockdown contributes to apoptosis caused by oxygen glucose deprivation in PC12 cells. *Mol. Med. Rep.*, **11**(1), pp. 719–723, 2015.

135. Hu, S. *et al.*, MicroRNA-210 as a novel therapy for treatment of ischemic heart disease. *Circulation*, **122**(1), pp. S124–S131, 2010.

136. Kim, H. W. *et al.*, Concomitant activation of miR-107/PDCD10 and hypoxamir-210/casp8ap2 and their role in cytoprotection during ischemic preconditioning of stem cells. *Antioxidants Redox Signaling*, **17**(8), pp. 1053–1065, 2012.

137. Chio, C.-C. *et al.*, MicroRNA-210 targets antiapoptotic Bcl-2 expression and mediates hypoxia-induced apoptosis of neuroblastoma cells. *Arch. Toxicol.*, **87**(3), pp. 459–468, 2013.

138. Qiu, J. *et al.*, Neuroprotective effects of microRNA-210 against oxygen-glucose deprivation through inhibition of apoptosis in PC12 cells. *Mol. Med. Rep.*, **7**(6), pp. 1955–1959, 2013.

139. Sun, Y. *et al.*, Hypoxia-induced autophagy reduces radiosensitivity by the HIF-1$\alpha$/miR-210/Bcl-2 pathway in colon cancer cells. *Int. J. Oncol.*, **46**(2), pp. 750–756, 2015.

140. Goda, N. *et al.*, Hypoxia-inducible factor 1$\alpha$ is essential for cell cycle arrest during hypoxia. *Mol. Cell. Biol.*, **23**(1), pp. 359–369, 2003.

141. Leone, G. *et al.*, E2F3 activity is regulated during the cell cycle and is required for the induction of S phase. *Genes Dev*, **12**(14), pp. 2120–2130, 1998.

142. Nakada, C. *et al.*, Overexpression of miR-210, a downstream target of HIF1$\alpha$, causes centrosome amplification in renal carcinoma cells. *J. Pathol.*, **224**(2), pp. 280–288, 2011.

143. Biswas, S. *et al.*, Hypoxia inducible microRNA 210 attenuates keratinocyte proliferation and impairs closure in a murine model of ischemic wounds. *P. Nat. Acad. Sci.*, **107**(15), pp. 6976–6981, 2010.

144. Tsuchiya, S. *et al.*, MicroRNA-210 regulates cancer cell proliferation through targeting fibroblast growth factor receptor-like 1 (FGFRL1). *J. Biol. Chem.*, **286**(1), pp. 420–428, 2011.

145. Zuo, J. *et al.*, MiR-210 links hypoxia with cell proliferation regulation in human laryngocarcinoma cancer. *J. Cell. Biochem.*, **116**(6), pp. 1039–1049, 2015.

146. Bodempudi, V. *et al.*, miR-210 promotes IPF fibroblast proliferation in response to hypoxia. *Am. J. Physiol. — Lung C.*, **307**(4), pp. L283–L294, 2014.

147. Hurlin, P. J., Quéva, C., and Eisenman, R. N., Mnt, a novel Max-interacting protein is coexpressed with Myc in proliferating cells and mediates repression at Myc binding sites. *Genes Dev.*, **11**(1), pp. 44–58, 1997.

148. Meroni, G. *et al.*, Rox, a novel bHLHZip protein expressed in quiescent cells that heterodimerizes with Max, binds a non-canonical E box and acts as a transcriptional repressor. *EMBO J.*, **16**(10), pp. 2892–2906, 1997.

149. Koshiji, M. *et al.*, HIF-1$\alpha$ induces cell cycle arrest by functionally counteracting Myc. *EMBO J.*, **23**(9), pp. 1949–1956, 2004.

150. Chen, W. Y. *et al.*, Induction, modulation and potential targets of miR-210 in pancreatic cancer cells. *Hepatobiliary Pancreat Dis. Int.*, **11**(3), pp. 319–324, 2012.

151. Shweiki, D. *et al.*, Vascular endothelial growth factor induced by hypoxia may mediate hypoxia-initiated angiogenesis. *Nature*, **359**(6398), pp. 843–845, 1992.

152. Lou, Y.-L. *et al.*, miR-210 activates notch signaling pathway in angiogenesis induced by cerebral ischemia. *Mol. Cell. Biochem.*, **370**(1), pp. 45–51, 2012.

153. Kuijper, S., Turner, C. J., and Adams, R. H., Regulation of angiogenesis by Eph–Ephrin interactions. *Trends Cardiovas. Med.*, **17**(5), pp. 145–151, 2007.

154. Wang, Z. *et al.*, MicroRNA-210 promotes proliferation and invasion of peripheral nerve sheath tumor cells targeting EFNA3. *Oncology Res.*, **21**(3), pp. 145–154, 2014.

155. Xiao, F. *et al.*, WSS25 inhibits Dicer, downregulating microRNA-210, which targets Ephrin-A3, to suppress human microvascular endothelial cell (HMEC-1) tube formation. *Glycobiology*, **23**(5), pp. 524–535, 2013.

156. Khong, T. L. *et al.*, Identification of the angiogenic gene signature induced by EGF and hypoxia in colorectal cancer. *BMC Cancer*, 2013. **13**, pp. 1–17, 2013.

157. Pulkkinen, K. *et al.*, Hypoxia induces microRNA miR-210 in vitro and in vivo: Ephrin-A3 and neuronal pentraxin 1 are potentially regulated by miR-210. *FEBS Lett.*, **582**(16), pp. 2397–2401, 2008.

158. Gomez-Maldonado, L. *et al.*, EFNA3 long noncoding RNAs induced by hypoxia promote metastatic dissemination. *Oncogene*, **34**(20), pp. 2609–2620, 2015.

159. Nakamura, Y. *et al.*, Role of Protein Tyrosine Phosphatase 1B in VEGF Signaling and Cell-Cell Adhesions in Endothelial Cells. *Circulation Res.*, **102**(10), pp. 1182–1191, 2008.

160. Liu, F. *et al.*, Upregulation of microRNA-210 regulates renal angiogenesis mediated by activation of VEGF signaling pathway under ischemia/perfusion injury in vivo and in vitro. *Kidney Blood Press Res.*, **35**(3), pp. 182–191, 2012.

161. Alaiti, M. A. *et al.*, Up-regulation of miR-210 by vascular endothelial growth factor in ex vivo expanded CD34+ cells enhances cell-mediated angiogenesis. *J. Cell. Mol. Med.*, **16**(10), pp. 2413–2421, 2012.

162. Zeng, L. *et al.*, MicroRNA-210 overexpression induces angiogenesis and neurogenesis in the normal adult mouse brain. *Gene Ther.*, **21**(1), pp. 37–43, 2014.

163. Foekens, J. A. *et al.*, Four miRNAs associated with aggressiveness of lymph node-negative, estrogen receptor-positive human breast cancer. *P. Natl. Acad. Sci.*, **105**(35), pp. 13021–13026, 2008.

164. Denko, N. C., Hypoxia, HIF1 and glucose metabolism in the solid tumour. *Nat. Rev. Cancer.*, **8**(9), pp. 705–713, 2008.

165. Chan, S. Y. *et al.*, MicroRNA-210 Controls Mitochondrial Metabolism during Hypoxia by Repressing the Iron-Sulfur Cluster Assembly Proteins ISCU1/2. *Cell Meta.*, **10**(4), pp. 273–284, 2009.

166. Chen, Z. *et al.*, Hypoxia-regulated microRNA-210 modulates mitochondrial function and decreases ISCU and COX10 expression. *Oncogene*, **29**(30), pp. 4362–4368, 2010.

167. Favaro, E. *et al.*, MicroRNA-210 regulates mitochondrial free radical response to hypoxia and Krebs cycle in cancer cells by targeting iron sulfur cluster protein ISCU. *PLoS ONE*, **5**(4), p. e10345, 2010.

168. Lee, D.-C. *et al.*, miR-210 targets iron-sulfur cluster scaffold homologue in human trophoblast cell lines: siderosis of interstitial trophoblasts as a novel pathology of preterm preeclampsia and small-for-gestational-age pregnancies. *Am. J. Pathol.*, **179**(2), pp. 590–602, 2011.

169. Yoshioka, Y. *et al.*, Micromanaging iron homeostasis: hypoxia-inducible micro-RNA-210 suppresses iron homeostasis-related proteins. *J. Biol. Chem.*, **287**(41), pp. 34110–34119, 2012.

170. Pugh, T. J. *et al.*, The genetic landscape of high-risk neuroblastoma. *Nat. Genet.*, **45**(3), pp. 279–284, 2013.

171. McCormick, R. I. *et al.*, miR-210 is a target of hypoxia-inducible factors 1 and 2 in renal cancer, regulates ISCU and correlates with good prognosis. *Br. J. Cancer.*, **108**(5), pp. 1133–1142, 2013.

172. Tong, W.-H., and Rouault, T. A., Functions of mitochondrial ISCU and cytosolic ISCU in mammalian iron-sulfur cluster biogenesis and iron homeostasis. *Cell. Meta.*, **3**(3), pp. 199–210, 2006.

173. Balsa, E. *et al.*, NDUFA4 Is a subunit of complex IV of the mammalian electron transport chain. *Cell Meta.*, **16**(3), pp. 378–386, 2012.

174. Pitceathly, Robert D. *et al.*, NDUFA4 mutations underlie dysfunction of a cytochrome c oxidase subunit linked to human neurological disease. *Cell Reports*, **3**(6), pp. 1795–1805, 2013.

175. Gottlieb, E., and Tomlinson, I. P. M., Mitochondrial tumour suppressors: a genetic and biochemical update. *Nat. Rev. Cancer.*, **5**(11), pp. 857–866, 2005.

176. Baysal, B. E. *et al.*, Mutations in SDHD, a mitochondrial Complex II Gene, in hereditary paraganglioma. *Science*, **287**(5454), pp. 848–851, 2000.

177. Kelly, T. J. *et al.*, A hypoxia-induced positive feedback loop promotes hypoxia-inducible factor 1a stability through miR-210 suppression of glycerol-3-phosphate dehydrogenase 1-like. *Mol. Cell. Biol.*, **31**(13), pp. 2696–2706, 2011.

178. Liu, S. C. *et al.*, CTGF increases vascular endothelial growth factor-dependent angiogenesis in human synovial fibroblasts by increasing miR-210 expression. *Cell Death Dis*, **5**, p. e1485, 2014.

179. Bunoust, O. *et al.*, Competition of electrons to enter the respiratory chain: A new regulatory mechanism of oxidative metabolism in saccharomyces cerevisiae. *J. Biol. Chem.*, **280**(5), pp. 3407–3413, 2005.

180. Warburg, O., On the origin of cancer cells. *Science*, **123**(3191), pp. 309–314, 1956.

181. Võsa, U. *et al.*, Meta-analysis of microRNA expression in lung cancer. *Int. J. Cancer.*, **132**(12), pp. 2884–2893, 2013.

182. Yang, W. *et al.*, Effects of knockdown of miR-210 in combination with ionizing radiation on human hepatoma xenograft in nude mice. *Radiation Oncology*, **8**(1), p. 102, 2013.

183. Redova, M. *et al.*, MiR-210 expression in tumor tissue and in vitro effects of its silencing in renal cell carcinoma. *Tumor Biol.*, **34**(1), pp. 481–491, 2013.

184. Cheng, A. M. *et al.*, Antisense inhibition of human miRNAs and indications for an involvement of miRNA in cell growth and apoptosis. *Nucleic Acids Res.*, **33**(4), pp. 1290–1297, 2005.

185. Chen, X. *et al.*, Characterization of microRNAs in serum: a novel class of biomarkers for diagnosis of cancer and other diseases. *Cell Research.*, **18**(10), pp. 997–1006, 2008.

186. Feng, G. *et al.*, Elevated serum-circulating RNA in patients with conventional renal cell cancer. *Anticancer Res.*, **28**(1A), pp. 321–326, 2008.

187. Gilad, S. *et al.*, Serum microRNAs are promising novel biomarkers. *PLoS ONE*, **3**(9), p. e3148, 2008.

188. Hunter, M. P. *et al.*, Detection of microRNA expression in human peripheral blood microvesicles. *PLoS ONE*, **3**(11), p. e3694, 2008.

189. Lawrie, C. H. *et al.*, Detection of elevated levels of tumour-associated microRNAs in serum of patients with diffuse large B-cell lymphoma. *Br. J. Haematol.*, **141**(5), pp. 672–675, 2008.

190. Mitchell, P. S. *et al.*, Circulating microRNAs as stable blood-based markers for cancer detection. *P. Nat. Acad. Sci.*, **105**(30), pp. 10513–10518, 2008.

191. Wong, T.-S. *et al.*, Mature miR-184 as potential oncogenic microRNA of squamous cell carcinoma of tongue. *Clinical Cancer Res.*, **14**(9), pp. 2588–2592, 2008.

192. Zhou, W. *et al.*, Cancer-Secreted miR-105 Destroys Vascular Endothelial Barriers to Promote Metastasis. *Cancer Cell*, **25**(4), pp. 501–515, 2014.

193. Melo, Sonia A. *et al.*, Cancer exosomes perform cell-independent microRNA biogenesis and promote tumorigenesis. *Cancer Cell*, **26**(5), pp. 707–721, 2014.

194. Hale, A. *et al.*, An Argonaute 2 switch regulates circulating miR-210 to coordinate hypoxic adaptation across cells. *Biochimica et Biophysica Acta (BBA) — Mole. Cell Res.*, **1843**(11), pp. 2528–2542, 2014.

195. Zhao, A. *et al.*, Serum miR-210 as a novel biomarker for molecular diagnosis of clear cell renal cell carcinoma. *Exp. Mol. Pathol.*, **94**(1), pp. 115–120, 2013.

196. Iwamoto, H. *et al.*, Serum miR-210 as a potential biomarker of early clear cell renal cell carcinoma. *Int. J. Oncol.*, **44**(1), pp. 53–58, 2014.

197. Ho, A. S. *et al.*, Circulating miR-210 as a novel hypoxia marker in pancreatic cancer. *Transl. Oncol.*, **3**(2), pp. 109–113, 2010.

198. Wang, J. *et al.*, MicroRNAs in plasma of pancreatic ductal adenocarcinoma patients as novel blood-based biomarkers of disease. *Cancer. Prev. Res.*, **2**(9), pp. 807–813, 2009.

199. Madhavan, D. *et al.*, Circulating miRNAs as surrogate markers for circulating tumor cells and prognostic markers in metastatic breast cancer. *Clin. Cancer Res.*, **18**(21), pp. 5972–5982, 2012.

200. Camacho, L., Guerrero, P., and Marchetti, D., MicroRNA and protein profiling of brain metastasis competent cell-derived exosomes. *PLoS ONE*, **8**(9), p. e73790, 2013.

201. Szabo, D. R. *et al.*, Analysis of circulating microRNAs in adrenocortical tumors. *Lab. Invest,* **94**(3), pp. 331–339, 2014.

202. Ono, S. *et al.*, A direct plasma assay of circulating microRNA-210 of hypoxia can identify early systemic metastasis recurrence in melanoma patients. *Oncotarget,* **6**(9), pp. 7053–7064, 2015.

203. Lai, N. *et al.*, Serum microRNA-210 as a potential noninvasive biomarker for the diagnosis and prognosis of glioma. *J. Cancer.,* **112**(7), pp. 1241–1246, 2015.

204. Koong, A. C. *et al.*, Pancreatic tumors show high levels of hypoxia. *Int. J. Radiat. Oncol. Biol. Phys.,* **48**(4), pp. 919–922, 2000.

205. Jung, E.-J. *et al.*, Plasma microRNA 210 levels correlate with sensitivity to trastuzumab and tumor presence in breast cancer patients. *Cancer,* **118**(10), pp. 2603–2614, 2012.

206. Pennisi, E., ENCODE project writes eulogy for junk DNA. *Science,* **337**(6099), pp. 1159–1161, 2012.

207. Fabbri, M. *et al.*, MicroRNAs bind to Toll-like receptors to induce prometastatic inflammatory response. *Proc Natl Acad Sci USA,* **109**(31), pp. E2110–E2116, 2012.

208. Kosaka, N. *et al.*, Neutral Sphingomyelinase 2 (nSMase2)-dependent exosomal transfer of angiogenic microRNAs regulate cancer cell metastasis. *J Biol Chem.* **288**(15), pp. 10849–10859, 2013.

209. Faraonio, R. *et al.*, A set of miRNAs participates in the cellular senescence program in human diploid fibroblasts. *Cell Death Differ,* **19**(4), pp. 713–721, 2012.

210. Fleischhacker, M., & Schmidt, B., Circulating nucleic acids (CNAs) and cancer--A survey. *Biochimica et Biophysica Acta (BBA) — Reviews on Cancer,* **1775**(1), pp. 181–232, 2007.

# Chapter 9

# Hypoxia-Induced Endoplasmic Reticulum Stress

Chih-Chien Chou, Rakesh Bam,
Zhifen Yang, Justin L. Bui, Dadi Jiang and Albert C. Koong*

*Department of Radiation Oncology,
Stanford University School of Medicine, Stanford, CA, USA
*akoong@stanford.edu*

## 1. Introduction

Hypoxia is an important tumor microenvironmental factor that induces endoplasmic reticulum (ER) stress. The presence of hypoxia regulates not only metabolism and proliferation but also genomic instability, invasion, and metastasis. Preclinical and clinical studies have demonstrated that hypoxia-induced ER stress activates the unfolded protein response (UPR), which is associated with poor patient survival in a variety of human cancers. The UPR is an adaptive signaling pathway activated by biochemical and physiological stimuli for ER homeostasis to promote tumor survival during ER stress. The inositol-requiring enzyme 1 (IRE1), protein ER kinase (PKR)-like ER kinase (PERK or EIF2AK3), and activating transcription factor 6 (ATF6) are three major UPR effectors through which different downstream signals emerge in response to ER stress. Although the details of UPR mechanisms have not been fully elucidated, recent studies suggest that UPR triggers prosurvival signals to prevent apoptosis in solid tumor cells under hypoxic conditions. Investigation of the molecular relationship between hypoxia and UPR is crucial and will lead to the development of cancer therapeutics targeting this pathway.

## 2.  Function of ER

In eukaryotic cells, ER is a complex organelle composed of a membrane-enclosed network of tubules, vesicles, and cisternae. This connected network sustained by the cytoskeleton is continuous from the cell membrane to the outer membrane of the nuclear envelope. The major role of ER is essential for the oligomerization, post-translational modification and folding of membrane and secretory proteins within the ER lumen, allowing proteins to assemble into their correct three-dimensional structures that are required for their normal physiological functions.[1] This complex process occurs in the rough ER (RER), which is studded with ribosomes on the outer surface. Not only necessary for protein synthesis and folding, the smooth ER (SER) which lacks associated ribosomes is responsible for calcium homeostasis, lipid metabolism, glucose metabolism, protein transportation, and detoxification of organic chemicals.[2] Thus, the ER plays a critical role in maintaining cellular function and homeostasis, and modulating cell signaling in this compartment is a promising therapeutic strategy.

## 3.  ER Stress

The ER is a highly dynamic organelle possessing complex functions and during physiological and pathological conditions may experience perturbations that disrupt ER homeostasis leading to "ER stress." For example, low oxygen concentration (hypoxia), lack of glucose (hypoglycemia), low pH in blood (acidosis), fluctuation in calcium homeostasis, accumulation of unfolded/misfolded proteins, and viral infection, are conditions that can disrupt ER homeostasis and impact proper functions of the ER.[3] Under ER stress, cells initiates an adaptive signaling pathway, known as the UPR, to relieve ER burden and restore ER homeostasis.[4] However, during prolonged ER stress, the adaptive and prosurvival of the UPR can paradoxically switch to proapoptotic signaling leading to cell death.

# 4. Unfolded Protein Response

As mentioned earlier, IRE1, PERK and ATF6 are three main UPR regulators, which are highly conserved transmembrane receptors localizing at the ER membrane (Fig. 1). They serve as critical sensors to transduce the signals from the ER to cytosol or the nucleus under ER stress in addition to monitoring the intensity and period of the stress stimuli from the microenvironment.[4] Currently, two models have been proposed to describe the activation of these stress transducers in response to ER stress. In the first model, with the absence of ER stress, the ER-resident chaperone glucose-regulated protein of 78 kDa (GRP78; also called Binding immunoglobulin Protein (BiP), directly binds to the intraluminal domains of these stress sensors to prevent dimerization and activation of IRE1 and PERK, or to prevent the translocation of ATF6 from the ER membrane to the golgi complex for proteolytic cleavage and activation.[5,6] GRP78 was originally identified as a protein that restricts the utilization of glucose under cellular stress conditions.[7] Later, GRP78 has been demonstrated as a chaperone belonging to the heat shock protein 70 (HSP70) family that is activated through transcriptional and translational regulation during ER stress.[8] Under ER stress, the accumulation of unfolded/misfolded proteins competes with GRP78 causing the dissociation of GRP78 from each stress sensors. Consequently, all of three stress sensors activate and trigger their downstream signaling cascades to meet the increased demand of protein folding. A second model has been characterized as a direct binding model in which unfolded/misfolded proteins directly interact with the intraluminal domains of the IRE1 receptor and allow the activation of the stress sensors in response to perturbation in ER homeostasis. Evidence for this model to date has largely come from the yeast system, and the data suggest that this model may represent a more efficient mechanism to activate the UPR by IRE1.[9]

# 5. IRE1 Signaling

IRE1 is the most evolutionarily conserved UPR protein among all of the stress sensors. It is a type I transmembrane protein composed of two major domains and a linker region. One domain is located on the N-terminal ER

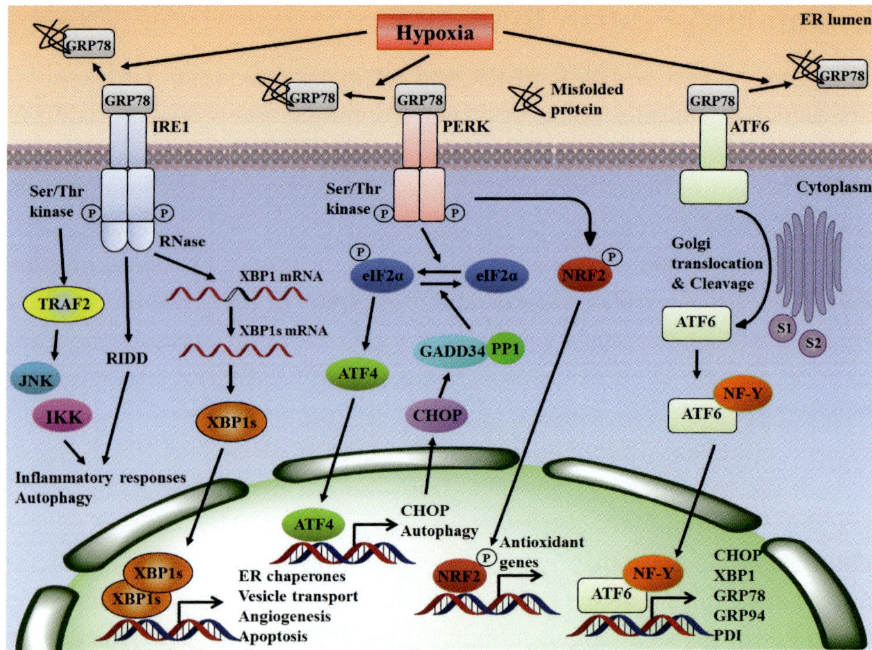



Fig. 1. Mechanisms of hypoxia induced UPR. The hypoxic microenvironment perturbs ER homeostasis through an increase in unfolded/misfolded proteins within the ER lumen, causing dissociation of GRP78 from all three major UPR sensors (IRE1, PERK, and ATF6). The RNase domain of IRE1 splices XBP1 mRNA, producing a transcription factor, XBP1s, which regulates expression of survival- and ERAD (ER associated degradation)-associated genes. The RNase domain of IRE1 also contains regulated IRE-1-dependent decay (RIDD) activity which degrades mRNAs associated with the ER. PERK activation attenuates global translation through the phosphorylation of translation initiation factor eIF2$\alpha$ and promotes apoptosis through ATF4-mediated CHOP expression. CHOP can also promote survival through association of GADD34 with PP1 and creating a feedback loop to dephosphorylate eIF2$\alpha$ and resume translation. PERK can phosphorylate the transcription factor NRF2 and induce the expression of anti-oxidant genes to control free radicals produced under hypoxia. After dissociation of GRP78, ATF6 translocates to the Golgi complex where it is cleaved by S1 and S2 enzymes. The cleaved form of ATF6, together with NF-Y, enters the nucleus and regulates the expression of survival-related genes, often establishing cross-talk with the IRE1 and PERK branches. Most importantly, the three ER sensors work in concert to determine cell fate, survival or apoptosis. Selective modulation of any of these pathways is an attractive therapeutic approach.

luminal side; the other is present on the cytoplasmic C-terminal end, which contains the transmembrane kinase and endoribonuclease (RNase) domain. There are two paralogs of *IRE1*: *IRE1α* which is ubiquitously expressed. *IRE1β* expression is restricted to epithelial cells of the gastrointestinal tract and lungs.[10] When unfolded/misfolded proteins dissociate GRP78 from IRE1α during ER stress, IRE1α undergoes dimerization/oligomerization and autophosphorylation by its kinase domain, leading to conformational change and activation of the endoribonuclease domain. Upon activation of the IRE1α endoribonuclease, two distinct pathways are initiated to counteract ER stress. When the active form of IRE1α excises a 26-nucleotide intron from the unique mRNA encoding the X-boxing binding protein 1-unspliced (XBP1u) leading to a frame-shift, it results in translation of a larger, more stable and more potent transcription factor called X-boxing binding protein 1-spliced (XBP1s).[11] XBP1 has been characterized as a basic leucine zipper protein (bZIP) and can heterodimerize with c-fos, as well as bZIP, to regulate the expression of major histocompatibility complex (MHC) class II molecules associated with cellular functions, such as phagocytosis and endocytosis.[12] Under ER stress conditions, activated XBP1s translocates to the nucleus where it functions as a transcriptional activator that, preferentially binds to a consensus sequence motif defined as TGACGTGG/A.[8,13] This motif is found in the regulatory regions of genes involved in protein folding, prosurvival signaling, glycosylation, adipogenesis, vesicular trafficking, and ER-associated degradation (ERAD).[14] For example, XBP1s regulates UPR targets, such as ER chaperones (DnaJ/Hsp40-like genes, p58[IPK], ERdj4, HEDJ, and PDI-P5), ER degradation-enhancing α-mannosidase-like protein (EDEM), and ribosome-associated membrane protein 4 (RAMP4).[15] In estrogen receptor alpha positive (ERα⁺) breast cancer cells, XBP1s increases NF-κB signaling and directly regulates the expression of p65/RelA to promote cancer progression.[16] Besides, in the early stage of adipogenesis, IRE1 α-XBP1 signaling transactivates a key adipogenic factor CCAAT/enhancer-binding protein α (C/EBPα), through activation of C/EBPβ to in adipocytes.[17] Based on microarray analysis in XBP1s-transduced fibroblasts, genes related to vesicular transport have been identified, such as archain 1 (*ARCN1*), lectin mannose-binding 1 (*LMAN1*), and vesicle-associated membrane protein 4 (*VAMP4*).[15]

Another function of the RNase activity of IRE1 $\alpha$ is to cleave and inactivate diverse groups of mRNAs or viral RNAs into inactive fragments, especially in order to decrease the demand of protein synthesis, restore ER homeostasis and provide a defense mechanism against the threatening stimuli in the microenvironment, such as inflammatory responses or pathogen infection. This unique process is called regulated IRE1-dependent mRNA decay (RIDD).[18] Depending on the context, RIDD may occur through oligomerization or dimerization of IRE1.[19,20] For instance, pathogen-activated IRE1α cleaves mRNAs to produce single-stranded mRNA fragments without 5′-caps or 3′ poly-tails which are the typical characteristics for cytosolic mRNAs. These single-stranded mRNA fragments further activate a specific anti-viral RNA helicase called retinoic acid-inducible gene 1 (RIG-I) to cause the physical interaction of RIG-I and mitochondrial anti-viral-signaling protein (MAVS). Activation of RIG-I/MAVS eventually leads to an inflammatory response via NF-$\kappa$B and IFN (interferon) pathways.[21] In the context of the tumor microenvironment, prolonged RIDD activation promotes apoptosis through degradation of multiple mRNAs. Activation of this pathway is context dependent and a complete understanding of this mechanism is yet to be elucidated. When activated by phosphorylation, IRE1α associates with TRAF2, an adaptor protein for c-Jun amino terminal kinase (JNK) and inhibitor of $\kappa$B kinase (IKK).[22] JNK and IKK are critical proteins that have been implicated in the inflammatory response.

## 6. PERK Signaling

PERK is also a type I transmembrane protein composed of a luminal domain which allows PERK dimerization and a cytoplasmic domain containing Ser/Thr kinase activity. Upon dissociation of GRP78 under ER stress conditions, PERK is activated through auto-phosphorylation, followed by homodimerization. With regards to regulating ER homeostasis, the major downstream target of activated PERK is eukaryotic initiation factor 2α (eIF2α). Phosphorylation of eIF2α at Ser51 by PERK causes inactivation of the eIF2α complex resulting in attenuation of global protein translation.[23] This process not only decreases the protein load on the ER, but PERK also selectively permits translation of a subset of genes involved in amino acid metabolism, autophagy, anti-oxidant responses, and apoptosis. For example, ATF4 is a downstream target of PERK signaling, which transcriptionaly regulates C/EBP homologous protein (CHOP; also called GADD153), a key transcription factor for apoptosis initiation during severe ER stress.[24] However, CHOP also induces the expression of growth arrest and DNA damage inducible protein 34 (GADD34) and enhances the interaction of GADD34 with protein phosphatase 1 (PP1). The complex of GADD34/PP1 can feedback and dephosphorylate eIF2$\alpha$, leading to the restoration of general mRNA translation.[25] Another example is a bZIP transcription factor, nuclear factor-erythroid 2-related factor 2 (NRF2). Upon PERK-mediated phosphorylation, followed by nuclear accumulation, NRF2 transcriptionally activates a subset of anti-oxidant genes, such as heme oxygenase 1 (HO-1), NADPH quinone oxidoreductase 1 (NQO1), and ATF3.[26] PERK–NRF2 signaling is crucial for preventing excessive accumulation of reactive oxygen species (ROS) during ER stress. Transmembrane protein 33 (TMEM33), a binding partner of PERK, increases the phosphorylation of eIF2 and IRE$\alpha$ and has been implicated in the regulation of autophagy and apoptosis in breast cancer cells.[27]

# 7. ATF6 Signaling

Unlike IRE$\alpha$ and PERK, which require oligomerization and phosphorylation for their kinase activities, ATF6, which has two isoforms ATF6$\alpha$ and ATF6$\beta$, is activated by proteolytic cleavage. Under ER stress, ATF6 dissociates from GRP78 and is translocated to the Golgi where it is cleaved by site-1 protease (S1) and site-2 protease (S2).[28] Consequently, the cytosolic bZIP domain of ATF6 is released from the Golgi and translocates to nucleus to promote transcription of protein folding genes, ER chaperones and ERAD components. The bZIP domain of nuclear ATF6 heterodimerizes with nuclear transcription factor Y (NF-Y; also called CCAAT-binding factor (CBF)) and binds to the ER stress response element (ERSE). The ERSE, defined as CCAAT-N$_9$-CCAGG, is responsible for regulating UPR target genes, such as *XBP1*, *GRP78*, *GRP94*, protein disulfide isomerase (*PDI*), *EDEM1*, and Calreticulin (*CALR*).[29,30] With respect to its downstream target genes, the ATF6 signaling is transient and generally characterized as a prosurvival pathway.[30] However, ATF6 has also been demonstrated that to upregulate the expression of CHOP and Bcl-2 family proteins associated with proapoptotic signaling during prolonged ER stress.[31] Moreover, studies have shown not only XBP1 but also ATF6 binds to ERSE II (ATTGG-N-CCACG), while the activation of ERSE II by ATF6 is NY-F dependent, its activation by XBP1 is independent of NY-F.[30] The promoter regions of several UPR-regulated genes have been identified to contain ERSE II, such as homocysteine-inducible ER stress protein (*HERP*), cationic amino acid transporter-1 (*CAT-1*) and arginine-rich, mutated in early stage of tumors (*ARMET*).[30,32] In contrast to the ubiquitous ATF6, several tissue-specific ATF6-like proteins such as Luman, CREB4, CREB3L1, and CREB3L2 have been discovered that are activated upon exposure to ER stress.[33] Luman (CREB3; also called LZIP), an ER transmembrane-bound transcription factor with structural similarity to ATF6, regulates *HERP* gene expression by directly binding to the second portion of ERSE II (CCACG).[34] The functions of these ATF6-like proteins are not entirely revealed but are believed to respond to various cellular stresses in tissue-specific conditions.

## 8. Hypoxia and the UPR Pathway

Due to fluctuations in pH, nutrient supply, and oxygen availability, the tumor microenvironment reflects a heterogeneous and dynamic compartment. In addition to the genetic and epigenetic disturbances, which promote tumor growth, changes in the microenvironment have also been proposed to impact the biologic behaviors of tumors including tumor progression and metastasis.[35,36] As tumor cells proliferate, hypoxia develops because of an imbalance between oxygen delivery and oxygen consumption. Tumors are well adapted to survive and proliferate even when they encounter hypoxic stress. The UPR is an adaptive response that enables tumor cells to survive under these conditions. However, under prolonged ER stress, signaling through the UPR can paradoxically result in apoptosis. Therefore, modulation of the UPR as a therapeutic strategy is complex and requires understanding the proper context for this signaling.

Recent *in vitro* and *in vivo* studies establish a strong relationship between hypoxia and activation of UPR.[37,38] In addition to hypoxia, other cellular stresses within the tumor microenvironment have been demonstrated to cause ER stress, including glucose and amino acid starvation, acidosis, ischemia-reperfusion and ROS production.[39] The major function of ER is essential for secreted and transmembrane proteins to process a series of post-translational modifications, such as glycosylation, formation of disulfide bonds, proteolytic cleavages, and assembling of multimetric proteins. These modifications are necessary for protein to fold properly and are required for their normal cellular functions. Investigators have shown that molecular oxygen act as a terminal in the process of disulfide bond formation mediated by FAD, Ero1, and PDI. In yeast, mutation of Ero1 increases the sensitivity of these cells to hypoxia.[40] In mammalian systems, several studies have linked hypoxia with activation of the UPR.[41–43] Thus, hypoxia is a critical regulator of the UPR within the tumor microenvironment and targeting this pathway is a promising anti-cancer therapeutic strategy. However, the exact mechanism of how hypoxia activates the UPR remains to be elucidated.

## 9. The Role of the UPR in Tumorigenesis

The development of hypoxia is a unique hallmark of the tumor microenvironment during tumor growth, resulting from perturbations in the delivery and consumption of oxygen and nutrients. Under severe hypoxic conditions, the UPR is activated in response to hypoxia and tumor microenvironment-induced ER stress. Initially, UPR promotes tumor cell survival but the prolonged activation of the UPR triggers proapoptotic signaling. Activation of the UPR under hypoxia is a HIF-1 $\alpha$-independent response that occurs under extremely low oxygen concentrations. These hypoxia-induced adaptive responses allow tumor cells to adapt to ER stress and also contribute to drug resistance. For example, *in vitro* studies have shown that inhibition of GRP78 by siRNA sensitizes cells to hypoxia. Conversely, ectopic expression of GRP78 increases resistance to chemotherapeutic agents, such as paclitaxel, bortezomib (also called PS341 or Velcade), and cisplatin.[44]

XBP1 is activated under hypoxia/anoxia, mediates survival under these conditions, and is required for tumor growth.[41] Under hypoxia, accumulation of unfolded/misfolded proteins induces phosphorylation of IRE1$\alpha$, which then processes XBP1u to XBP1s through its RNase activity.

XBP1s colocalizes with hypoxia markers, such as carbonic anhydrase 9 (CA9).[45] XBP1 is robustly activated in triple-negative breast cancers (TNBCs), and targeting this pathway in TNBCs may represent a therapeutic opportunity.[45] TNBCs are characterized by the lack of expression of estrogen receptor (ER), progesterone receptor (PR) and human epithelial growth factor receptor 2 (HER2).[46] This subtype of breast cancer behaves aggressively, and there are few effective therapies. Although the expression of HIF-$1\alpha$ in TNBCs is relatively higher than other breast cancer subtypes, XBP1 splicing occurs independently of HIF-$1\alpha$. In addition, XBP1s interacts directly with HIF-$1\alpha$ in the nucleus and binds to the hypoxia response element (HRE), facilitating expression of hypoxia target genes.[45] Moreover, knockdown of XBP1 causes loss of HIF-$1\alpha$ mediated mammosphere formation under hypoxia in TNBCs.[45]

In lung carcinoma, the IRE1 pathway is essential for upregulation of vascular endothelial growth factor-A (VEGF-A) under hypoxic or hypoglycemic conditions. Furthermore, A549 IRE1 dominant-negative (DN) tumors were observed to have lower number of neovascular vessels compared to control tumors. In tumor development and angiogenesis studies, U87 IRE1 DN cell-derived tumors exhibited significant inhibition of XBP1 mRNA splicing, low cellularity and low microvascular density in contrast to U87 pCDNA3 cell-derived control tumors in mouse brain model.[47] In addition, in human pancreatic adenocarcinomas, expression of XBP1 correlates with increased microvessel density to suggest that XBP1 is also a critical regulator of angiogenesis.[48] Finally, the significance of the IRE1/XBP1 pathway is supported by the clinical observation that high XBP1 levels correlate with better response to the proteasomal inhibitor, bortezomib in human myeloma cells. These cells typically reside in the hypoxic microenvironment of bone marrow.[49]

During tumor development, hypoxia not only triggers HIF pathways to activate various cellular activities, such as erythropoiesis, angiogenesis, glucose metabolism and epithelial-to-mesenchymal transition (EMT), but also causes the reduction of cell proliferation and downregulation of global protein synthesis.[50] A critical step of protein synthesis is phosphorylation of eIF$2\alpha$ on Ser51, which is mediated through activation of PERK upon hypoxia. In PERK knockout mouse embryonic fibroblasts (MEFs) model, both phosphorylation of eIF$2\alpha$ and the rate of protein synthesis in cells expressing a DN PERK construct were significantly reduced. In clonogenic assays, *PERK–/–* MEFs, compared to wild-type MEFs, were more sensitive to prolonged exposure to hypoxia.[42,43] These results indicate that cells activate adaptive responses to hypoxia-induced ER stress through PERK, thus providing a direct link between the UPR, hypoxia, and cell survival. For example, carbonic anhydrase 9 (CA9), a tumor-associated enzyme, plays a critical role in regulating ion transport and pH maintenance in a variety of tumor types. This gene contains an HRE in its promoter region that regulates its activation by HIF-1$\alpha$ during hypoxia.[51] However, another mechanism for regulating CA9 expression occurs through the PERK/eIF2$\alpha$/ATF4-dependent pathway during hypoxia. In a chromatin immunoprecipitation (ChIP) assay, ATF4 was shown to bind directly to the CA9 promoter and induce CA9 expression in response to PERK-dependent phosphorylation of eIF2$\alpha$ during hypoxia.[52] Moreover, CA9 expression is correlated with a poor prognosis and an aggressive tumor phenotype. Therefore, CA9 could be a putative target for anti-cancer therapy in hypoxic regions of tumors.[53]

In mammalian cells, cellular stresses, such as ER stress, nutrient deprivation and oxidative stress, induce ATF4 expression through PERK and other eIF2$\alpha$ kinase, e.g. general control non-derepressible 2 (GCN2), in order to activate target genes involved in ER folding capacity, translation recovery and apoptosis. Therefore, the eIF2$\alpha$-ATF4 axis integrates all types of stress signals and facilitates downstream cellular responses either to maintain normal physiological functions or promote cell death.[54] This pathway is referred to as the integrated stress response (ISR). For example, PERK knockout or eIF2$\alpha$ S51A mutation leading to inactivation of ISR has been shown to increase cell sensitivity to hypoxia/anoxia and level of apoptosis both *in vitro* and *in vivo*.[43] During hypoxia, mitochondria are the primary sites for the production of ROS, which has been demonstrated as a critical factor to activate the ISR for energy homeostasis and activation of the UPR.[55] One study has also shown that activation of the PERK/eIF2$\alpha$ signaling under severe hypoxia stimulates glutathione (GSH) synthesis and reduces ROS production, thereby increasing autophagic capacity and promotion of survival rate of tumor cells.[56] Recent reports have shown that tumor hypoxia activates autophagy in the result of promoting cell survival through UPR induction. Several autophagy-related genes, such as microtubule-associated protein 1 light chain 3β (*MAP1LC3B*) and autophagy-related gene 5 (*ATG5*), required for phagophore expansion and autophagosome formation, have been shown to be upregulated by ATF4 and CHOP, respectively.[57] Moreover, lysosomal-associated membrane protein 3 *(LAMP3)*, a novel metastasis-associated gene, is also induced upon activation of the PERK/eIF2α/ATF4 signaling under hypoxia.[58] These findings suggest that the PERK/eIF2α/ATF4 signaling branch of UPR plays a central role in mediating hypoxia-induced autophagy, metastasis, and apoptosis.

Although the regulation of ATF6 by hypoxia is an important factor integrating stress signaling with maintenance of ER homeostasis, direct evidence for activation of ATF6 by hypoxia is still lacking. In a primary cardiac myocyte model, ischemia-induced nutrient and oxygen starvation increases the nuclear fractions of ATF6 that bind to the GRP78 promoter containing the ERSE sequence for transcriptional activation. Additional experiments also demonstrate that inhibition of ATF6 blocks ischemia (0.1% Oxygen)-mediated GRP78 induction and promotes cardiac myocyte death.[59] A recent microarray data revealed that the Derlin-3 (*Derl3*) gene, which encodes one of the ERAD machinery components, was strongly induced by ATF6 and may play a protective role in ischemic mouse cardiac cells.[60] However, both *in vivo* and *in vitro* studies indicated that under severe hypoxia (0.1% Oxygen), cleavage of ATF6 and caspase-12 was induced, which drives apoptotic signaling in neonatal hypoxic-ischemic encephalopathy (HIE).[61] In cancer, several studies also show a link between ATF6 and hypoxia in terms of tumorigenesis. For example, a disintegrin and metalloproteinase (ADAM17), a tumor-associated protein has been found to overexpress in several human cancers, including breast, gastric and prostate cancer, showed the correlation with UPR and hypoxia.[62] Although HIF-1α is necessary to maintain the basal expression of ADAM17 mRNA under hypoxic conditions, the induction of ADAM17 requires the PERK/eIF2α/ATF4 and ATF6 branches upon severe hypoxia. Activation of ADAM17 causes the release of tumor necrosis factor receptor 1 (TNFR1) from the cell membrane, which contributes to the resistance to ER stress and promotes survival in response to hypoxia and inflammation.[62] Additional evidence demonstrates that hypoxia not only activates UPR signaling to modulate ER homeostasis and cell survival but also promotes EMT towards tumor metastasis. In human gastric cancer cells, severe hypoxia or treatment with thapsigargin, a $Ca^{2+}$-ATPase inhibitor that potently induces ER stress, results in activation of the PERK/eIF2$\alpha$/ATF4 and ATF6 branches and initiation of EMT.[63] All of these studies provide a putative link between ATF6 and hypoxia, which needs to be further investigated for the development of UPR targeted cancer therapies.

## 10. Therapeutic Targeting of the UPR in Disease

Numerous *in vitro* and *in vivo* findings point to the importance of the UPR in a variety of diseases, such as neurodegenerative and metabolic diseases, tissue ischemia, diabetes, inflammatory diseases and cancer.[64] Targeting various elements of the UPR is an attractive therapeutic strategy, considerable efforts have been made to develop pharmacologic modulators of this pathway. In some diseases, selective activation of the UPR is desired and in other disease states, inhibition is required. Thus, understanding the biological processes that regulate the UPR is critical for developing drugs that target this complex signaling pathway.

Two major strategies have been adopted to modulate the UPR for therapeutic purposes. The first strategy focuses on increasing the adaptive capacity of cells under ER stress to reduce the accumulation of misfolded proteins and restore ER homeostasis (Table 1). This strategy provides therapeutic benefits by promoting ER stress-induced cell survival pathways in neurodegenerative diseases and metabolic disorders. For example, salubrinal, an inhibitor of eIF2$\alpha$ phosphatase, indirectly increases eIF2$\alpha$ phosphorylation by inactivating the eIF2$\alpha$ phosphatase complex GADD34-PP1 and constitutive regulator of eIF2$\alpha$ phosphorylation (CReP).[65] Increased eIF2$\alpha$ phosphorylation attenuates global protein translation and activates ATF4 signaling in order to maintain normal cellular functions. Salubrinal has been shown to increase neuronal survival during excitotoxic neuronal injury and also extends survival in the pre-clinical models of Parkinson's disease and amyotrophic lateral sclerosis (ALS).[66,67] 4-phenylbutyrate (4-PBA) and tauroursodeoxycholic acid (TUDCA) are chemical chaperones that can stabilize protein folding and reduce abnormal protein aggregation to improve ER function in primary biliary cirrhosis and urea cycle disorders, respectively.[68,69] In addition,

Table 1.   Therapeutic compounds modulating the UPR.

| Molecule | Type | Target | Readout | Refs. |
| --- | --- | --- | --- | --- |
| **Improves ER function** | | | | |
| Salubrinal | Inhibitor | GADD34-PP1C and CReP | Increases eIF2$\alpha$ phosphorylation | 65–67 |
| 4-PBA | Chemical chaperones | Misfolded proteins | Decreases misfolded protein and protein aggregation | 68 |
| TUDCA | Chemical chaperones | Misfolded proteins | Decreases misfolded protein and protein aggregation | 69 |
| BIX | Inducer | ATF6 pathway | Induces GRP78 expression | 71, 72 |
| **Inhibits UPR pro-survival signaling** | | | | |
| Salicyaldehydes | Inhibitor | IRE1$\alpha$ RNase domain | Blocks XBP1 mRNA splicing | 73 |
| 4$\mu$8C | Inhibitor | IRE1$\alpha$ RNase domain | Blocks XBP1 mRNA splicing | 74 |
| STF-083010 | Inhibitor | IRE1$\alpha$ RNase domain | Blocks XBP1 mRNA splicing | 75 |
| MKC-3946 | Inhibitor | IRE1$\alpha$ RNase domain | Blocks XBP1 mRNA splicing | 49 |
| Hydroxy aryl aldehydes | Inhibitor | IRE1$\alpha$ RNase domain | Blocks XBP1 mRNA splicing | 85 |
| Sunitinib | Inhibitor | IRE1$\alpha$ kinase domain | Inhibits IRE1 activity | 76 |
| APY29 | Inhibitor | IRE1$\alpha$ kinase domain | Inhibits IRE1 activity | 77 |
| Compound 3 | Inhibitor | IRE1$\alpha$ kinase domain | Inhibits IRE1 activity | 78 |
| GSK2606416 | Inhibitor | PERK | Inhibits PERK and eIF2$\alpha$ phosphorylation | 79 |
| ISRIB | Inhibitor | eIF2$\alpha$ | Inhibits eIF2$\alpha$ phosphorylation | 80 |
| Bortezomib | Inhibitor | 26S proteasome | Activation of UPR | 81 |
| MG132 | Inhibitor | 26S proteasome | Activation of UPR | 81 |
| Eeyarestatin | Inhibitor | VCP | Accumulation of polyubiquitinated proteins | 82 |
| ML240 | Inhibitor | VCP | Accumulation of polyubiquitinated proteins | 83 |
| DBeQ | Inhibitor | VCP | Accumulation of polyubiquitinated proteins | 84 |

chemical chaperones have also been reported to improve insulin sensitivity and glucose homeostasis by reducing ER stress in mouse models of obesity.[70] Another strategy to improve ER folding capacity was shown by the identification of BiP inducer X (BIX), identified through a compound library screen as a molecule that increases GRP78 (BiP) expression.[71] BIX has cytoprotective effects in several diseases including cerebral artery occlusion and kidney ischaemia.[72]

A second major strategy for modulating the UPR therapeutically is based on inhibiting UPR pro-survival signaling and switching the UPR towards ER stress-induced cell death (Table 1). This approach is a promising anti-cancer therapeutic strategy. MEFs that are deficient in either *Xbp1* or *Perk* have diminished potential to grow as tumor xenografts, suggesting that pharmacologic inhibition of these pathways could be an effective cancer therapy.[41,43] As discussed above, IRE1$\alpha$ contains two enzymatic domains located on the C-terminal cytoplasmic portion of this ER transmembrane protein: the RNase and the ER transmembrane kinase. Both of these domains may be targets for drug discovery to inhibit IRE1$\alpha$ activity, thereby promoting proapoptosis signals by inhibiting the ER homeostasis signaling aspects of the UPR. Several molecules, such as salicyaldehydes, 4$\mu$8C, STF-083010, and MKC-3946, have been developed, that target the catalytic core of IRE1$\alpha$'s RNase domain.[39] For example, salicyaldehydes and 4$\mu$8C block XBP1 splicing and RIDD in multiple myeloma, and STF-083010 and MKC-3946 show significant suppression of tumor growth in human multiple myeloma-bearing mouse model.[49,73–75] Kinase inhibitors such as sunitinib, APY29 and compound 3 were demonstrated to interact with the ATP binding pocket of IRE1$\alpha$ *in vitro* and *in vivo*.[76–78] With regards to the PERK branch of UPR, GSK2606416, a structurally-based inhibitor, blocks PERK and eIF2$\alpha$ phosphorylation in pancreatic cancer, whereas ISRIB, a potent inhibitor of eIF2$\alpha$ phosphorylation, impairs ER homeostasis without altering PERK activity.[79,80] These strategies show considerable promise in preclinical cancer models.

When unfolded/misfolded proteins accumulate in the ER, IRE1$\alpha$ also regulates ERAD a pathway stimulates ubiquitination and degradation of ER proteins. Thus, disruption of ERAD is another strategy to reduce protein clearance and thereby increase ER stress in tumor cells that ultimately results in apoptosis. Two categories of small molecules may be utilized to inhibit ERAD: the 26S proteasome inhibitors, such as bortezomib and MG132; valosin-containing protein (VCP; also called p97) ATPase inhibitors such as eeyarestatin, ML240 and DBeQ.[81–84] VCP, an AAA+ATPase (ATPases associated with diverse cellular activities), modulates ERAD by facilitating protein degradation of polyubiquitinated ERAD substrates through the ubiquitin–proteasome system in the cytoplasm. Eeyarestatin, a VCP inhibitor, blocks ERAD to result in inhibition of tumor proliferation in cervical cancer.[81]

Combination strategies to simultaneously inhibit multiple branches of the UPR are yet to be attempted, but in theory this approach may by highly synergistic since there is considerable redundancy in UPR signaling and overlap in the regulation of common genes. However, normal tissue toxicity with complete inhibition of the UPR may limit the feasibility of this approach.

## 11. Concluding Remarks

In the field of tumor biology, significant progress has been made towards understanding the role of the IRE1$\alpha$ and PERK pathways in tumor progression. A growing body of evidence provides multidirectional views in exploring the role of UPR under a variety of tumor microenvironmental conditions, such as inflammation, metabolic stress, hypoxia, and pH fluctuations. Tumor cells have been highly adapted to survive and proliferate under these microenvironmental conditions. Therefore, to increase the efficacy of current anti-cancer treatments, it is critical to identify the downstream effectors of the UPR that regulate tumor growth in the context of the tumor microenvironment. Thus, genetic manipulation of UPR-related genes and inhibition of major UPR effectors by pharmacologic methods are important biologic tools that can be used to dissect out the complexities of UPR signaling in tumors. Ultimately, a complete mechanistic understanding of how these networks function is essential to developing therapies that target these pathways.

## References

1. Ron, D., and Walter, P., Signal integration in the endoplasmic reticulum unfolded protein response, *Nat. Rev. Mol. Cell Biol.*, **8**, pp. 519–529, 2007.

2. Boelens, J., Lust, S., Offner, F. *et al.*, Review. The endoplasmic reticulum: a target for new anticancer drugs, *In Vivo*, **21**, pp. 215–226, 2007.

3. Kim, I., Xu, W., and Reed, J. C., Cell death and endoplasmic reticulum stress: disease relevance and therapeutic opportunities, *Nat. Rev. Drug Discov.*, **7**, pp. 1013–1030, 2008.

4. Bernales, S., Papa, F. R., and Walter, P., Intracellular signaling by the unfolded protein response, *Annu Rev Cell Dev. Biol.*, **22**, pp. 487–508, 2006.

5. Bertolotti, A., Zhang, Y., Hendershot, L. M. *et al.*, Dynamic interaction of BiP and ER stress transducers in the unfolded-protein response, *Nat. Cell Biol.*, **22**, pp. 326–332, 2000.

6. Shen, J., Chen, X., Hendershot, L., and Prywes R., ER stress regulation of ATF6 localization by dissociation of BiP/GRP78 binding and unmasking of Golgi localization signals, *Dev. Cell.*, **3**, pp. 99–111, 2002.

7. Stein, I., Neeman, M., Shweiki, D. *et al.*, Stabilization of vascular endothelial growth factor mRNA by hypoxia and hypoglycemia and coregulation with other ischemia-induced genes, *Mol. Cell. Biol.*, **15**, pp. 5363–5368, 1995.

8. Yoshida, H., Haze, K., Yanagi, H. *et al.*, Identification of the cis-acting endoplasmic reticulum stress response element responsible for transcriptional induction of mammalian glucose-regulated proteins. Involvement of basic leucine zipper transcription factors, *J. Biol. Chem.*, **273**, pp. 33741–33749, 1998.

9. Gardner, B. M., and Walter, P., Unfolded proteins are Ire1-activating ligands that directly induce the unfolded protein response, *Science.*, **333**, pp. 1891–1894, 2011.

10. Tirasophon, W., Welihinda, A. A., and Kaufman, R. J., A stress response pathway from the endoplasmic reticulum to the nucleus requires a novel bifunctional protein kinase/endoribonuclease (Ire1p) in mammalian cells, *Genes Dev.*, **12**, pp. 1812–1824, 1998.

11. Yoshida, H., Matsui, T., Yamamoto, A. *et al.*, XBP1 mRNA is induced by A TF6 and spliced by IRE1 in response to ER stress to produce a highly active transcription factor, *Cell*, **107**, pp. 881–891, 2001.

12. Ono, S. J., Liou, H. C., Davidon, R. *et al.*, Human X-box-binding protein 1 is required for the transcription of a subset of human class II major histocompatibility genes and forms a heterodimer with c-fos, *P. Natl. Acad. Sci. USA*, **88**, pp. 4309–4312, 1991.

13. Yamamoto, K., Yoshida, H., Kokame, K. *et al.*, Differential contributions of ATF6 and XBP1 to the activation of endoplasmic reticulum stress-responsive cis-acting elements ERSE, UPRE and ERSE-II, *J. Biochem.*, **136**, pp. 343–350, 2004.

14. Hampton, R. Y. ER-associated degradation in protein quality control and cellular regulation, *Curr. Opin. Cell. Biol.*, **14**, pp. 476–482, 2002.

15. Sriburi, R., Jackowski, S., Mori, K., and Brewer, J. W., XBP1: a link between the unfolded protein response, lipid biosynthesis, and biogenesis of the endoplasmic reticulum, *J. Cell. Biol.*, **167**, pp. 35–41, 2004.

16. Hu, R., Warri, A., Jin, L. *et al.*, NF-$\kappa$B signaling is required for XBP1 (unspliced and spliced)-mediated effects on antiestrogen responsiveness and cell fate decisions in breast cancer, *Mol. Cell. Biol.*, **35**, pp. 379–390, 2015.

17. Sha H, He Y, Chen. H. *et al.*, The IRE1 $\alpha$-XBP1 pathway of the unfolded protein response is required for adipogenesis, *Cell. Metab.*, **9**, pp. 556–564, 2009.

18. Fung, T. S., Liao, Y., and Liu, D. X., The endoplasmic reticulum stress sensor IRE1$\alpha$ protects cells from apoptosis induced by the coronavirus infectious bronchitis virus, *J. Virol.*, **88**, pp. 12752–12764, 2014.

19. Han, D., Lerner, A. G., Vande Walle, L. *et al.*, IRE1$\alpha$ kinase activation modes control alternate endoribonuclease outputs to determine divergent cell fates, *Cell*, **138**, pp. 562–575, 2009.

20. Tam, A. B., Koong, A. C., and Niwa, M., Ire1 has distinct catalytic mechanisms for XBP1/HAC1 splicing and RIDD, *Cell. Rep.*, **9**, pp. 850–858, 2014.

21. Lencer, W. I., DeLuca, H., Grey, M. J., and Cho, J. A., Innate immunity at mucosal surfaces: the IRE1-RIDD-RIG-I pathway, *Trends Immunol.*, **36**, pp. 401–409, 2015.

22. Hu, P., Han, Z., Couvillon, A. D. *et al.*, Autocrine tumor necrosis factor $\alpha$ links endoplasmic reticulum stress to the membrane death receptor pathway through IRE1$\alpha$-mediated NF-kappaB activation and down-regulation of TRAF2 expression, *Mol. Cell. Biol.*, **26**, pp. 3071–3084, 2006.

23. Harding, H. P., Zhang, Y., and Ron, D., Protein translation and folding are coupled by an endoplasmic-reticulum-resident kinase, *Nature*, **397**, pp. 271–274, 1999.

24. Harding, H. P., Novoa, I., Zhang, Y. *et al.*, Regulated translation initiation controls stress-induced gene expression in mammalian cells, *Mol Cell.*, **6**, pp. 1099–1108, 2000.

25. Novoa, I., Zeng, H., Harding, H. P., and Ron, D., Feedback inhibition of the unfolded protein response by GADD34-mediated dephosphorylation of eIF2 $\alpha$, *J Cell Biol.*, **153**, pp. 1011–1022, 2001.

26. Qaisiya, M., Coda Zabett,a C. D., Bellarosa, C., and Tiribelli, C., Bilirubin mediated oxidative stress involves antioxidant response activation via Nrf2 pathway, *Cell Signal.*, **26**, pp. 512–520, 2014.

27. Sakabe, I., Hu, R., Jin, L. *et al.*, TMEM33: a new stress-inducible endoplasmic reticulum transmembrane protein and modulator of the unfolded protein response signaling, *Breast Cancer Res Treat.*, **153**, pp. 285–297, 2015.

28. Haze, K., Yoshida, H., Yanagi, H. *et al.*, Mammalian transcription factor ATF6 is synthesized as a transmembrane protein and activated by proteolysis in response to endoplasmic reticulum stress, *Mol Biol Cell.*, **10**, pp. 3787–3799, 1999.

29. Yoshida, H., Okada, T., Haze, K. *et al.*, ATF6 activated by proteolysis binds in the presence of NF-Y (CBF) directly to the cis-acting element responsible for the mammalian unfolded protein response, *Mol Cell Biol.*, **20**, pp. 6755–6767, 2000.

30. Kokame, K., Kato, H., and Miyata, T., Identification of ERSE-II, a new cis-acting element responsible for the ATF6-dependent mammalian unfolded protein response, *J Biol Chem.*, **276**, pp. 9199–9205, 2001.

31. Manga, P., Bis, S., Knoll, K. *et al.*, The unfolded protein response in melanocytes: activation in response to chemical stressors of the endoplasmic reticulum and tyrosinase misfolding, *Pigment Cell Melanoma Res.*, **23**, pp. 627–634, 2010.

32. Huang, C. C., Li, Y., Lopez, A. B. *et al.*, Temporal regulation of Cat-1 (cationic amino acid transporter-1) gene transcription during endoplasmic reticulum stress, *Biochem J.*, **429**, pp. 215–224, 2010.

33. Balogh, A., Németh, M., Koloszár, I. *et al.*, Overexpression of CREB protein protects from tunicamycin-induced apoptosis in various rat cell types, *Apoptosis.*, **19**, pp. 1080–1098, 2014.

34. Liang, G., Audas, T. E., Li, Y. *et al.*, Luman/CREB3 induces transcription of the endoplasmic reticulum (ER) stress response protein Herp through an ER stress response element, *Mol Cell Biol.*, **26**, pp. 7999–8010, 2006.

35. Heddleston, J. M., Li, Z., Lathia, J. D. *et al.*, Hypoxia inducible factors in cancer stem cells, *Br J Cancer.*, **102**, pp. 789–795, 2010.

36. Patiar, S. and Harris, L. A. Role of hypoxia-inducible factor-1$\alpha$ as a cancer therapy target. *Endocr Relat Cancer.*, **13**, pp. S61–S75, 2006.

37. Feldman, D. E., Chauhan, V., and Koong, A. C., The unfolded protein response: a novel component of the hypoxic stress response in tumors, *Mol Cancer Res.*, **3**, pp. 597–605, 2005.

38. Schönenberger, M. J., and Kovacs, W. J., Hypoxia signaling pathways: modulators of oxygen-related organelles, *Front Cell Dev Biol.*, **3**, pp. 1–19, 2015.

39. Jiang, D., Niwa, M., and Koong, A. C., Targeting the IRE1$\alpha$-XBP1 branch of the unfolded protein response in human diseases, *Semin Cancer Biol.*, **33**, pp. 48–56, 2015.

40. Tu, B. P., and Weissman, J. S., The FAD- and O(2)-dependent reaction cycle of Ero1-mediated oxidative protein folding in the endoplasmic reticulum, *Mol Cell.*, **10**, pp. 983–994, 2002.

41. Romero-Ramirez, L., Cao, H., Nelson, D. *et al.*, XBP1 is essential for survival under hypoxic conditions and is required for tumor growth, *Cancer Res.*, **64**, pp. 5943–5947, 2004.

42. Koumenis, C., Naczki, C., Koritzinsky, M. *et al.*, Regulation of protein synthesis by hypoxia via activation of the endoplasmic reticulum kinase PERK and phosphorylation of the translation initiation factor eIF2$\alpha$, *Mol Cell Biol.*, **22**, pp. 7405–7416, 2002.

43. Bi, M., Naczki, C., Koritzinsky, M. *et al.*, ER-stress-regulated translation increases tolerance to extreme hypoxia and promotes tumor growth, *EMBO J.*, **24**, pp. 3470–3481, 2005.

44. Pi, L., Li, X., Song, Q. *et al.*, Knockdown of glucose-regulated protein 78 abrogates chemoresistance of hypopharyngeal carcinoma cells to cisplatin induced by unfolded protein in response to severe hypoxia, *Oncol Lett.*, **7**, pp. 685–692, 2013.

45. Chen, X., Iliopoulos, D., Zhang, Q. *et al.*, XBP1 promotes triple-negative breast cancer by controlling the HIF1 $\alpha$ pathway, *Nature.*, **508**, pp. 103–107, 2014

46. Chacón, R. D., and Costanzo, M. V., Triple-negative breast cancer, *Breast Cancer Res.*, **12**, pp. 1–9, 2010.

47. Drogat, B., Auguste, P., Nguyen, D. T. *et al.*, IRE1 signaling is essential for ischemia-induced vascular endothelial growth factor-A expression and contributes to angiogenesis and tumor growth *in vivo*, *Cancer Res.*, **67**, pp. 6700–6707, 2007.

48. Romero-Ramirez, L., Cao, H., Regalado, M. P. *et al.*, X box-binding protein 1 regulates angiogenesis in human pancreatic adenocarcinomas, *Transl. Oncol.*, **2**, pp. 31–38, 2009.

49. Mimura, N., Fulciniti, M., Gorgun, G. *et al.*, Blockade of XBP1 splicing by inhibition of IRE1$\alpha$ is a promising therapeutic option in multiple myeloma, *Blood.*, **119**, 5772–5781, 2012.

50. Majmundar, A. J., Wong, W. J., and Simon, M. C., Hypoxia-inducible factors and the response to hypoxic stress, *Mol Cell.*, **40**, pp. 294–309, 2010.

51. Wykoff, C. C., Beasley, N. J., Watson, P. H. *et al.*, Hypoxia-inducible expression of tumor-associated carbonic anhydrases, *Cancer Res.*, **60**, pp. 7075–7083, 2000.

52. van den Beucken, T., Koritzinsky, M., Niessen, H. *et al.*, Hypoxia-induced expression of carbonic anhydrase 9 is dependent on the unfolded protein response, *J Biol Chem.*, **28**, pp. 24204–24212, 2009.

53. Benej, M., Pastorekova, S. and Pastorek, J. Carbonic anhydrase IX: regulation and role in cancer, *Subcell Biochem.*, **75**, pp. 199–219, 2014.

54. Fels, D. R., and Koumenis, C., The PERK/eIF2$\alpha$/ATF4 module of the UPR in hypoxia resistance and tumor growth, *Cancer Biol Ther.*, **5**, pp. 723–728, 2006.

55. Liu, L., Wise, D. R., Diehl, J. A., and Simon, M. C., Hypoxic reactive oxygen species regulate the integrated stress response and cell survival, *J Biol Chem.*, **283**, pp. 31153–31162, 2008.

56. Rouschop, K. M., Dubois, L. J., Keulers, T. G. *et al.*, PERK/eIF2 $\alpha$ signaling protects therapy resistant hypoxic cells through induction of glutathione synthesis and protection against ROS, *Proc Natl Acad Sci USA.*, **110**, pp. 4622–4627, 2013.

57. Rouschop, K. M., van den Beucken, T., Dubois, L. *et al.*, The unfolded protein response protects human tumor cells during hypoxia through regulation of the autophagy genes MAP1LC3B and ATG5, *J Clin Invest.*, **120**, pp. 127–141, 2010.

58. Mujcic, H., Rzymski, T., Rouschop, K. M. *et al.*, Hypoxic activation of the unfolded protein response (UPR) induces expression of the metastasis-associated gene LAMP3, *Radiother Oncol.*, **92**, pp. 450–459, 2009.

59. Doroudgar, S., Thuerauf, D. J., Marcinko, M. C. *et al.*, Ischemia activates the ATF6 branch of the endoplasmic reticulum stress response, *J Biol Chem.*, **284**, pp. 29735–29745, 2009.

60. Belmont, P. J., Chen, W. J., San Pedro, M. N. *et al.*, Roles for endoplasmic reticulum-associated degradation and the novel endoplasmic reticulum stress response gene Derlin-3 in the ischemic heart, *Circ Res.*, **106**, pp. 307–316, 2010.

61. Liu, L., Liu, C., Lu, Y. *et al.*, ER stress related factor ATF6 and caspase-12 trigger apoptosis in neonatal hypoxic-ischemic encephalopathy, *Int J Clin Exp Pathol.*, **8**, pp. 6960–6966, 2015.

62. Rzymski, T., Petry, A., Kračun, D. *et al.*, The unfolded protein response controls induction and activation of ADAM17/TACE by severe hypoxia and ER stress, *Oncogene.*, **31**, pp. 3621–3634, 2012.

63. Shen, X., Xue, Y., Si, Y. *et al.*, The unfolded protein response potentiates epithelial-to-mesenchymal transition (EMT) of gastric cancer cells under severe hypoxic conditions, *Med Oncol.*, **32**, p. 447, 2015.

64. Wang, S., and Kaufman, R. J., The impact of the unfolded protein response on human disease, *J Cell Biol.*, **197**, pp. 857–867, 2012.

65. Boyce, M., Bryant, K. F., Jousse, C. *et al.*, A selective inhibitor of eIF2 aplpha dephosphorylation protects cells from ER stress, *Science.*, **307**, pp. 935–939, 2005.

66. Colla, E., Coune, P., Liu, Y. *et al.*, Endoplasmic reticulum stress is important for the manifestations of α-synucleinopathy *in vivo*, *J Neurosci.*, **32**, pp. 3306–3320, 2012.

67. Saxena, S., Cabuy, E., and Caroni, P. A role for motoneuron subtype-selective ER stress in disease manifestations of FALS mice, *Nat Neurosci.*, **12**, pp. 627–636, 2009.

68. Lindquist, S. L., and Kelly, J. W., Chemical and biological approaches for adapting proteostasis to ameliorate protein misfolding and aggregation diseases: progress and prognosis, *Cold Spring Harb Perspect Biol.*, **3**, pp. 1–34, 2011.

69. Seyhun, E., Malo, A., Schäfer, C. *et al.*, Tauroursodeoxycholic acid reduces endoplasmic reticulum stress, acinar cell damage, and systemic inflammation in acute pancreatitis, *Am J Physiol Gastrointest Liver Physiol.*, **301**, pp. G773–782, 2011.

70. Ozcan, U., Yilmaz, E., Ozcan, L. *et al.*, Chemical chaperones reduce ER stress and restore glucose homeostasis in a mouse model of type 2 diabetes, *Science.*, **313**, pp. 1137–1140, 2006.

71. Kudo, T., Kanemoto, S., Hara, H. *et al.*, A molecular chaperone inducer protects neurons from ER stress, *Cell Death Differ.*, **15**, pp. 364–375, 2008.

72. Prachasilchai, W., Sonoda, H., Yokota-Ikeda, N. *et al.*, The protective effect of a newly developed molecular chaperone-inducer against mouse ischemic acute kidney injury, *J Pharmacol Sci.*, **109**, pp. 311–314, 2009.

73. Volkmann, K., Lucas, J. L., Vuga, D. *et al.*, Potent and selective inhibitors of the inositol-requiring enzyme 1 endoribonuclease, *J Biol Chem.*, **286**, pp. 12743–12755, 2011.

74. Cross, B. C., Bond, P. J., Sadowski, P. G. *et al.*, The molecular basis for selective inhibition of unconventional mRNA splicing by an IRE1-binding small molecule, *P. Natl. Acad. Sci. USA.*, **109**, pp. E869–E878, 2012.

75. Papandreou, I., Denko, N. C., Olson, M. *et al.*, Identification of an Ire1 α endonuclease specific inhibitor with cytotoxic activity against human multiple myeloma, *Blood*, **117**, pp. 1311–1314, 2011.

76. Ali, M. M., Bagratuni, T., Davenport, E. L. *et al.*, Structure of the Ire1 auto-phosphorylation complex and implications for the unfolded protein response, *EMBO J.*, **30**, pp. 894–905, 2011.

77. Bouchecareilh, M., Higa, A., Fribourg, S. *et al.*, Peptides derived from the bifunctional kinase/RNase enzyme IRE1α modulate IRE1α activity and protect cells from endoplasmic reticulum stress, *FASEB J.*, **25**, pp. 3115–3129, 2011.

78. Wang, L., Perera, B. G., Hari, S. B. *et al.*, Divergent allosteric control of the IRE1α endoribonuclease using kinase inhibitors, *Nat. Chem. Biol.*, **8**, pp. 982–989, 2012.

79. Axten, J. M., Medina, J. R., Feng, Y. *et al.*, Discovery of 7-methyl-5-(1-{[3-(trifluoromethyl)phenyl]acetyl}-2,3-dihydro-1H-indol-5-yl)-7H-pyrrolo[2,3-d] pyrimidin-4-amine (GSK2606414), a potent and selective first-in-class inhibitor of protein kinase R (PKR)-like endoplasmic reticulum kinase (PERK), *J Med. Chem.*, **55**, pp. 7193–7207, 2012.

80. Sidrauski, C., Acosta-Alvear, D., Khoutorsky, A. *et al.*, Pharmacological brake-release of mRNA translation enhances cognitive memory, *Elife.*, **2**, pp. 1–22, 2013.

81. Kisselev, A. F., van der Linden, W. A., and Overkleeft, H. S. Proteasome inhibitors: an expanding army attacking a unique target, *Chem. Biol.*, **19**, pp. 99–115, 2012.

82. Brem, G. J., Mylonas, I., and Brüning, A., Eeyarestatin causes cervical cancer cell sensitization to bortezomib treatment by augmenting ER stress and CHOP expression, *Gynecol. Oncol.*, **128**, pp. 383–390, 2013.

83. Chou, T. F., Li, K., Frankowski, K. J. *et al.*, Structure-activity relationship study reveals ML240 and ML241 as potent and selective inhibitors of p97 ATPase, *Chem. Med. Chem.*, **8**, pp. 297–312, 2013.

84. Chou, T. F., Brown, S. J., Minond, D. *et al.*, Reversible inhibitor of p97, DBeQ, impairs both ubiquitin-dependent and autophagic protein clearance pathways, *P. Natl. Acad. Sci. USA.*, **108**, pp. 4834–4839, 2011.

# Chapter 10

# The Hypoxic Tumor Microenvironment and the Anti-cancer Immune Response

Joseph Barbi[*,†] and Fan Pan[*,‡]

*Immunology and Hematopoiesis Division, Department
of Oncology, Sidney Kimmel Comprehensive Cancer Center,
Johns Hopkins University School of Medicine,
Baltimore, MD 21287, USA
†Department of Immunology,
Roswell Park Cancer Institute,
Buffalo, NY 14263, USA
‡fpan1@jhmi.edu

Oxygen is often scarce in inflamed, infected, or injured tissues. Therefore the ability of leukocytes to adapt to and function under these hypoxic conditions is central to the immune response. Solid tumors are also notorious for harboring regions of extreme oxygen deprivation making hypoxia highly relevant to the cancer-immune system interface. Hypoxia inducible factors (HIFs) have been well characterized as sensors of low oxygen stress, and they regulate the significant genetic reprogramming needed for cellular adaptation to hypoxia. These molecules have also been recently shown to be critical regulators of immune cell differentiation and function. Here, we summarize the growing body of literature describing the relationship between hypoxia and critical participants in the anti-tumor immune response. A central theme to this relationship is the capacity for immune modulation by the hypoxic tumor microenvironment. While this theme arises from numerous examples of immune impotency in the face of tumor hypoxia, understanding the mechanisms of hypoxia-enforced immune modulation and how they may be targeted therapeutically will pave the way for new and potent treatment strategies.

# 1. Introduction

Hypoxia is a hallmark trait of inflamed tissues along with acidosis, nutrient scarcity and an abundance of free oxygen radicals. Inflammation-associated injury to the microvasculature can compromise regional supplies of oxygen, and elevated consumption by invading microbes and activated leukocytes accumulating at inflammatory loci can result in oxygen levels as low as 0.5–3% by volume (compared to ~11% for normoxic tissues and ~20% for standard *in vitro* culture conditions).[16,97] Solid tumors are also known to encompass regions of extreme oxygen deprivation (hypoxic or anoxic zones). In tumors, the rapid growth of densely packed malignant cells outpaces the ability of the local circulation to deliver oxygen, and the aberrant and disorganized neovascularization induced by tumor cells accounts for zones of chronic and cycling hypoxia in tumor microenvironments.[28]

Tumor cells respond to hypoxia by upregulating gene products that support their survival, growth and spread. These gene expression changes are coordinated in large part by the oxygen sensor and transcriptional regulators known as HIFs. HIF-regulated genes (which number in the hundreds) include those responsible for promoting cancer cell metabolic function (glycolysis), angiogenesis, metastasis, and resistance to therapy.[118] More recently, the immunomodulatory qualities of hypoxia and HIFs have also been brought to light.

Indeed, it is clear now that hypoxic microenvironments found within tumors work in concert with a number of immunomodulatory factors (e.g. cytokines, metabolic byproducts, etc.) that ultimately work to impede the productive anti-tumor immunity. Understanding how hypoxia and the cellular response to the condition influence the function of immune cells engaged in the anti-tumor response is necessary for the design of therapies capable of breaking tumor-enforced tolerance and unleashing the destructive potential of the immune system to combat malignant threats.

## 1.1.  Oxygen dependent regulation of HIF-1

HIF is expressed across a remarkable range of species, and it is responsible for the cell's metabolic adaption to low oxygen status.[80] This oxygen sensor is a heterodimeric transcription factor comprised of a constitutively expressed HIF-1$\beta$ subunit (also known as the aryl hydrocarbon receptor nuclear translocator (ARNT) and an alpha subunit (either HIF-1$\alpha$ or HIF-2$\alpha$) that is tightly regulated at the protein level. While HIF-1 and HIF-2 are similar in their regulation, as well as the target genes they regulate in response to hypoxia, they are not identical in either respect. A 3rd molecule, HIF-3$\alpha$ has also been described as a negative feedback mechanism for inhibiting the activity of HIF-1$\alpha$.[113] Both HIF-1$\alpha$ and HIF-1$\beta$ contain basic-helix-loop-helix (bHLH) and PER–ARNT–SIM (PAS) domains, which are involved in DNA binding and hetreodimerization, respectively.[58]

Under normoxic conditions, HIF-1 expression is tightly regulated in an oxygen-dependent manner.[139] Here HIF-1 is rapidly downregulated at the protein level through the ubiquitin-proteasome pathway (Fig.1a). This process begins when HIF-1$\alpha$ protein is hydroxylated at prolines 402 and 564 by members of a family of prolyl hydroxylases domain proteins (PHD1, 2, and 3), which require oxygen for their function. These modifications permit the recruitment of the von Hippel–Lindau (VHL) tumor suppressor— ubiquitin E3 ligase complex (including elongin B/C, RBX1, and cullin2). Subsequent polyubiquitination of HIF-1$\alpha$ by the VHL complex marks the molecule for degradation by way of the 26S proteasome.[113]

In contrast, under low-oxygen conditions, or hypoxia, inactive PHDs do not modify HIF-1$\alpha$ subunits, which in, turn, fail to interact with VHL, and are therefore spared from degradation. Upon translocation to the nucleus, HIF subunit dimerization occurs, and the HIF complex can interact with cofactors such as p300 in order to bind the promoters of HIF-1-target genes at defined five-nucleotide sequences termed hypoxia response elements (HREs, 5'-[A/G]CGTG-3') (Fig. 1b). Among the many genes regulated by HIF-1 are those central to processes needed for hypoxia adaptation

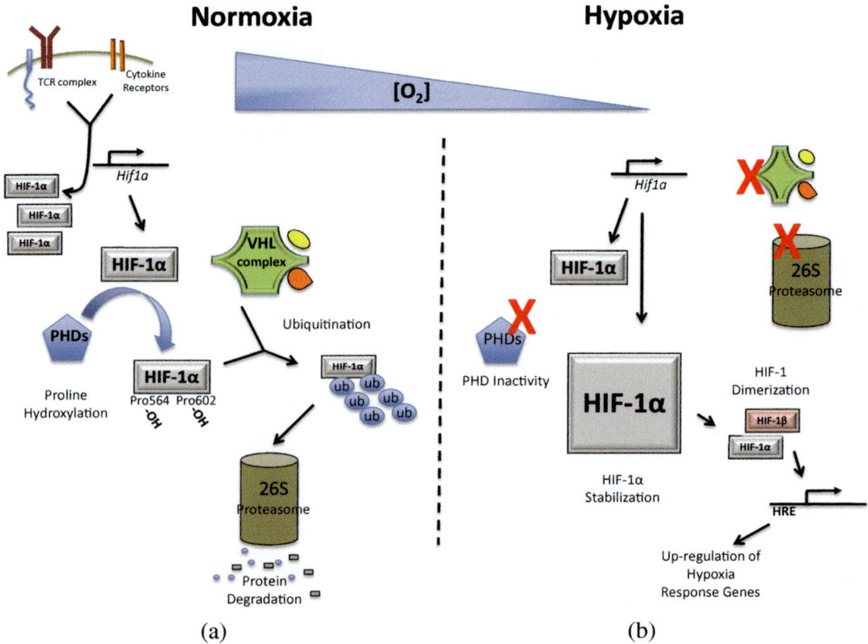



Fig. 1.   Regulation of HIF expression and function by oxygen levels. HIF is regulated at the protein level by oxygen-dependent mechanisms. HIF subunits are readily transcribed, however, in the presence of oxygen 1(a), proline residues of the HIF-1$\alpha$ subunit are hydroxylated by PHD enzymes (which are inactive under hypoxic conditions). Modified HIF-1 molecules then interact with the VHL/E3ligase complex, become polyubiquitinated, and are then degraded by the 26S proteasome. Under hypoxic conditions, HIF $\alpha$ subunits accumulate and associate with $\beta$ subunits to form an active transcription-regulating complex 1(b). In immune cells, and particularly T cells, HIF-1 expression can be transcriptionally upregulated even in the presence of oxygen in response to stimuli triggering TLR, TCR, and costimulation.

including metabolism, angiogenesis and apoptosis to name a few.[113,115] Importantly, HIF-1 can be up-regulated by a number of other stimuli capable of enhancing transcription of the *Hif1a* gene. These factors include cytokines, Toll-like receptor (TLR) ligands as well as triggers of T cell receptors (TCR) and mammelian target of rapamycin (mTOR) signaling.[10,94,129]

In the following sections, we will discuss the effects of hypoxia and HIFs on certain cells of the immune system that are highly relevant in determining the outcome of the leukocyte–tumor interaction.

## 2. Neutrophils

Neutrophils are granulocytic myeloid cells that constitute the first wave of immune system mobilization to various threats. Within hours of insult, these cells, recruited from the circulation, migrate into peripheral tissues where they encounter, environmental "danger signals" and stresses including microbial products, inflammatory cytokines and chemokines and, often, low oxygen levels. In this inhospitable microenvironment, these cells destroy invading pathogens in a "suicide-run" fashion by engulfing them (phagocytosis), releasing anti-microbial peptides and other cytotoxic molecules stored pre-formed in characteristic granules. Neutrophils also deploy a deadly oxidative burst and ensnare pathogens in a net-like matrix.[12,15]

There is ample evidence that both hypoxia and pathogen-induced stabilization of HIF levels significantly impacts neutrophil biology. In one study, HIF-1$\alpha$ was found to be crucial for expression of the anti-microbial molecule cathelicidin-related antimicrobial peptide (CRAMP) as well as cathepsin G activity in response to bacterial infection. Indeed, myeloid restricted knockout of HIF reduced the ability of mice to control infection.[104]

Other studies have shown an effect of hypoxia on, the mechanics of neutrophil recruitment. Specifically, HIF has been shown to mediate leukocyte adhesion under hypoxia by inducing $\beta$-2 integrin expression allowing adhesion to activated endothelium[64] suggesting a role for HIF-1 in the recruitment of neutrophils and other myeloid cells to regions of inflammation and hypoxia. Importantly, hypoxia can upregulate tumor and stromal cell production of CXCL8 — an important neutrophil chemoattractant — allowing for the accumulation of these cells in hypoxic tumor tissues.[131]

Hypoxic conditions also affect neutrophil longevity in a HIF-1-dependent fashion. Since a neutrophil's inflammatory potential is limited by its relatively short life span (6–8 hours in circulation),[128] mechanisms for staving off apoptosis can enhance the overall contribution of these cells to an immune response. Walmsely *et al.* used HIF-1$\alpha$ deficient neutrophils to demonstrate that HIF prolongs the survival of these cells in hypoxia through an NF$k$B-dependent mechanism.[137] This suggests that neutrophils entering the hypoxic zones at inflammatory sites as well as tumors may survive longer than their counterparts in circulation or healthy tissues.

Despite their cytotoxic and proinflammatory reputation, the accumulation and extended lifespan of neutrophils in hypoxic tumors can play a tumor-promoting role. This appears to be the case despite the potential for tumor-associated neutrophils (TANs) to positively contribute to an effective anti-tumor immune response (either by direct killing[20] *or* by collaborating with CD8+ T cells).[42] Neutrophils can constitute a major portion of the immune cells found associated with cancerous tissues, and indeed they display an activated phenotype in the early stages of lung cancer (stages, I, II) and can stimulate CD4+ and CD8+ T cell proliferation *ex vivo*.[33] Interestingly, during the early stages of lung carcinoma and mesothelioma mouse tumor models, neutrophils have been reported to chiefly accumulate in the presumably less hypoxic periphery of tumors. Moreover these early stage neutrophils were demonstrated to be more cytotoxic and proinflammatory than their late stage counterparts. With the progression of tumors, neutrophils take on a more promoting phenotype.[89]

As tumors progress, elements of the tumor microenvironment (e.g. the cytokine TGF$\beta$) have been reported to polarize TANs into tumor-abetting phenotypic subsets.[42] Indeed significant modulation of neutrophil function has been attributed to cancer cells.[47] These late stage TANs are decidedly less inflammatory with reduced killing ability, producing less TNF$\alpha$, NO, and $H_2O_2$ than early stage TANs.[89] Since hypoxic and necrotic regions become more prominent as tumors grow, and hypoxia and HIF-1 –regulated genes are enriched in TANs and other myeloid residents of tumors,[32] it is very likely that hypoxia contributes to this functional shift from a tumor-fighting to a tumor-promoting cell.

TANs, like macrophages residing in tumors, promote angiogenesis and have immunosuppressive function.[132] Angiogenesis is enhanced by TANs through the antagonism of anti-angiogenesis factors and the induction of vascular endtolhelial growth factor (VEGF).[66,101] These cells have also been reported to promote neovascularization by VEGF-independent[121] and chemokine-mediated pathways.[81] TAN-mediated immune suppression has been proposed to depend upon the release of arginase-1,[110] which suppresses T cell proliferation by depleting the extracellular pools of arginine, an amino acid required for T cell activity.[13,91]

In addition to promoting angiogenesis and having immune-dampening potential of their own, TANs have the capacity to recruit other suppressor cell types to the tumor microenvironment. Compared to circulatory neutrophils in blood, TANs upregulate the chemokines CCL2 and CCL17 that are capable of attracting regulatory T cells and immunosuppressive macrophage subsets in liver cancer.[152] Indeed, production of these cytokines and the presence of the regulatory cells they attract are enhanced under hypoxia, suggesting that early cellular recruits to the hypoxic tumor microenvironment facilitate the bolstering of the suppressor cell population there.

TAN have also been linked to the proliferation and survival of tumors. Also these cells can potentiate the metastatic capacity of tumor cells. Modulation of integrin expression by TANs can facilitate circulating tumor cell (CTC) adhesion to vascular endothelium promoting tumor cell metastasis.[54] Neutrophil production of collagenase-IV and heparanase — enzymes capable of digesting basement membranes and releasing tumor cells have also been thought for some time to contribute to tumor spreading.[143] In light of these multiple, potentially tumor-aiding roles that may be influenced by hypoxia, it is not surprising that an abundance of TANs has been linked to poor patient prognosis in many cancers.[119]

## 3. Myeloid-derived Suppressor Cells

Immature myeloid cells are generated in the bone marrow, and, under normal conditions, these precursor cells differentiate into the diverse populations of the myeloid lineage (e.g. macrophages, dendritic cells or "DCs", neutrophils). In the cancer setting, however, this course of differentiation is subverted and instead these cells give rise to myeloid-derived suppressor cell (MDSC) populations.[67] While cells of this heterogeneous population can show phenotypic shades of the different myeloid classes, MDSCs are incompletely differentiated (immature) and primarily suppress immune responses rather than prime them.

MDSCs are generally identifiable in mice by the surface markers CD11b and Gr-1. These cells are further subdivided based on their granulocytic traits (marked as CD11b + /Ly6G + /Ly6Clow expression) or monocytic character (the typically less abundant subset defined as CD11b + / Ly6C + /Ly6G-). Human MDSCs are CD11b + /CD33 + but lack expression of maturation markers and the class II MHC molecule, HLA-DR.[3,29,93,149]

These cells, relatively scarce under normal conditions, can be expanded significantly in tumor-bearing mice as well as cancer patients.[68]

MDSCs suppress T cell activation and expansion in response to antigen. This is accomplished through several mechanisms. One depends upon their metabolism of the amino acid L-arginine, the absence and products of which (resulting from the action of arginase or nitric-oxide synthase) down-modulate T cell activation.[13] Additionally, depletion of extracellular pools of cysteine, another amino acid necessary for T cell activation and proliferation contributes to the suppressive capacity of MDSCs.[125] Production of reactive oxygen species (ROS) and anti-inflammatory cytokines are also important mechanisms for MDSC-mediated suppression.[44,130] These suppressive mechanisms can be applied differentially across MDSC subsets.

Humans MDSC populations have been observed in most cancers[67] and tumor hypoxia has been implicated as a major influence on the differentiation and function of MDSCs in this setting. Corzo *et al.* found that MDSCs accumulating in the spleens of tumor-bearing mice exhibited the ability to suppress antigen-specific T cell activation in an ROS-dependent manner. Meanwhile their counterparts in the tumor microenvironment favored production of NO and arginase 1 activity and suppressed T cells in a non-antigen dependent manner.[22]

These findings suggested that the hypoxic tumor microenvironment modulates MDSC function. In support of this, stabilizing HIF-1 expression in splenic MDSCs by either hypoxic culture or treatment with deferrioxamine (an iron chelator and hypoxia mimetic) recapitulated the functional changes seen between the spleen and tumor derived MDSCs. Furthermore, exposure of MDSCs to hypoxia resulted in higher expression of IL-10, arginase I, nitric oxide synthase (iNOS) and IL-6 by the resulting macrophages.[22]

Hypoxia also appears to be important for the suppressive function of MDSCs in the tumor microenvironment mediated by inhibitory coreceptor signaling. It was recently revealed that HIF-1 binds and activates the promoter of the gene encoding programmed death-ligand 1(PD-L1, or B7H1). Blockade of PD-L1 alleviated the suppressive control of MDSCs over T cells and this was attributed to reduced production of IL-10 and IL-6 in the absence of PD1-PD-L1 signaling.[99] Ablation of HIF-1$\alpha$ also was found to undermine the ability of MDSCs to suppress T cells.[22] MDSCs under hypoxic conditions also upregulate chemokines including macrophage migration inhibitory factor (MIF), which can augment the immunosuppressive cellular presence in the tumor microenvironment through the recruitment of additional MDSCs.[153]

An aspect of MDSC biology that is highly relevant to the tumor-immune system interface is their ability to differentiate into tumor-associated macrophages (TAMs). Suggesting that tumor hypoxia promotes conversion to the TAM stage, in tumors tissue sections, mature macrophages (F480 + / GR1+ cells) were found enriched in zones of hypoxia (detected by the chemical hypoxia indicator pimonidazole). Furthermore, exposure of MDSCs to hypoxia resulted in higher expression of IL-10, arginase I, iNOS and IL-6 by the resulting macrophages[22] suggesting that hypoxia drives an immunosuppressive phenotype in mature TAMs.

The HIF-1 dependent nature of hypoxia-enhanced MDSC suppression was demonstrated using conditional, myeloid-restricted HIF-1 knockout mice. MDSCs from these mice were less effective suppressors than wild-type cells *in vitro* and *in vivo* and they showed lower expression of arginase I and iNOS, as well. HIF-1-deficient MDSCs also were much less likely to acquire the macrophage marker F480 than cells from wild-type mice. This defective TAM presence was notably linked to slower tumor growth.[22]

These results indicate that the hypoxic tumor microenvironment drives conversion of MDSCs to TAMs capable of promoting tumor growth rather than slowing it. In the following section, we will discuss the distinct roles played by hypoxia and HIFs in the broader biology of macrophages in- and outside the tumor microenvironment.

## 4. Macrophages

Macrophages residing in the peripheral tissues or derived from recruited monocyte precursors are critical for the triggering of an immune response and its subsequent execution. Through phagocytosis, release of anti-microbial peptides and ROS and NO, tissue resident macrophages patrol and defend peripheral tissues and facilitate the killing of pathogens. They also remove dead/dying host cells. Additionally macrophages are capable of presenting antigen to T cells, and along with the DCs they bridge the innate and adaptive immune responses.

Hypoxia has been shown to induce HIF in macrophages and have dramatic effects on the behavior of these cells.[77] Phagocytosis has been reported to increase in hypoxic macrophages, likely due to phagocytic receptor upregulation.[1] This enhancement is lost upon siRNA knockdown of HIF while, conversely, over-expression of HIF results in increased phagocytosis compared to control cells.[4] It has also been reported that under hypoxic conditions, macrophages display enhanced levels of the Th1-promoting cytokines IFN$\gamma$ and IL-12 compared to normoxic cells. HIF-1$\alpha$ binding to the *Ifng* promoter was crucial in this induction. Additionally antigen presentation was more efficient under hypoxia due to enhanced immune synapse formation.[1] In response to hypoxia HIF-1 binds the promoter of the gene encoding TLR4 and drives its upregulation[62] enhancing the sensitivity of macrophages to inflammatory triggers like LPS.

Reflecting a proinflammatory role for HIF-1 in macrophages, the molecule has been shown to be necessary for efficient killing of several clinically important bacterial pathogens by macrophages (and neutrophils as well). After demonstrating that bacterial infection of macrophages results in significant HIF induction, even under normoxic *in vitro* conditions, Peyssonnaux *et al.* used myeloid specific HIF1 deficient mice to evaluate the importance of the molecule in the anti-microbial action of macrophages against MRSA, *Salmonella typhimurium*, *Pseudomonas aeruginosa*, and group A Streptococcus. They found that HIF1-deficient bone marrow derived macrophages killed intracellular bacteria far less efficiently than wild-type cells.[104] Hypoxia-treated macrophages (both human and murine) were also more resistant to infection by parasitic protozoa when cocultured *in vitro* compared to normoxic controls.[21] These findings suggest that hypoxic conditions can actually promote the killing of engulfed pathogens by macrophages.

## 4.1. Macrophage polarization

The capacity of macrophages to become functionally specialized has gained wide appreciation. This so-called polarization is influenced heavily by cytokines in the microenvironment. "M1" or Classically Activated

Macrophages stimulated by TLR ligands (e.g. LPS) or inflammatory cytokines (such as IFNγ, GM-CSF, TNFα) upregulate their ability to kill microbial threats and drive proinflammatory immune responses. These cells are marked by high expression of iNOS and the heightened production of inflammatory cytokines (e.g. IL-12 and IL-23).[34] "M2" or alternatively activated macrophages (AAM), on the other hand, arise from exposure to the Th2-associated cytokines IL-4 and IL-13, or IL-10, TGFβ, M-CSF, and glucocorticoids. These cells have been noted for their high levels of IL-10 and production of arginase I. In stark contrast to their M1 counterparts, they can suppress inflammation and promote tissue repair. Importantly, M2 cells also have tumor-promoting functions as well.[34] These include the promotion of angiogenesis and metastasis and the suppression of anti-tumor immunity.[76]

The HIFs play significant roles in macrophage polarization. HIF-1α is induced in macrophages by Th1-associated cytokines. HIF-1α also appears to be required for macrophage maturation[37,102] and the promotion of a classical or M1-styled polarization. As mentioned in the previous section, HIF-1 appears necessary for effective microbicidal action, and HIF-1 deficiencies lead to less robust killing.[104] HIF-1 also promotes proinflammatory cytokine gene expression and effective immune synapse development.[1] Similar to the metabolic functions of HIF-1 in other cells of the immune system, this molecule's ability to promote glycolysis as a means to fuel activated, effector cells appears to be involved in the activation of macrophages.[23]

HIF-2α expression, on the other hand, can be upregulated in macrophages by Th2 cytokines. This factor, which is less involved in regulating glycolysis and apparently less critical for classical macrophage activation, is still readily detected *in vivo* in bone marrow by macrophages. Importantly, HIF-2 has been shown to be highly expressed by macrophages in tumor (TAMs) and is likely key to their protumor functions. Interestingly, the same cannot be said for HIF-1 as its deletion in macrophages actually enhances the acquisition of a TAM or M2-like phenotype[144] suggesting antagonistic cross-regulation between HIF-1 and HIF-2 in determining the polarization phenotype of macrophages. HIF-2 deficiency, on the other hand, has been associated with reduced TAM presence and impaired tumor progression in murine carcinoma models.[56]

## 4.2. Tumor associated macrophages

Macrophages tend to preferentially accumulate in hypoxic zones in tumors.[92] Indeed, TAMs are found across a diversity of human cancers, and these cells tend to display a decidedly M2 phenotype.[133] The prevalence of HIF-2+ TAMs is negatively associated with patient prognosis[61] reflecting the role played by these cells in tumor-promoting processes.

TAMs are either recruited to hypoxic zones or they differentiate there from monocyte precursors drawn to these tissues. Tumors release the chemokines CCL2 and CCL5, as well as the cytokine M-CSF, which recruits CCR2+ monocytes from the circulation, and TAM numbers positively correlate with these chemokine levels. Hypoxia does not appear to promote this element TAM. However retention of TAMs in hypoxic zones may involve the down-regulation of this chemokine–chemokine receptor axis.[92]

The chemokine receptor CXCR4 is stably upregulated in various cell types under hypoxia (including monocytes, macrophages, endothelial cells, and cancer cells). This apparently is dependent on HIF-1$\alpha$.[112] HIF-2 also induces the expression of CXCR4, and HIF-2 deficiency has been associated with reduced TAM recruitment and stymied (in fact, hypoxia can down-regulate CCL2 and its receptor) tumor progression in mice.[56] Furthermore the CXCR4 ligand CXCL12 (or Stromal Derived Factor 1-$\alpha$, SDF-1) is expression under hypoxic conditions[111] and is regulated by HIF-2 as well.[84] These observations suggest hypoxia potentiates TAM trafficking through this chemokine–chemokine receptor axis.

Elevated Eotaxin and Oncostatin M expression within the hypoxic zones of human breast cancer tissue has been linked to increased M2-type macrophage presence. Furthermore, blocking these factors can prevent the recruitment of macrophages as well as their polarization towards an M2-polarized phenotype. Importantly, this blockade slows tumor progression in a murine model of breast-cancer improving the anti-tumor effects of Bevacizumab, an anti-angiogenesis drug.[133]

Indeed promoting angiogenesis is a major tumor-abetting function of TAMs. Reflecting this, the specific presence of HIF-2-expressing TAMs is associated with increased tumor vascularity.[76] TAM enhanced angiogenesis appears to depend upon their ability to produce pro-angiogenic factors including factors stimulating endothelial migration, proliferation and growth (FGF-2, VEGF, G-CSF, GM-CSF, and CXCL8), as well as their ability to liberate pro-angiogenic factors through the degradation of the extracellular matrix. TAMs also mediate immune suppression. This can involve their production of the anti-inflammatory cytokines TGF$\beta$ and IL-10, as well as the metabolism of L-arginine by TAM-derived arginase I.[69]

One of these pro-angiogenesis factors, (VEGF) can have a multifaceted impact on hypoxic tumor niches. Levels of this well-known mediator of both normal and (pathologic) cancer-induced neovascularization are typically elevated in many tumors — especially in zones of hypoxia.[38] Indeed, VEGF is perhaps one of the most recognized genes activated in the HIF-mediated cellular response to hypoxia. Besides promoting the growth of new blood vessels in the tumor vicinity, VEGF can act as a chemotactic factor. Monocytes and macrophages migrate in response to VEGF *in vitro*,[92] and their presence in the breast cancer microenvironment correlates with VEGF expression there.[75] Importantly, in addition to potentially suppressive myeloid cells, Regulatory T cells (Tregs) can also detect and respond to VEGF as they express the VEGF receptor. As with TAMs, Treg levels have also been correlated with VEGF expression. These suppressor cells also express VEGF themselves,[35,36] suggesting that the prevalence of the molecule can reflect a feed-forward regulation of both neovascularization and immune suppression in hypoxic tumors.

Analysis of TAM gene expression revealed that while these macrophages can share some functional similarity with the M2/AAM subset, they display distinct patterns of gene regulation[40] suggesting elements of the tumor microenvironment may impart unique aspects to the TAM phenotype. As mentioned above, MDSCs can also differentiate into TAMs. Hypoxia has been shown to be critical for this transition.[22] Others contend that the hypoxic tumor microenvironment does not skew TAM subsets, but rather it determines the angiogenic potential of certain TAM populations.[70]

These findings demonstrate the important role played by hypoxia and HIF in the subversion of macrophages from potential instigators of tumor cell destruction to tumor-aiding cells.

## 5. Dendritic Cells

DCs are professional antigen-presenting cells. They play a crucial part in the detection of antigens and danger signals in the tissue microenvironment, and they are very important in the priming of T cell responses. The effects of hypoxia, and particularly, the hypoxic tumor microenvironment, on the behavior of DCs is less clear than with other immune cells at present.

In some studies, hypoxia appears to enhance their antigen-presenting capacity to stimulate T cell activation. Exposing human DCs to hypoxic conditions leads to the upregulation of various receptors (including toll-like receptors, C-type lectin receptors and Fc-receptors) that are capable of triggering well-known pathways of DC activation.[11,105] Indeed, LPS-induced activation of DCs under hypoxic culture conditions results in enhanced upregulation of MHC II, costimulatory molecules, proinflammatory cytokines and priming of T cell proliferation. This improved DC function was found to be HIF-$1\alpha$ dependent.[9,57]

Despite these reported stimulatory effects of hypoxia on DC function, it is well established that the tumor microenvironment has a decidedly negative impact on the immune-priming function of DCs. For instance, VEGF produced by tumors can inhibit the functional maturation of DCs.[43] Also, HIF-$1\alpha$ upregulation by human DCs in the hypoxic tumor environment induces adenosine receptor-mediated immune modulation (to be discussed in the following section). This favors development of Th2 cells over those of the Th1 lineage, and since the latter cell population is comprised of the more potent mediators of anti-tumor immunity,[148] this could certainly undermine the ability to target malignant cells. Additionally, lactic acid (a byproduct of hypoxic metabolism) produced by tumors has been linked to impaired DC function.[46] Hypoxia has also been reported to negatively impact human DC survival.[95] Other reports present a mixed message concerning hypoxia's effect on DC maturation and function. Hypoxia can increase proinflammatory cytokine production by DCs while preventing the upregulation of several maturation markers post-activation. Limited expression of the chemokine CCR7 in hypoxic DCs also suggests a negative role for hypoxia in DC trafficking to the sites of T cell priming.[83]

Future work will no doubt clarify our concept of the interplay between hypoxia and other inputs unique to the tumor microenvironment (metabolic products, cytokines, etc.) and their ultimate effects on DC function in the anti-tumor immune response.

# 6. T cells

The negative effects of hypoxia on T cell activation and function have been appreciated for some time.[5] Hypoxic culture of T cells dampens their proliferation in response to polyclonal stimuli — an effect attributed to negative regulation by HIF-1. On the other hand, knocking out HIF-1 has been linked to elevated proinflammatory cytokine production and NF$\kappa$B activity.[96]

A significant way in which hypoxia impacts the anti-tumor T cell response hinges upon the accumulation of extracellular adenosine in the hypoxic tumor microenvironment. Surges in the extracellular adenosine pool are a hallmark of inflamed tissues which affords a degree of protection from overzealous immune activation.[103]

Hypoxia can lead to the upregulation of adenine nucleotide-metabolizing ecto-enzymes CD39 and CD73, which facilitate the breakdown of tri- and diadenosine phosphate (ATP and AMP) to free adenosine. HIF-1 is capable of directly upregulating CD73 leading to increased adenosine production. Hypoxia also inhibits the action of adenosine kinase and that of adenosine deaminase, which catalyze the generation of AMP from adenosine.[82,123] Furthermore, adenosine uptake by cells is also inhibited under hypoxia due to the down-modulation of nucleoside transporters.[17]

By interacting with A2A receptors, which are expressed on multiple immune cell types, adenosine triggers an accumulation of cAMP and protein kinase A activity leading to suppression of T cell activation.[82,123] Adenosine can also activate suppressive Treg cells[103] and negatively impact the ability of DCs to prime T cell activation.[100]

This potent mechanism of T cell activation suppression ties hypoxia to the inhibition of T cell activation. Interestingly, hypoxia and HIF-1 have recently been shown to influence the differentiation of naïve T cells into functionally specialized lineages as well.

## 6.1. CD4+ T cell differentiation

Upon activation, naïve CD4+ T cells are capable of acquiring remarkably specialized effector functions in response to lineage-driving cytokines in the microenvironment. Signaling events downstream of the cytokine–cytokine receptor interaction activate the expression of "master regulator" transcription factors responsible for establishing and enforcing specific gene expression programs. These, in turn, underlie similarly unique T helper lineage-defining functions.[154]

T helper (Th) 1 cells, for instance, produce interferon-$\gamma$ (IFN$\gamma$) under the control of the transcription factor T-bet and drive cell-mediated immunity to protect against intracellular viral, bacterial, and parasitic infection. The Th1 response is also beneficial for anti-tumor immunity. Th2 cells produce interleukin-4 (IL-4), and are critical for controlling extracellular parasites such as helminthes. In these cells, GATA3 is a critical regulator of Th2-accociated gene expression. Th17 cell differentiation is driven by cytokines utilizing the STAT3 signaling pathway (e.g. IL-6) and the transcriptional regulator ROR$\gamma$t, and these cells are responsible for expelling extracellular bacteria and fungi through secretion of IL-17a, IL-17f, and IL-22. However, these cells, with their considerable inflammatory potential, are perhaps better known for their contribution to autoimmune disease and immune pathology.[154]

Naïve T cells can also acquire the ability to suppress the activation of other immune cells including the aforementioned effector subsets. By upregulating the transcription factor Foxp3 in response to signaling triggered by the cytokine TGF$\beta$ in conjunction with IL-2 and moderate TCR activation, naïve T cells can differentiate into induced (i)Tregs or peripheral (p)Tregs.[59]

Interestingly, the functionally opposite proinflammatory Th17 lineage and the immune-suppressing iTregs share common elements in their differentiation pathways. Specifically, the cytokine TGF$\beta$, for instance is required for both Th17 and iTreg generation.[74] High concentrations of TGF$\beta$ (among other factors) can sustain Foxp3 expression and commitment to an iTreg fate. The presence of STAT3-activating cytokines (such as IL-6, IL-21, and IL-23), in contrast, promotes the upregulation of the Th17-promoting transcription factor ROR$\gamma$t and the characteristic cytokine IL-17.[8,74] Since Foxp3 expression has been noted in the early stages of both subsets, and Foxp3 is known to actively suppress ROR$\gamma$t driven expression of Th17-associated genes,[151] timely down-regulation of Foxp3 activity from cells poised at the crossroads of these divergent lineages is likely necessary for optimal commitment to the Th17 fate.

Since STAT3-dependent signaling stabilizes HIF-1 expression in non-T cells,[60,147] we suspected such a pathway might be operative in developing T cells, influencing the relative balance between Th17 and Treg generating processes. In our studies, we found that during Th17 differentiation, HIF-1 is indeed induced in naïve CD4+ T cells, even in the presence of oxygen in a STAT3-dependent manner. Suggesting that HIF-1 is important for Th17 differentiation, HIF-1$\alpha$-deficient naïve CD4+ T cells (from CD4cre+/HIF-1$\alpha^{\text{flox/flox}}$ mice) display stunted upregulation of Th17 genes, including those encoding ROR$\gamma$t and IL-17 compared to wild-type cells. Further investigation would reveal that HIF-1 promotes expression of several Th17-linked genes through the activation of ROR$\gamma$t expression and function. Furthermore, we found that subjecting differentiating CD4+ T cells to periodic hypoxia also enhances Th17 commitment.[25]

Interestingly, in the absence of HIF-1, T cells show reciprocal upregulation of Foxp3 protein — but not its transcript[25] suggesting a HIF-1 dependent mechanism for the rapid down-regulation of Foxp3 protein at the crossroads of Th17 and iTreg differentiation. Reflecting an impaired commitment to the Th17 fate in favor of an iTreg one, T cell-specific HIF-1 deficient mice were protected from the more severe disease seen in wild-type mice in the EAE model of MS. The influence of HIF-1 on the reciprocal differentiation of Th17 and iTregs was independently observed by Shi *et al*. In their study, HIF-1's part in shaping the nature of the T cell response was tied to the molecule's role as a regulation of glycolytic metabolism.[120]

In T cells, as in cells of the tumor, HIF-1 drives expression of a number of genes necessary for the shift to a glycolysis-dominated metabolism.[117,136] In order to differentiate from uncommitted naïve CD4+ precursors into specialized effectors (Th1, Th2, Th17, etc.), proper upregulation of glucose metabolism is an absolute requisite. An inability to do so inhibits T effector cell differentiation both *in vitro* and *in vivo*.[45] Glycolytic inadequacies or forced utilization of fatty acid metabolism instead result in either T cell anergy or the commitment to the iTreg lineage.[26,88]

Reflecting this, in the study by Shi *et al.*, disrupting HIF-1 in T cells results in stunted expression of several glycolysis genes including those encoding Glut1, a glucose transporter; hexokinase 2; glucose-6-phosphate isomerase; enolase 1; pyruvate kinase muscle; and lactate dehydrogenase along side the Th17-associated factors IL-23R, IL-21, IL-22, and IL-17.

Supporting an important role for HIF-1 in the metabolic reprogramming necessary for Th17 differentiation, blocking glycolysis with the inhibitory glucose analog 2-DG recapitulated the results of genetic HIF-1 ablation in CD4+ T cells — as did the mTOR inhibiting drug rapamycin. These results suggest that HIF-1 is an important player, along with mTOR and PI3K/AKT, in a metabolic reprogramming pathway capable of shaping the nature of the T cell response.[120]

HIF-1 has also been implicated as a factor sustaining inflammatory Th17 cells and their function. Kryczek *et al.* found that long-lived and highly plastic human Th17 cells can be recovered from numerous types of diseased tissues. In their study, they found that Th17 cells express heightened levels of HIF-1 message compared to other T cell subsets, in agreement with the aforementioned mouse studies.[25,120] Suspecting that the ability of Th17 cells to survive in various inflamed tissues was mediated by HIF-1, the authors tested the effects of HIF-1 inhibition (echinomycin treatment) on the *in vivo* persistence of these cells. Supporting a role for HIF-1 in promoting the longevity of Th17 cells, inhibiting the molecule promoted the *in vivo* apoptosis of Th17 cells — an effect attributed to HIF-1s control of Notch signaling and anti-apoptotic gene expression.[65]

While these studies do not directly address the effects of tumor hypoxia on the T cell response, they are nevertheless relevant to the development of potential anti-cancer immunotherapies that take advantage of HIF-1's role in T cell immunity. Targeting HIF-1 in cancer (a therapeutic strategy already being pursued in order to disrupt tumor cell metabolism) should yield direct, negative effects on tumor cell growth. Such a treatment strategy should also undermine a tumor-abetting immune cell population. Since IL-17-producing cells have tumor-promoting functions[141] down-modulating a major cellular source of IL-17 is likely to eliminate this aid. The potential benefits of this strategy must, however, be weighed against the possible loss of the anti-tumor effects attributed to Th17 cells at later stages of tumor progression.[145]

## 6.2. Regulatory T cells

While HIF-1 drives commitment of naïve CD4+ T cells to a Th17 fate, it does so apparently at the expense of reciprocal induction of Foxp3+ Tregs. Naïve CD4+ T cells lacking HIF-1 preferentially up-regulate Foxp3 under Th17-inducing conditions, *in vitro*.[25,120] Interestingly, this effect of disrupting HIF-1 function occurred at the protein level as Foxp3 message was not markedly altered between wild-type and HIF-1-deficient CD4+ T cells.[25] It was also demonstrated that HIF-1 and Foxp3 physically interact, and HIF-1 promotes the proteasomal degradation of Foxp3 through the same pathway responsible for its own oxygen-dependent regulation in cell lines and developing iTregs.[25] Whether or not HIF-1 and Foxp3 can be codegraded in complex together remains to be elucidated, as do the precise molecular events involved in this process.

Interestingly, others have reported that hypoxia and HIF-1 can positively affect expression of Foxp3 primarily by enhancing transcription of the *Foxp3* gene.[7,19] Indeed the ability to activate transcription at the HIF-responsive *Foxp3* and *Ctla4* loci in established Tregs appears to be important for their fitness and their function in the inhospitable setting of the inflamed colon.[19] It is tempting to speculate that elements of the hypoxic response induce distinct protein- and transcript-level regulatory mechanisms that may have opposite effects. These may allow for negative feedback control or highly responsive fine-tuning mechanisms to up- or down-modulate the suppressive function of Tregs. This hypothetical tug-of-war may provide for context-dependent regulation of T cell development. For instance, under prolonged hypoxia, the transcriptional output of HIF-1 activity may prevail, while cycling levels of hypoxia, or intermittent hypoxic stress (in which the HIF-1 turnover machinery is still active) may facilitate the loss of Foxp3 protein from developing and committed Tregs. More study will be needed to evaluate this potentially complex relationship between hypoxia and Tregs.

Nevertheless, Foxp3+ Tregs are frequently found enriched systemically in cancer patients and also in close association with tumor tissues where zones of hypoxia are common. This association may be, however, quite complex.

Evidence is mounting that Tregs, while enriched in the tumor microenvironment do not differentiate there, and instead these suppressor cells are recruited from elsewhere including tumor-draining lymph nodes.[134,138] In line with the notion that Tregs may accumulate, but do not arise in hypoxic zones, imaging leukocyte migration in tumor tissues revealed that most Tregs migrate close to blood vessels, where one might expect relatively less hypoxic zones.[31] Also expression levels of HIF-1 and Foxp3 have been negatively correlated in a form of cutaneous T cell lymphoma an observation seemingly at odds with a general association between Tregs and hypoxia.[2]

In contrast, gastric tumors witness increased levels of both HIF-1 and Foxp3. Importantly, hypoxic tumor cells of this type have been shown to up-regulate systemic levels of TGF-$\beta$. Widespread elevation of this pro-Treg cytokine could result enhanced generation of Foxp3+ T cells, especially in the lymphoid tissues proximal to hypoxic tumors.[27] In this way, tumor hypoxia may have anatomically far-reaching effects on Treg induction.

The trafficking of Tregs to tumors also appears to be highly responsive to the oxygen levels there,[53] and indeed, HIF-1 has been implicated in the guiding of Tregs to the tumor site. Tumor hypoxia has been shown to induce high expression of the chemokine CCL28, which is responsible for recruiting CCR10+ Tregs.[36] In ovarian cancer, TAMs, which also accumulate in hypoxic tumors, produce CCL22.[24] This chemokine, which is also produced by tumor cells themselves can facilitate the recruitment of a subpopulation of Tregs referred to as activated or effector Tregs that express the receptor CCR4. These CCR4+ Tregs are known to be potent suppressors that preferentially home to and accumulate in tumors.[6,126] CCL17, another CCR4 ligand, also promotes Treg accumulation in tumors.[85,90] Importantly, both CCL17[79] and CCL22 are induced by hypoxia.[63]

In addition to Treg recruitment, hypoxia has also been reported to promote the expansion of Tregs.[49] All these findings suggest that multiple aspects of Foxp3+ Treg biology are influenced by hypoxia. Moreover, they suggest that different subsets of Tregs (i.e. activated/effector, established, or developing Tregs) may respond uniquely to hypoxia and the products of the hypoxic tumor microenvironment.

A similarly complex role for hypoxia and HIF-1 in the programming of a distinct regulatory T cell subset, the Tr1 cells, was recently brought to light.[86] These cells, which do not express Foxp3, are characterized by their ready production of the anti-inflammatory cytokine IL-10. Like their Foxp3+ counterparts, Tr1 are important in the maintenance of immune homeostasis and are capable of limiting inflammatory damage in a number of disease models including those for neuroinflammation and IBD.[106,108,109]

In this study, hypoxia inhibited Tr1 generation and specifically, HIF-1 upregulation (a hallmark of hypoxia), negatively impacted the differentiation of Tr1 cells. This antagonism of Tr1 generation by high HIF-1 levels was found to stem from the negative effects of HIF-1 on both the protein pool and activity of a key player in the Tr1 differentiation program — the aryl hydrocarbon receptor (AHR). This was linked to a competition for HIF-1$\beta$/ARNT subunits between its potential binding partners HIF-1$\alpha$ and AHR, the latter requiring ARNT to activate expression of key Tr1-associated genes like *Il10*, *Il21*, and *Entpd1*.[86] Interestingly, HIF-1 was also found to play a positive role in the early differentiation of Tr1 by promoting an aerobic glycolysis-dominated metabolic profile necessary for the Tr1 phenotype — suggesting that HIF-1 plays a duplicitous role in the biology of this unique Treg subset.

## 6.3. Dynamic regulation of T cells by hypoxia

The duration and extent of hypoxic stress may have significant consequences for the shaping of the T cell response. These variables also likely influence the anti-tumor immune response. It has been shown that Th17 skewing can be boosted by short-term, HIF-1-inducing, hypoxic culture. Importantly, however, optimal Th17 commitment was seen only when cells were primed with a brief period of hypoxia followed by re-oxygenation. This boost in Th17 differentiation, which was not observed for other Th cell lineages, was found to be HIF-1-dependent as it was not seen in T cells lacking HIF-1 expression.[55]

Another study confirmed that not only does short-term hypoxic priming enhance IL-17 upregulation by naïve CD4+ T cells, such treatment actually resulted in more robust HIF-1 levels than prolonged hypoxic culture. Correspondingly, the upregulation of IL-17 under extended hypoxia was less robust than after transient hypoxia/re-oxygenation. These observations were explained by the discovery of a hypoxia/HIF-1-dependent upregulation of a microRNA (miR210) capable of targeting HIF-1's own transcript.[140] Short-term hypoxic priming apparently avoids this built-in mechanism for negative feedback control of HIF-1 activity as it fails to induce high miR210 levels. In this study, knocking out miR210 resulted in even higher levels of HIF-1 and HIF-1-dependent Th17 differentiation following hypoxic priming compared to that seen in wild-type T cells.[140]

Also, speaking on the issues of hypoxia duration and the extent of HIF-1 induction (HIF-1 "dose"), a pair of recent studies explored the consequences of an overly robust HIF-1 pool on Treg function and phenotypic stability. In one study, deletion of Deltex (DTX1) — a promoter of HIF-1 protein turnover, in mice predictably result in high and apparently stable HIF-1 expression. DTX1-deficient Tregs were shown to be less effective suppressors than their wild-type counterparts *in vivo* (using models of airway inflammation and colitis). This was linked to unstable expression of Foxp3, which was observed in parallel with bolstered HIF-1 levels. DTX1 expression could prevent a hypoxia-induced reduction of the Foxp3 protein pool in T cells. Importantly, the authors showed that simultaneous HIF-1- and DTX1-deficiency in Tregs restored their *in vivo* Foxp3 expression level, which largely rescued the ability of DTX1-deficient Tregs to function *in vivo*.[52]

In the other study, conditional, Foxp3-driven knockout of VHL, the E3 ligase complex responsible for HIF degradation, caused a sustained elevation in HIF levels in Tregs. This undermined the suppressive phenotype of Tregs as evidenced by both the spontaneous inflammation and early mortality seen in Foxp3Cre[+]/VHL[fl/fl] mice. Furthermore these mice showed signs of high-baseline levels of T cell activation, and Tregs isolated from these mice show reduced Foxp3 expression, especially in Tregs isolated from tissues reputed to be hypoxic.[72] These phenotypically unstable and ineffective Tregs were further shown to acquire an abhorrent, Th1 effector-like phenotype driven by HIF-1s transcriptional regulation of effect T cell genes (i.e. *Ifng*) and metabolic genes encoding the machinery needed for glycolysis[72] — a metabolic lifestyle incompatible with the suppressive phenotype of Tregs.[88]

These studies suggest that very high levels HIF-1 expression or activity can negatively impact Treg phenotype. Taken with the observation that established Tregs can be less effective *in vivo* without HIF-1, one comes away with the notion that to some degree, HIF-1 can stabilize Tregs, but "too much of a good thing" can have the opposite effect. These findings also suggest that the relationship between HIF-1 expression and Treg stability may be complex.

## 7. CD8+ T cells

HIF-1 also plays important, and somewhat complex roles in the CD8+ T cell compartment. Insights into these roles may improve our understanding of CD8+ T cells behavior in hypoxic tumor niches.

## 7.1.  HIF-1 and CD8+ T cell metabolism

Resting CD8+ T cells, like their CD4+ counterparts are fueled by fatty acid oxidation while quiescent. However, following activation, these cells adopt a glycolysis-dominated metabolism needed to support their proliferation and differentiation into effector and memory subsets.[41,45,107,135] The triggering of TCR signaling and costimulation through CD28 induces expression of Myc and expression of Myc-dependent genes that are critical for the initial activation and expansion of T cells. Another wave of TCR-triggered genes including AP4, IRF4, and HIF-1 is thought to continue the cellular commitment to glycolysis by facilitating the upregulation of enzymes involved in glycolysis and glutaminolysis.[18] Effector CD8+ T cells are characteristically short-lived and their numbers contract with the waning of the immune response. Memory CD8+ T cells, on the other hand, persist[146] and can respond to antigenic re-challenge with rapid kinetics.[87] Among the effector and memory CD8+ T cell subsets are those with defining killing capacity that are known as cytotoxic T lymphocytes (CTLs).

CTLs are crucial mediators of cell-mediated immunity. Activation of these cells can trigger the killing of infected or altered (malignant) host cells mediated by production and release of perforin and granzymes. CTLs are also capable of driving proinflammatory immune responses by producing cytokines including TNF$\alpha$ and IFN$\gamma$.[48]

Finlay *et al.* identified HIF-1 as a major facilitator of the metabolic shift in newly activated CD8+ T cells. These authors found that upon encountering their cognate antigen in the presence of IL-2, CD8+ T cells show enhanced mTORC1 activity, which leads to robust levels of HIF-1$\alpha$ and $\beta$ subunits and isolated CTLs also showed high expression of HIF-1 as well. Upregulation of HIF-1 by mTORC1 in these activated CD8+ T cells was found to promote glucose uptake and glycolysis through the upregulation of numerous glycolytic enzymes and the glucose transporter Glut1. On the other hand, HIF-1-deficiency resulted in the downregulation of CTL effector molecules (granzymes and perforin).[39] Importantly, these authors also found that hypoxic culture conditions could enhance the expression of metabolic and effector molecules (perforin and Glut1) in CTLs[39] clearly linking HIF-1 to the metabolic lifestyle of activated, effector CD8+ T cells.

While antigen-mediated activation of CTLs potentiates their cytotoxic and proinflammatory potential, scenarios of persistent antigen exposure (i.e. chronic infection, cancer) dampen the intensity of CTL responses.[146] Using a model for chronic viral infection, specifically a lymphocytic choriomeningitis virus (LCMV) model, Doedens *et al.* found that high levels of HIF-1 activity resulted in a bolstered, sustained CTL phenotype.

Deletion of the VHL complex, which mediates the degradation of HIFs in the presence of oxygen, has been shown to enhance levels of HIF-1 and HIF-2 in activated CD8+ T cells and may partially mimic hypoxia. This in turn resulted in a more intense and sustained effector phenotype in CD8+ T cells marked by elevated expression of genes related to glycolysis, CTL effector function, and T cell activation. Furthermore, in this study, stabilization of HIF-1 levels by hypoxic culture could recapitulate the effects of VHL-knockout. Specifically, hypoxic culture resulted in a HIF-1-dependent enhancement of granzyme B, activation-induced surface markers (i.e. LAG3, CTLA-4) while transcription factors involved in T cell differentiation (i.e. T-bet and TCF-1) were downregulated by hypoxia as they were in T cells genetically lacking VHL.[30] The results of these studies suggest that under hypoxic conditions, CD8+ T cells may be enhanced in their ability to function as proinflammatory agents of cell-mediated immunity.

Interestingly, however, hypoxia and HIF-1 may make tumor cells a tougher target, for these HIF-1 dependent CTLs. Hypoxia has also been shown to render tumor cells resistant to killing by CTLs. This occurs from the cooperative activity of HIF-1 and STAT3 signaling in the malignant target cell.[98] Hypoxia also induces a shedding of MHC I molecules, making them less detectible to immune surveillance.[122]

HIF-1 also plays a role in memory CD8+ T cells, which persist beyond the immune response's contraction phase, outlasting their terminally differentiated effector counterparts. Like naïve T cells, these cells are quiescent, but they can respond to antigenic re-challenge with accelerated kinetics comparable to cells of the innate immune system. This functional shift is accompanied by an "immediate early" upregulation of glycolytic metabolism.

Stabilized HIF-1 expression, resulting either from hypoxia or other means, might therefore be expected to optimize the killing and inflammatory potential of the memory CD8+ T cell compartment as well as that of effector counterparts. Interestingly, however, Sukumar *et al.* found that while chemical inhibition of glycolysis (and HIF-1 expression) reduced commitment to a short-lived effector CD8+ T cell fate, these conditions led instead to an enhanced, memory-like population (identifiable as KLRG1[low]/CD62L[high]). Also, artificially enforcing glycolytic metabolism in CD8+ T cells could restrict the generation of memory cells in this study.[127] Interestingly, these memory CD8+ accumulating upon glycolysis-blockade and HIF-1 downregulation were actually more effective at combating tumor growth than control cells more inclined to become short-lived effectors.[127] These results suggest that HIF-1 (and potentially the hypoxic tumor microenvironment) may suppress the generation of potent tumor-killing CD8+ T cells.

## 8.  B cells

B cells can contribute to the anti-tumor immune response.[78] However, recently characterized, immune-suppressing B cell subsets (so-called Regulatory B cells or Bregs) are found in tumor bearing mice and humans. These cells can produce anti-inflammatory cytokines such as IL-10 or they can mediate the expansion and generation of Tregs to antagonize the anti-tumor immune response.[51] It is not clear, at present, how tumor hypoxia impacts this suppressor cell subset. However, there appears to be a metabolic component to Breg accumulation in the cancer setting.[142] Given that the hypoxia response machinery (i.e. HIFs) are actively involved in the metabolic programming of immune cells, it seems likely that hypoxic tumors or the products of these microenvironments can influence the generation, expansion or function of suppressive B cells. Continued work will no doubt shed light on this topic.

## 9.  Summary and Discussion

The immunomodulatory potential of hypoxia is considerable. As we have discussed here, a variety of immune cell types are susceptible to modulation by the low oxygen levels they are likely to encounter in the tumor microenvironment and tumor associated tissues. These examples of regulation-by-hypoxia include the processes of cellular differentiation, function, trafficking, fitness and in some cases the acquisition of tumor-aiding

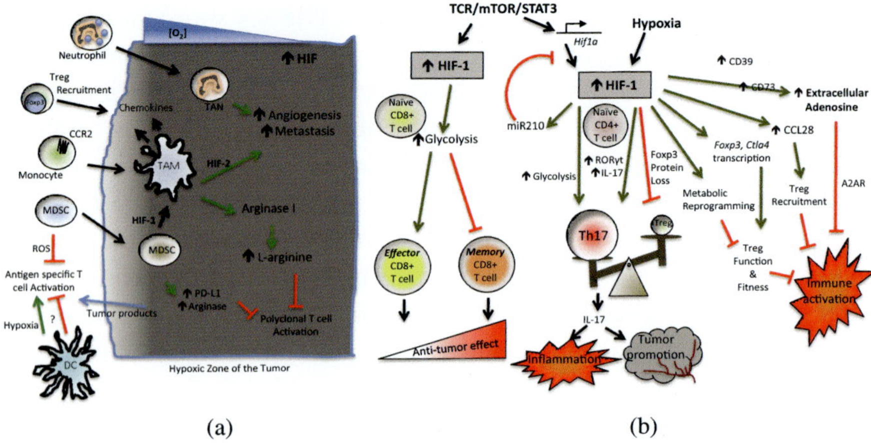

(a)                                                      (b)

Fig. 2. Multifaceted immune modulation by the hypoxic tumor microenvironment. Hypoxia has numerous effects on the leukocyte populations involved in the anti-tumor immune response. Myeloid cell types can take on immune-suppressing and pro-angiogenic function in the tumor microenvironment. They can also mediate the recruitment of suppressor cell subsets including Tregs (a). CD4+ and CD8+ T cells are also significantly impacted by hypoxia and HIF-1 upregulation. Examples of HIF-modified T cell biology include skewed Thelper cell differentiation, altered T cell recruitment and function and metabolic reprogramming events that impact both Tregs and effector T cells (b).

properties. This appears to be the case for myeloid (Fig. 2(a)) and well various T cell populations involved in the immune response to tumors (Fig. 2(b)). As should be clear from our discussion, there are still many unanswered questions left to be addressed before we can boast a comprehensive grasp on the effects of tumor hypoxia on the immune system.

The influence of low oxygen levels specifically on the interface of tumors and the immune system is not only a fascinating example of the complex interplay between immunity and the microenvironment, it is also of great interest to those seeking to develop novel therapies to bolster the armory of cancer fighting weapons.

## 10. Therapeutic Implications

With the hypoxic tumor microenvironment having such a profound impact on the anti-tumor immune response (summarized in Fig. 2), it is not surprising that treatment strategies counteracting hypoxia and targeting HIF-1 activity are being looked to as potential cancer-fighting immunotherapies.

Thermal therapy is a promising approach with the capacity to undermine tumor growth and alleviate the suppressive effects of the hypoxic tumor on various immune cells. In tumors, hypoxic zones result from the combined action of tumor cell metabolism, the growth rate of these cells that outpaces regional microcirculation, the density of the resulting cell pack, and the disorganized and largely ineffectual nature of tumor-induced neovascularization. Tumor cells in these hypoxic zones can be resistant to chemotherapy based on their limited contact with drugs in circulation.

Historically, high temperatures were explored as a means to directly kill cancer cells, however, implementing this modality stalled. Current thermal therapies, which subject patients to mild-to-moderate hyperthermia at or near the fever range (fever-range, 39–41°C) have proven effective at enhancing the vascular perfusion of hypoxic tumors, elevating oxygen levels which improve the effectiveness of other anti-cancer measures. By increasing circulatory access to tumor cells, thermal interventions improve the effectiveness of chemotherapies. Importantly, these approaches can also reverse some of the immune suppression associated with hypoxia. Mild hyperthermia also enhances the ability of the immune system to detect malignant threats (due to increased *MHC* I expression on tumor cells), increases the mobilization and activation of leukocytes and triggers the release of heat shock factors capable of stimulating effective anti-tumor immunity.[124] Encouragingly, use of thermal therapy in conjunction with other regiments has shown promise in clinical trials.[71]

Recently, the notion that tumor hypoxia can be countered by whole-body respiratory hyperoxia (supplemental oxygen) treatment was also tested. Supplying tumor-bearing mice with supplemental oxygen alleviated intratumoral hypoxia as well as immune-suppressing extracellular adenosine pools. Hyperoxia also increased the prevalence of pro-inflammatory cytokines while decreasing that of suppressive cytokines. CD8+ T cells in oxygen-supplemented mice were enhanced in their activation while frequency and potency of Tregs were reduced. These immunological enhancements were associated with increased survival of hyperoxia-treated mice which also had reduced incidence of metastasis.[50] This astonishingly

    *Tumor Hypoxia*

straightforward means to simultaneously undermine the tumor growth and immune suppression tied to hypoxia appears to be a promising avenue for future cancer-fighting regiments.

Therapies targeting one of the most central players in the hypoxia response also hold promise. HIF-1 has for some time been a molecular target in the sites of cancer biologists since it regulates genes important for the tumor cell adaptation to hypoxia. Since these include factors key to the processes of immortalization and de-differentiation, glucose metabolism, pH regulation, survival, angiogenesis, metastatic growth, and resistance to chemotherapy, HIF-1 inhibition has been explored as a multi-pronged strategy of attack on tumors. Correspondingly, numerous compounds inhibiting HIF-1 function and/or expression have been characterized,[114,116] and some have proven effective at suppressing *in vivo* tumor progression in mouse models.[73,150]

Discoveries suggesting that HIF-1 targeting, may undermine potentially tumor-abetting IL-17-producing cells,[25,120,141] MDSCs and TAMs[22] while encouraging the development of highly tumoricidal memory CD8+ T cells,[127] reveal another enticing aspect of potential HIF-1-targeting therapies — an immunotherapeutic one.

While HIF-1 inhibitors can interfere with the tumor-promoting processes of angiogenesis and cancer cell metabolism while negating the pro-tumor effects of IL-17, they may, as suggested by the previous work of our group and others, also elevate the frequency of immune suppressive Treg cells. In cancer, these cells tend to be enriched, either locally in developing tumors or systemically at advanced stages, and the immune-suppressing nature of these cells hampers the anti-tumor response permitting tumor growth.[14] Sabotaging Tregs or blocking their function has been explored as an immunotherapeutic measure to enhance the anti-tumor immune response and increase the effectiveness of anti-cancer therapies including tumor-vaccines. Therefore the anti-tumor efficacy of HIF-1 inhibition should be evaluated in combination with additional agents aimed at counteracting potential suppressor cell accumulation such as the drugs used to deplete Treg cells. Such a combinational approach, should in theory, simultaneously neutralize two tumor-promoting T cell populations.

Additional insights gleaned from studying the machinery of the cellular hypoxic response (i.e. HIF-1) suggest considerable complexity exists at the interface of hypoxic environments and immune cells. For instance,

HIF-1 and hypoxia may have decidedly different effects on a cell type that are stage or subset-specific (as is the case for effector and memory CD8+ T cells). Also, hypoxia and the complex milieu produced in the tumor microenvironment may trigger regulatory mechanisms poised in opposition to each other (as may be the case in Tregs). Lastly, dynamic changes in oxygen levels (re-oxygenation post-hypoxia and the much more recently appreciated "cycling hypoxia" phenomenon) may have significant implications for the role played by HIF-1 in regulating the immune response. Indeed this is illustrated by the relationship between interrupted hypoxia and Th17 development). These points should be regarded as both notes of caution and guideposts in the ongoing and future development of therapies exploiting the insights gained by studying hypoxic in the cancer setting.

## Acknowledgments

The authors declare no financial conflicts of interest. Funding support comes from grants from the Melanoma Research Alliance, the National Institutes of Health (RO1AI099300 and RO1AI089830), "Kelly's Dream" Foundation, the Janey Fund, and the Seraph Foundation, and gifts from Bill and Betty Topecer and Dorothy Needle. FP is a Stewart Trust Scholar, JB was supported by a Crohn's and Colitis Foundation of America Research Fellowship.

## References

1. Acosta-Iborra, B., Elorza, A., Olazabal, I. M., Martin-Cofreces., N. B., Martin-Puig, S., Miro. M. Calzada, M. J, Aragones, J., Sanchez-Madrid, F., and Landazuri, M. O., Macrophage oxygen sensing modulates antigen presentation and phagocytic functions involving IFN-gamma production through the HIF-1 alpha transcription factor. *J. Immunol.*, **182**, pp. 3155–3164, 2009.
2. Alcantara-Hernandez, M., Torres-Zarate, C., Perez-Montesinos, G., Jurado-Santacruz, F., Dominguez-Gomez, M.A., Peniche-Castellanos, A., Ferat-Osorio, E., Neri, N., Nambo, M. J, Alvarado-Cabrero, I., Moreno-Lafont, M., Huerta-Yepez, S., and Bonifaz, L. C., Overexpression of hypoxia-inducible factor 1 alpha impacts FoxP3 levels in mycosis fungoides — cutaneous T-cell lymphoma: clinical implications. *Int J. Cancer.*, **134**, pp. 2136–2145, 2014.

3. Almand, B., Clark, J. I., Nikitina, E., van Beynen, J., English, N. R., Knight, S. C., Carbone, D. P., and Gabrilovich, D. I., Increased production of immature myeloid cells in cancer patients: a mechanism of immunosuppression in cancer. *J. Immunol.*, **166**, pp. 678–689, 2001.

4. Anand, R. J., Gribar, S. C., Li, J., Kohler, J. W., Branca, M. F., Dubowski, T., Sodhi, C. P., and Hackam, D. J., Hypoxia causes an increase in phagocytosis by macrophages in a HIF-1alpha-dependent manner. *J. Leukoc. Biol.*, **82**, pp. 1257–1265, 2007.

5. Atkuri, K. R., and Herzenberg, L. A., Culturing at atmospheric oxygen levels impacts lymphocyte function. *P. Natl. Acad. Sci., USA,* **102**, pp. 3756–3759, 2005.

6. Baatar, D., Olkhanud, P., Sumitomo, K., Taub, D., Gress, R., and Biragyn, A., Human peripheral blood T regulatory cells (Tregs), functionally primed CCR4+ Tregs and unprimed CCR4- Tregs, regulate effector T cells using FasL. *J. Immunol.*, **178**, pp. 4891–4900, 2007.

7. Ben-Shoshan, J., Maysel-Auslender, S., Mor, A., Keren, G., and George, J. Hypoxia controls CD4+CD25+ regulatory T-cell homeostasis via hypoxia-inducible factor-1alpha. *Eur. J. Immunol.*, **38**, pp. 2412–2418, 2008.

8. Bettelli, E., Carrier, Y., Gao, W., Korn, T., Strom, T. B., Oukka, M., Weiner H. L., and Kuchroo, V. K., Reciprocal developmental pathways for the generation of pathogenic effector TH17 and regulatory T cells. *Nature*, **441**, pp. 235–238, 2006.

9. Bhandari, T., Olson, J., Johnson, R. S., and Nizet, V., HIF-1alpha influences myeloid cell antigen presentation and response to subcutaneous OVA vaccination. *J. Mol. Med. (Berl),* **91**, pp. 1199–1205, 2013.

10. Blouin, C. C., Page, E. L., Soucy, G. M., and Richard, D. E., Hypoxic gene activation by lipopolysaccharide in macrophages: implication of hypoxia-inducible factor 1alpha. *Blood*, **103**, pp. 1124–1130, 2004.

11. Bosco, M. C., Pierobon, D., Blengio, F., Raggi, F., Vanni, C., Gattorno, M., Eva, A., Novelli, F., Cappello, P., Giovarelli, M., and Varesio, L., Hypoxia modulates the gene expression profile of immunoregulatory receptors in human mature dendritic cells: identification of TREM-1 as a novel hypoxic marker *in vitro* and *in vivo*. *Blood*, **117**, pp. 2625–2639, 2011.

12. Brinkmann, V., Reichard, U., Goosmann, C., Fauler, B., Uhlemann Y., Weiss, D. S., Weinrauch, Y., and Zychlinsky A., Neutrophil extracellular traps kill bacteria. *Science*, **303**, pp. 1532–1535, 2004.

13. Bronte, V., and Zanovello, P., Regulation of immune responses by L-arginine metabolism. *Nat. Rev. Immunol.*, **5**, pp. 641–654, 2005.

14. Byrne, W. L., Mills, K. H, Lederer, J. A., and O'Sullivan, G. C., Targeting regulatory T cells in cancer. *Cancer. Res.*, **71**, pp. 6915–6920, 2011.

15. Campanelli, D., Detmers, P. A., Nathan, C. F., and Gabay, J. E., Azurocidin and a homologous serine protease from neutrophils. Differential antimicrobial and proteolytic properties. *J. Clin. Invest.*, **85**, pp. 904–915, 1990.

16. Carreau, A., El Hafny-Rahbi, B., Matejuk, A., Grillon, C., and Kieda, C., Why is the partial oxygen pressure of human tissues a crucial parameter? Small molecules and hypoxia. *J. Cell. Mol. Med.*, **15**, pp. 1239–1253, 2011.

17. Casanello, P., Torres, A., Sanhueza, F., Gonzalez, M., Farias, M., Gallardo, V., Pastor-Anglada, M., San Martin, R., and Sobrevia, L., Equilibrative nucleoside transporter 1 expression is downregulated by hypoxia in human umbilical vein endothelium. *Circ. Res.*, **97**, pp. 16–24, 2005.

18. Chisolm, D. A., and Weinmann, A. S., TCR-Signaling events in cellular metabolism and specialization. *Front. Immunol.*, **6**, p. 292, 2015.

19. Clambey, E. T., McNamee, E. N., Westrich, J. A., Glover, L. E., Campbell, E. L., Jedlicka, P., de Zoeten, E. F., Cambier, J. C., Stenmark, K. R., Colgan, S. P., and Eltzschig, H. K., Hypoxia-inducible factor-1 alpha-dependent induction of FoxP3 drives regulatory T-cell abundance and function during inflammatory hypoxia of the mucosa. *P. Natl. Acad. Sci., USA,* **109**, pp. E2784–2793, 2012.

20. Clark, R. A., and Klebanoff, S. J., Neutrophil-mediated tumor cell cytotoxicity: role of the peroxidase system. *J. Exp. Med.*, **141**, pp. 1442–1447, 1975.

21. Colhone, M. C., Arrais-Silva, W. W., Picoli, C., and Giorgio, S., Effect of hypoxia on macrophage infection by Leishmania amazonensis. *J. Parasitol.*, **90**, pp. 510–515, 2004.

22. Corzo, C. A., Condamine, T., Lu, L., Cotter, M. J., Youn, J. I., Cheng, P., Cho H. I., Celis, E., Quiceno, D. G., Padhya, T., McCaffrey, T. V., McCaffrey, J. C., and Gabrilovich, D. I., HIF-1$\alpha$ regulates function and differentiation of myeloid-derived suppressor cells in the tumor microenvironment. *J. Exp. Med.*, **207**, pp. 2439–2453, 2010.

23. Cramer, T., Yamanishi, Y., Clausen, B. E., Forster, I., Pawlinski, R., Mackman, N., Haase, V. H., Jaenisch, R., Corr, M., Nizet, V., Firestein, G. S., Gerber, H. P., Ferrara, N., and Johnson, R. S., HIF-1alpha is essential for myeloid cell-mediated inflammation. *Cell*, **112**, pp. 645–657, 2003.

24. Curiel, T. J., Coukos, G., Zou, L., Alvarez, X., Cheng, P., Mottram, P., Evdemon-Hogan, M., Conejo-Garcia, J. R., Zhang, L., Burow, M., Zhu, Y., Wei, S., Kryczek, I., Daniel, B., Gordon, A., Myers, L., Lackner, A., Disis, M. L., Knutson, K. L., Chen, L., and Zou, W., Specific recruitment of

regulatory T cells in ovarian carcinoma fosters immune privilege and predicts reduced survival. *Nat. Med.*, **10**, pp. 942–949, 2004.

25. Dang, E. V., Barbi, J., Yang, H. Y., Jinasena, D., Yu, H., Zheng, Y., Bordman, Z., Fu, J., Kim, Y., Yen, H. R., Luo, W., Zeller, K., Shimoda, L., Topalian, S. L., Semenza, G. L., Dang, C. V., Pardoll, D. M., and Pan, F., Control of T(H)17/T(reg) balance by hypoxia-inducible factor 1. *Cell*, **146**, pp. 772–784, 2011.

26. Delgoffe, G. M., Pollizzi, K. N., Waickman, A. T., Heikamp, E., Meyers, D. J., Horton, M. R., Xiao, B., Worley, P. F., and Powell, J. D., The kinase mTOR regulates the differentiation of helper T cells through the selective activation of signaling by mTORC1 and mTORC2. *Nat. Immunol.*, **12**, pp. 295–303, 2011.

27. Deng, B., Zhu, J. M., Wang, Y., Liu, T. T., Ding, Y. B., Xiao, W. M., Lu, G. T., Bo, P., and Shen, X. Z., Intratumor hypoxia promotes immune tolerance by inducing regulatory T cells via TGF-beta1 in gastric cancer. *PLoS One*, **8**, p. e63777, 2013.

28. Dewhirst, M. W., Cao, Y., and Moeller, B., Cycling hypoxia and free radicals regulate angiogenesis and radiotherapy response. *Nat. Rev. Cancer*, **8**, pp. 425–437, 2008.

29. Diaz-Montero, C. M., Salem, M. L., Nishimura, M. I., Garrett-Mayer, E., Cole, D. J., and Montero, A. J., Increased circulating myeloid-derived suppressor cells correlate with clinical cancer stage, metastatic tumor burden, and doxorubicin-cyclophosphamide chemotherapy. *Cancer Immunol. Immunother.*, **58**, pp. 49–59, 2009.

30. Doedens, A. L., Phan, A. T., Stradner, M. H., Fujimoto, J. K., Nguyen, J. V., Yang, E., Johnson, R. S., and Goldrath, A. W., Hypoxia-inducible factors enhance the effector responses of CD8(+) T cells to persistent antigen. *Nat. Immunol.*, **14**, pp. 1173–1182, 2013.

31. Egeblad, M., Ewald, A. J., Askautrud, H. A., Truitt, M. L., Welm, B. E., Bainbridge, E., Peeters, G., Krummel, M. F., and Werb, Z., Visualizing stromal cell dynamics in different tumor microenvironments by spinning disk confocal microscopy. *Dis. Model. Mech.*, **1**, pp. 155–167, 2008 discussion 165.

32. Elpek, K. G., Cremasco, V., Shen, H., Harvey, C. J., Wucherpfennig, K. W., Goldstein, D. R., Monach, P. A., and Turley, S. J., The tumor microenvironment shapes lineage, transcriptional, and functional diversity of infiltrating myeloid cells. *Cancer Immunol. Res.*, **2**, pp. 655–667, 2014.

33. Eruslanov, E. B., Bhojnagarwala, P. S., Quatromoni, J. G., Stephen, T. L., Ranganathan, A., Deshpande, C., Akimova, T., Vachani, A., Litzky, L., Hancock, W. W., Conejo-Garcia, J. R., Feldman, M., Albelda, S. M., and

Singhal, S., Tumor-associated neutrophils stimulate T cell responses in early-stage human lung cancer. *J. Clin. Invest.*, **124**, pp. 5466–5480, 2014.

34. Escribese, M. M., Casas, M., and Corbi, A. L., Influence of low oxygen tensions on macrophage polarization. *Immunobiology*, **217**, pp. 1233–1240, 2012.

35. Facciabene, A., Motz, G. T., and Coukos, G., T-regulatory cells: key players in tumor immune escape and angiogenesis. *Cancer. Res.*, **72**, pp. 2162–2171, 2012.

36. Facciabene, A., Peng, X., Hagemann, I. S., Balint, K., Barchetti, A., Wang, L. P., Gimotty, P. A., Gilks, C. B., Lal, P., Zhang, L., and Coukos, G., Tumour hypoxia promotes tolerance and angiogenesis via CCL28 and T(reg) cells. *Nature*, **475**, pp. 226–230, 2011.

37. Fang, H. Y., Hughes, R., Murdoch, C., Coffelt, S. B., Biswas, S. K., Harris, A. L., Johnson, R. S., Imityaz, H. Z., Simon, M. C., Fredlund, E., Greten, F. R., Rius, J., and Lewis, C. E., Hypoxia-inducible factors 1 and 2 are important transcriptional effectors in primary macrophages experiencing hypoxia. *Blood*, **114**, pp. 844–859, 2009.

38. Ferrara, N., and Davis-Smyth, T., The biology of vascular endothelial growth factor. *Endocr. Rev.*, **18**, pp. 4–25, 1997.

39. Finlay, D. K., Rosenzweig, E., Sinclair, L. V., Feijoo-Carnero, C., Hukelmann, J. L., Rolf, J., Panteleyev, A. A., Okkenhaug, K., and Cantrell, D. A., PDK1 regulation of mTOR and hypoxia-inducible factor 1 integrate metabolism and migration of CD8+ T cells. *J Exp. Med.*, **209**, pp. 2441–2453, 2012.

40. Franklin, R. A., Liao, W., Sarkar, A., Kim, M. V., Bivona, M. R., Liu, K., Pamer, E. G., and Li, M. O., The cellular and molecular origin of tumor-associated macrophages. *Science*, **344**, pp. 921–925, 2014.

41. Frauwirth, K. A and Thompson, C. B. Regulation of T lymphocyte metabolism. *J Immunol.*, **172**, pp. 4661–4665, 2004.

42. Fridlender, Z. G., Sun, J., Kim, S., Kapoor, V., Cheng, G., Ling, L., Worthen, G. S., and Albelda, S. M., Polarization of tumor-associated neutrophil phenotype by TGF-beta: "N1" versus "N2" TAN. *Cancer Cell*, **16**, pp. 183–194, 2009.

43. Gabrilovich, D. I., Chen, H. L., Girgis, K. R., Cunningham, H. T., Meny, G. M., Nadaf, S., Kavanaugh, D., and Carbone, D. P., Production of vascular endothelial growth factor by human tumors inhibits the functional maturation of dendritic cells. *Nat. Med.*, **2**, pp. 1096–1103, 1996.

44. Gabrilovich, D. I., and Nagaraj, S., Myeloid-derived suppressor cells as regulators of the immune system. *Nat Rev Immunol.*, **9**, pp. 162–174, 2009.

45. Gerriets, V. A., and Rathmell, J. C., Metabolic pathways in T cell fate and function. *Trends Immunol.*, **33**, pp. 168–173, 2012.

46. Gottfried, E., Kunz-Schughart, L. A., Ebner, S., Mueller-Klieser, W., Hoves, S., Andreesen, R., Mackensen, A., and Kreutz, M., Tumor-derived lactic acid modulates dendritic cell activation and antigen expression. *Blood*, **107**, pp. 2013–2021, 2006.

47. Gregory, A. D., and Houghton, A. M., Tumor-associated neutrophils: new targets for cancer therapy. *Cancer Res.*, **71**, pp. 2411–2416, 2011.

48. Harty, J. T., Tvinnereim, A. R., and White, D. W., CD8+ T cell effector mechanisms in resistance to infection. *Annu. Rev. Immunol.*, **18**, pp. 275–308, 2000.

49. Hasmim, M., Noman, M. Z., Messai, Y., Bordereaux, D., Gros, G., Baud, V., and Chouaib, S., Cutting edge: Hypoxia-induced Nanog favors the intratumoral infiltration of regulatory T cells and macrophages via direct regulation of TGF-beta1. *J. Immunol.*, **191**, pp. 5802–5806, 2013.

50. Hatfield, S. M., Kjaergaard, J., Lukashev, D., Schreiber, T. H., Belikoff, B., Abbott, R., Sethumadhavan, S., Philbrook, P., Ko, K., Cannici, R., Thayer, M., Rodig, S., Kutok, J. L., Jackson, E. K., Karger, B., Podack, E. R., Ohta, A., and Sitkovsky, M. V., Immunological mechanisms of the antitumor effects of supplemental oxygenation. *Sci. Transl. Med.*, **7**, pp. 277–230, 2015.

51. He, Y., Qian, H., Liu, Y., Duan, L., Li, Y., and Shi, G. The roles of regulatory B cells in cancer. *J. Immunol. Res.*, **2014**, p. 215471, 2014.

52. Hsiao, H. W., Hsu, T. S., Liu, W. H., Hsieh, W. C., Chou, T. F., Wu, Y. J., Jiang, S. T., and Lai, M. Z., Deltex1 antagonizes HIF-1alpha and sustains the stability of regulatory T cells *in vivo*. *Nat. Commun.*, **6**, p. 6353, 2015.

53. Huang, J. H., Cardenas-Navia, L. I., Caldwell, C. C., Plumb, T. J., Radu, C. G., Rocha, P. N., Wilder, T., Bromberg, J. S., Cronstein, B. N., Sitkovsky, M., Dewhirst, M. W., and Dustin, M. L., Requirements for T lymphocyte migration in explanted lymph nodes. *J. Immunol.*, **178**, pp. 7747–7755, 2007.

54. Huh, S. J., Liang, S., Sharma, A., Dong, C., and Robertson, G. P., Transiently entrapped circulating tumor cells interact with neutrophils to facilitate lung metastasis development. *Cancer Res.*, **70**, pp. 6071–6082, 2010.

55. Ikejiri, A., Nagai, S., Goda, N., Kurebayashi, Y., Osada-Oka, M., Takubo, K., Suda, T., and Koyasu, S., Dynamic regulation of Th17 differentiation by oxygen concentrations. *Int. Immunol.*, **24**, pp. 137–146, 2012.

56. Imtiyaz, H. Z., Williams, E. P., Hickey, M. M., Patel, S. A., Durham, A. C., Yuan, L. J., Hammond, R., Gimotty, P. A., Keith, B., and Simon, M. C., Hypoxia-inducible factor 2alpha regulates macrophage function in mouse models of acute and tumor inflammation. *J. Clin. Invest.*, **120**, pp. 2699–2714, 2010.

57. Jantsch, J., Chakravortty, D., Turza, N., Prechtel, A. T., Buchholz, B., Gerlach, R. G., Volke, M., Glasner, J., Warnecke, C., Wiesener, M. S., Eckardt, K. U., Steinkasserer, A., Hensel, M., and Willam, C., Hypoxia and hypoxia-inducible factor-1 alpha modulate lipopolysaccharide-induced dendritic cell activation and function. *J. Immunol.*, **180**, pp. 4697–4705, 2008.

58. Jiang, B. H., Rue, E., Wang, G. L., Roe, R., and Semenza, G. L., Dimerization, DNA binding, and transactivation properties of hypoxia-inducible factor 1. *J. Biol., Chem.*, **271**, pp. 17771–17778, 1996.

59. Josefowicz, S. Z., Lu, L. F., and Rudensky, A. Y., Regulatory T cells: mechanisms of differentiation and function. *Annu. Rev. Immunol.*, **30**, pp. 531–564, 2012.

60. Jung, J. E., Lee, H. G., Cho, I. H., Chung, D. H., Yoon, S. H., Yang, Y. M., Lee, J. W., Choi, S., Park, J. W., Ye, S. K., and Chung, M. H., STAT3 is a potential modulator of HIF-1-mediated VEGF expression in human renal carcinoma cells. *FASEB J.*, **19**, pp. 1296–1298, 2005.

61. Kawanaka, T., Kubo, A., Ikushima, H., Sano, T., Takegawa, Y., and Nishitani, H., Prognostic significance of HIF-2alpha expression on tumor infiltrating macrophages in patients with uterine cervical cancer undergoing radiotherapy. *J. Med. Invest.*, **55**, pp. 78–86, 2008.

62. Kim, S. Y., Choi, Y. J., Joung, S. M., Lee, B. H., Jung, Y. S., and Lee, J. Y., Hypoxic stress up-regulates the expression of Toll-like receptor 4 in macrophages via hypoxia-inducible factor. *Immunology*, **129**, pp. 516–524, 2010.

63. Kohler, T., Reizis, B., Johnson, R. S., Weighardt, H., and Forster, I., Influence of hypoxia-inducible factor 1alpha on dendritic cell differentiation and migration. *Eur J Immunol.*, **42**, pp. 1226–1236, 2012.

64. Kong, T., Eltzschig, H. K., Karhausen, J., Colgan, S. P., and Shelley, C. S., Leukocyte adhesion during hypoxia is mediated by HIF-1-dependent induction of beta2 integrin gene expression. *P. Natl. Acad. Sci. USA*, **101**, pp. 10440–10445, 2004.

65. Kryczek, I., Zhao, E., Liu, Y., Wang, Y., Vatan, L., Szeliga, W., Moyer, J., Klimczak, A., Lange, A., and Zou ,W., Human TH17 cells are long-lived effector memory cells. *Sci. Transl. Med.*, **3**, p. 104ra100, 2011.

66. Kuang, D. M., Zhao, Q., Wu, Y., Peng, C., Wang, J., Xu, Z., Yin, X. Y., and Zheng, L., Peritumoral neutrophils link inflammatory response to disease progression by fostering angiogenesis in hepatocellular carcinoma. *J. Hepatol.*, **54**, pp. 948–955, 2011.

67. Kumar, V., and Gabrilovich, D. I., Hypoxia-inducible factors in regulation of immune responses in tumour microenvironment. *Immunology*, **143**, pp. 512–519, 2014.

68. Kusmartsev, S., and Gabrilovich, D. I., Role of immature myeloid cells in mechanisms of immune evasion in cancer. *Cancer Immunol. Immunother.*, **55**, pp. 237–245, 2006.

69. Lamagna, C., Aurrand-Lions, M., and Imhof, B. A., Dual role of macrophages in tumor growth and angiogenesis. *J. Leukoc. Biol.*, **80**, pp. 705–713, 2006.

70. Laoui, D., Van Overmeire, E., Di Conza, G., Aldeni, C., Keirsse, J., Morias, Y., Movahedi, K., Houbracken, I., Schouppe, E., Elkrim, Y., Karroum, O., Jordan, B., Carmeliet, P., Gysemans, C., De Baetselier, P., Mazzone, M., and Van Ginderachter, J. A., Tumor hypoxia does not drive differentiation of tumor-associated macrophages but rather fine-tunes the M2-like macrophage population. *Cancer Res.*, **74**, pp. 24–30, 2014.

71. Lee, C. T., Mace, T., and Repasky, E. A., Hypoxia-driven immunosuppression: a new reason to use thermal therapy in the treatment of cancer? *Int. J. Hyperthermia*, **26**, pp. 232–246, 2010.

72. Lee, J. H., Elly, C., Park, Y., and Liu, Y. C., E3 Ubiquitin Ligase VHL Regulates Hypoxia-Inducible Factor-1alpha to Maintain Regulatory T Cell Stability and Suppressive Capacity. *Immunity.*, **42**, pp. 1062–1074, 2015.

73. Lee K, Zhang H, Qian, D. Z., Rey S, Liu, J. O., and Semenza, G. L., Acriflavine inhibits HIF-1 dimerization, tumor growth, and vascularization. *P. Natl. Acad. Sci.*, *USA,* **106**, pp. 17910–17915, 2009.

74. Lee, Y. K., Mukasa, R., Hatton, R. D., and Weaver, C. T., Developmental plasticity of Th17 and Treg cells. *Curr. Opin. Immunol.*, **21**, pp. 274–280, 2009.

75. Leek, R. D., Hunt, N. C., Landers, R. J., Lewis, C. E., Royds, J. A., and Harris, A. L., Macrophage infiltration is associated with VEGF and EGFR expression in breast cancer. *J. Pathol.*, **190**, pp. 430–436, 2000.

76. Leek, R. D., Talks, K. L., Pezzella, F., Turley, H., Campo, L., Brown, N. S., Bicknell, R., Taylor, M., Gatter, K. C., and Harris, A. L., Relation of hypoxia-inducible factor-2 alpha (HIF-2 alpha) expression in tumor-infiltrative macrophages to tumor angiogenesis and the oxidative thymidine phosphorylase pathway in Human breast cancer. *Cancer Res.*, **62**, pp. 1326–1329, 2002.

77. Lewis, J. S., Lee, J. A., Underwood, J. C., Harris, A. L., and Lewis, C. E., Macrophage responses to hypoxia: relevance to disease mechanisms. *J. Leukoc. Biol.*, **66**, pp. 889–900, 1999.

78. Li, Q., Lao, X., Pan, Q., Ning, N., Yet, J., Xu, Y., Li, S., and Chang, A. E., Adoptive transfer of tumor reactive B cells confers host T-cell immunity and tumor regression. *Clin Cancer Res.*, **17**, pp. 4987–4995, 2011.

79. Liu, L. B., Xie, F., Chang, K. K., Shang, W. Q., Meng, Y. H., Yu, J. J., Li, H., Sun, Q., Yuan, M. M., Jin, L. P., Li, D. J., and Li, M. Q., Chemokine CCL17 induced by hypoxia promotes the proliferation of cervical cancer cell. *Am. J. Cancer Res.*, **5**, pp. 3072–3084, 2015.

80. Loenarz, C., Coleman, M. L., Boleininger, A., Schierwater, B., Holland, P. W., Ratcliffe, P. J., and Schofield, C. J., The hypoxia-inducible transcription factor pathway regulates oxygen sensing in the simplest animal, Trichoplax adhaerens. *EMBO Rep.*, **12**, pp. 63–70, 2011.

81. Loukinova, E., Dong, G., Enamorado-Ayalya, I., Thomas, G. R., Chen, Z., Schreiber, H., and Van Waes, C., Growth regulated oncogene-alpha expression by murine squamous cell carcinoma promotes tumor growth, metastasis, leukocyte infiltration and angiogenesis by a host CXC receptor-2 dependent mechanism. *Oncogene*, **19**, pp. 3477–3486, 2000.

82. Lukashev, D., Ohta, A., and Sitkovsky, M., Hypoxia-dependent anti-inflammatory pathways in protection of cancerous tissues. *Cancer Metastasis Rev.*, **26**, pp. 273–279, 2007.

83. Mancino, A., Schioppa, T., Larghi, P., Pasqualini, F., Nebuloni, M., Chen, I. H., Sozzani, S., Austyn, J. M., Mantovani, A., and Sica, A., Divergent effects of hypoxia on dendritic cell functions. *Blood*, **112**, pp. 3723–3734, 2008.

84. Martin, S. K., Diamond, P., Williams, S. A., To, L. B., Peet, D. J., Fujii, N., Gronthos, S., Harris, A. L., and Zannettino, A. C., Hypoxia-inducible factor-2 is a novel regulator of aberrant CXCL12 expression in multiple myeloma plasma cells. *Haematologica*, **95**, pp. 776–784, 2010.

85. Maruyama, T., Kono, K., Izawa, S., Mizukami, Y., Kawaguchi, Y., Mimura, K., Watanabe, M., and Fujii, H., CCL17 and CCL22 chemokines within tumor microenvironment are related to infiltration of regulatory T cells in esophageal squamous cell carcinoma. *Dis Esophagus*, **23**, pp. 422–429, 2010.

86. Mascanfroni, I. D., Takenaka, M. C., Yeste, A., Patel, B., Wu, Y., Kenison, J. E., Siddiqui, S., Basso, A. S., Otterbein, L. E., Pardoll, D. M., Pan, F., Priel, A., Clish, C. B., Robson, S. C., and Quintana, F. J., Metabolic control of type 1 regulatory T cell differentiation by AHR and HIF1-alpha. *Nat. Med.*, **21**, pp. 638–646, 2015.

87. Masopust, D., and Picker, L. J., Hidden memories: frontline memory T cells and early pathogen interception. *J. Immunol.*, **188**, pp. 5811–5817, 2012.

88. Michalek, R. D., Gerriets, V. A., Jacobs, S. R., Macintyre, A. N., MacIver, N. J., Mason, E. F., Sullivan, S. A., Nichols, A. G., and Rathmell, J. C., Cutting edge: distinct glycolytic and lipid oxidative metabolic programs are

essential for effector and regulatory CD4+ T cell subsets. *J. Immunol.*, **186**, pp. 3299–3303, 2011.

89. Mishalian, I., Bayuh, R., Levy, L., Zolotarov, L., Michaeli, J., and Fridlender, Z. G., Tumor-associated neutrophils (TAN) develop pro-tumorigenic properties during tumor progression. *Cancer Immunol. Immunother.*, **62**, pp. 1745–1756, 2013.

90. Mizukami Y, Kono K, Kawaguchi Y, Akaike H, Kamimura K, Sugai H., and Fujii H., CCL17 and CCL22 chemokines within tumor microenvironment are related to accumulation of Foxp3+ regulatory T cells in gastric cancer. *Int. J. Cancer*, **122**, pp. 2286–2293, 2008.

91. Munder, M., Schneider, H., Luckner, C., Giese, T., Langhans, C. D., Fuentes, J. M., Kropf, P., Mueller, I., Kolb, A., Modolell, M., and Ho, A. D., Suppression of T-cell functions by human granulocyte arginase. *Blood*, **108**, pp. 1627–1634, 2006.

92. Murdoch, C., Giannoudis, A., and Lewis, C. E., Mechanisms regulating the recruitment of macrophages into hypoxic areas of tumors and other ischemic tissues. *Blood*, **104**, pp. 2224–2234, 2004.

93. Nagaraj, S., Youn, J. I., Weber, H., Iclozan, C., Lu, L., Cotter, M. J., Meyer, C., Becerra, C. R., Fishman, M., Antonia, S., Sporn, M. B., Liby, K. T., Rawal, B., Lee, J. H., and Gabrilovich, D. I., Anti-inflammatory triterpenoid blocks immune suppressive function of MDSCs and improves immune response in cancer. *Clin. Cancer Res.*, **16**, pp. 1812–1823, 2010.

94. Nakamura, H., Makino, Y., Okamoto, K., Poellinger, L., Ohnuma, K., Morimoto, C., and Tanaka, H., TCR engagement increases hypoxia-inducible factor-1 alpha protein synthesis via rapamycin-sensitive pathway under hypoxic conditions in human peripheral T cells. *J. Immunol.*, **174**, pp. 7592–7599, 2005.

95. Naldini, A., Morena, E., Pucci, A., Miglietta, D., Riboldi, E., Sozzani, S., and Carraro, F., Hypoxia affects dendritic cell survival: role of the hypoxia-inducible factor-1alpha and lipopolysaccharide. *J. Cell Physiol.*, **227**, pp. 587–595, 2012.

96. Neumann, A. K., Yang, J. Biju, M. P., Joseph, S. K., Johnson, R. S., Haase, V. H., Freedman, B. D., and Turka, L. A., Hypoxia inducible factor 1 alpha regulates T cell receptor signal transduction. *P. Natl. Acad. Sci., USA*, **102**, pp. 17071–17076, 2005.

97. Nizet, V., and Johnson, R. S., Interdependence of hypoxic and innate immune responses. *Nat. Rev. Immunol.*, **9**, pp. 609–617, 2009.

98. Noman, M. Z., Buart, S., Van Pelt, J, Richon, C., Hasmim, M., Leleu, N., Suchorska, W. M., Jalil, A., Lecluse, Y., El Hage, F., Giuliani, M., Pichon,

C., Azzarone, B., Mazure, N., Romero, P., Mami-Chouaib F., and Chouaib, S., The cooperative induction of hypoxia-inducible factor-1 alpha and STAT3 during hypoxia induced an impairment of tumor susceptibility to CTL-mediated cell lysis. *J. Immunol.*, **182**, pp. 3510–3521, 2009.

99. Noman, M. Z., Desantis, G., Janji, B., Hasmim, M., Karray, S., Dessen, P., Bronte, V., and Chouaib, S., PD-L1 is a novel direct target of HIF-1alpha, and its blockade under hypoxia enhanced MDSC-mediated T cell activation. *J. Exp. Med.*, **211**, pp. 781–790, 2014.

100. Novitskiy, S. V., Ryzhov, S., Zaynagetdinov, R., Goldstein, A. E., Huang, Y., Tikhomirov, O. Y., Blackburn, M. R., Biaggioni, I., Carbone, D. P., Feoktistov, I., and Dikov, M. M., Adenosine receptors in regulation of dendritic cell differentiation and function. *Blood*, **112**, pp. 1822–1831, 2008.

101. Nozawa, H., Chiu, C., and Hanahan, D., Infiltrating neutrophils mediate the initial angiogenic switch in a mouse model of multistage carcinogenesis. *P. Natl. Acad. Sci., USA*, **103**, pp. 12493–12498, 2006.

102. Oda, T., Hirota, K., Nishi, K., Takabuchi, S., Oda, S., Yamada, H., Arai, T., Fukuda, K., Kita, T., Adachi, T., Semenza, G. L., and Nohara, R., Activation of hypoxia-inducible factor 1 during macrophage differentiation. *Am J Physiol. Cell Physiol.*, **291**, pp. C104–113, 2006.

103. Ohta, A., and Sitkovsky, M., Extracellular adenosine-mediated modulation of regulatory T cells. *Front Immunol.*, **5**, p. 304, 2014.

104. Peyssonnaux, C., Datta, V., Cramer, T., Doedens, A., Theodorakis, E. A., Gallo, R. L., Hurtado-Ziola, N., Nizet, V., and Johnson, R. S., HIF-1alpha expression regulates the bactericidal capacity of phagocytes. *J. Clin. Invest.*, **115**, pp. 1806–1815, 2005.

105. Pierobon, D., Bosco, M. C., Blengio, F., Raggi, F., Eva, A., Filippi, M., Musso, T., Novelli, F., Cappello, P., Varesio, L., and Giovarelli, M., Chronic hypoxia reprograms human immature dendritic cells by inducing a proinflammatory phenotype and TREM-1 expression. *Eur. J. Immunol.*, **43**, pp. 949–966, 2013.

106. Pot, C., Apetoh, L., and Kuchroo, V. K., Type 1 regulatory T cells (Tr1) in autoimmunity. *Semin, Immunol.*, **23**, pp. 202–208, 2011.

107. Powell, J. D., and Pollizzi, K., Fueling memories. *Immunity*, **36**, pp. 3–5, 2012.

108. Roncarolo, M. G., Gregori, S., Bacchetta, R., and Battaglia, M., Tr1 cells and the counter-regulation of immunity: natural mechanisms and therapeutic applications. *Curr. Top Microbiol. Immunol.*, **380**, pp. 39–68, 2014.

109. Roncarolo, M. G., Gregori, S., Battaglia, M., Bacchetta, R., Fleischhauer, K., and Levings, M. K., Interleukin-10-secreting type 1 regulatory T cells in rodents and humans. *Immunol. Rev.*, **212**, pp. 28–50, 2006.

110. Rotondo, R., Barisione, G., Mastracci, L., Grossi, F., Orengo, A. M., Costa, R., Truini, M., Fabbi, M., Ferrini, S., and Barbieri, O., IL-8 induces exocytosis of arginase 1 by neutrophil polymorphonuclears in nonsmall cell lung cancer. *Int. J. Cancer*, **125**, pp. 887–893, 2009.

111. Santiago, B., Calonge, E., Del Rey, M.J., Gutierrez-Canas, I., Izquierdo, E., Usategui, A., Galindo, M., Alcami, J., and Pablos, J. L., CXCL12 gene expression is upregulated by hypoxia and growth arrest but not by inflammatory cytokines in rheumatoid synovial fibroblasts. *Cytokine*, **53**, pp. 184–190, 2011.

112. Schioppa, T., Uranchimeg, B., Saccani, A., Biswas, S. K., Doni, A., Rapisarda, A., Bernasconi, S., Saccani, S., Nebuloni, M., Vago, L., Mantovani, A., Melillo, G., and Sica, A., Regulation of the chemokine receptor CXCR4 by hypoxia. *J. Exp. Med.*, **198**, pp. 1391–1402, 2003.

113. Semenza, G. L., Defining the role of hypoxia-inducible factor 1 in cancer biology and therapeutics. *Oncogene*, **29**, pp. 625–634, 2010.

114. Semenza, G. L., Evaluation of HIF-1 inhibitors as anticancer agents. *Drug Discov. Today*, **12**, pp. 853–859, 2007.

115. Semenza, G. L., HIF-1 and human disease: one highly involved factor. *Genes Dev.*, **14**, pp. 1983–1991, 2000.

116. Semenza, G. L., HIF-1 inhibitors for cancer therapy: from gene expression to drug discovery. *Curr. Pharm. Des.*, **15**, pp. 3839–3843, 2009.

117. Semenza, G. L., HIF-1 mediates metabolic responses to intratumoral hypoxia and oncogenic mutations. *J. Clin. Invest.*, **123**, pp. 3664–3671, 2013.

118. Semenza, G. L., Hypoxia-inducible factors: mediators of cancer progression and targets for cancer therapy. *Trends Pharmacol. Sci.*, **33**, pp. 207–214, 2012.

119. Shen, M., Hu, P., Donskov, F., Wang, G., Liu, Q., and Du, J., Tumor-associated neutrophils as a new prognostic factor in cancer: a systematic review and meta-analysis. *PLoS One*, **9**, p. e98259, 2014.

120. Shi, L. Z., Wang, R., Huang, G., Vogel, P., Neale, G., Green, D. R., and Chi, H., HIF1alpha-dependent glycolytic pathway orchestrates a metabolic checkpoint for the differentiation of TH17 and Treg cells. *J. Exp. Med.*, **208**, pp. 1367–1376, 2011.

121. Shojaei, F., Wu, X., Malik, A. K., Zhong, C., Baldwin, M. E., Schanz, S., Fuh, G., Gerber, H.P., and Ferrara, N., Tumor refractoriness to anti-VEGF treatment is mediated by CD11b+Gr1+ myeloid cells. *Nat. Biotechnol.*, **25**, pp. 911–920, 2007.

122. Siemens, D. R., Hu, N., Sheikhi, A. K., Chung, E., Frederiksen, L. J., Pross, H., and Graham, C. H., Hypoxia increases tumor cell shedding of

MHC class I chain-related molecule: role of nitric oxide. *Cancer Res*, **68**, pp. 4746–4753, 2008.

123. Sitkovsky, M. V., Kjaergaard, J., Lukashev, D., and Ohta, A., Hypoxia-adenosinergic immunosuppression: tumor protection by T regulatory cells and cancerous tissue hypoxia. *Clin. Cancer Res.*, **14**, pp. 5947–5952, 2008.

124. Skitzki, J. J., Repasky, E. A., and Evans, S. S., Hyperthermia as an immuno-therapy strategy for cancer. *Curr. Opin. Investig. Drugs*, **10**, pp. 550–558, 2009.

125. Srivastava, M. K., Sinha, P., Clements, V. K., Rodriguez, P., and Ostrand-Rosenberg, S., Myeloid-derived suppressor cells inhibit T-cell activation by depleting cystine and cysteine. *Cancer Res.*, **70**, pp. 68–77, 2010.

126. Sugiyama, D., Nishikawa, H., Maeda, Y., Nishioka, M., Tanemura, A., Katayama, I., Ezoe, S., Kanakura, Y., Sato, E., Fukumori, Y., Karbach, J., Jager, E., and Sakaguchi, S., Anti-CCR4 mAb selectively depletes effector-type FoxP3+CD4+ regulatory T cells, evoking antitumor immune responses in humans. *P. Natl. Acad. Sci. USA*, **110**, pp. 17945–17950, 2013.

127. Sukumar, M., Liu, J., Ji, Y., Subramanian, M., Crompton, J. G., Yu, Z., Roychoudhuri, R., Palmer, D. C., Muranski, P., Karoly, E. D., Mohney, R. P., Klebanoff, C. A., Lal, A., Finkel, T., Restifo, N. P., and Gattinoni, L., Inhibiting glycolytic metabolism enhances CD8+ T cell memory and anti-tumor function. *J. Clin. Invest.*, **123**, pp. 4479–4488, 2013.

128. Summers, C., Rankin, S. M., Condliffe, A. M., Singh, N., Peters, A. M., and Chilvers, E. R., Neutrophil kinetics in health and disease. *Trends Immunol.*, **31**, pp. 318–324, 2010.

129. Takeda, N., O'Dea, E. L., Doedens, A., Kim, J. W., Weidemann, A., Stockmann, C., Asagiri, M., Simon, M. C., Hoffmann, A., and Johnson, R. S., Differential activation and antagonistic function of HIF-{alpha} iso-forms in macrophages are essential for NO homeostasis. *Genes. Dev.*, **24**, pp. 491–501, 2010.

130. Talmadge, J. E., Pathways mediating the expansion and immunosuppressive activity of myeloid-derived suppressor cells and their relevance to cancer therapy. *Clin. Cancer Res.*, **13**, pp. 5243–5248, 2007.

131. Tazzyman, S., Lewis, C. E., and Murdoch, C., Neutrophils: key mediators of tumour angiogenesis. *Int. J. Exp. Pathol.*, **90**, pp. 222–231, 2009.

132. Tazzyman, S., Niaz, H., and Murdoch, C., Neutrophil-mediated tumour angiogenesis: subversion of immune responses to promote tumour growth. *Semin Cancer Biol.*, **23**, pp. 149–158, 2013.

133. Tripathi, C., Tewari, B. N., Kanchan, R. K., Baghel, K. S., Nautiyal, N., Shrivastava, R., Kaur, H., Bhatt, M. L., and Bhadauria, S., Macrophages are

recruited to hypoxic tumor areas and acquire a pro-angiogenic M2-polarized phenotype via hypoxic cancer cell derived cytokines Oncostatin M and Eotaxin. *Oncotarget*, **5**, pp. 5350–5368, 2014.

134. Valzasina, B., Piconese, S., Guiducci, C., and Colombo, M. P., Tumor-induced expansion of regulatory T cells by conversion of CD4+CD25- lymphocytes is thymus and proliferation independent. *Cancer Res.*, **66**, pp. 4488–4495, 2006.

135. van der Windt, G. J., and Pearce, E. L., Metabolic switching and fuel choice during T-cell differentiation and memory development. *Immunol. Rev.*, **249**, pp. 27–42, 2012.

136. Waickman, A. T., and Powell, J. D., mTOR, metabolism, and the regulation of T-cell differentiation and function. *Immunol Rev.*, **249**, pp. 43–58, 2012.

137. Walmsley, S. R., Print, C., Farahi, N., Peyssonnaux, C., Johnson, R. S., Cramer, T., Sobolewski, A., Condliffe, A. M., Cowburn, A. S., Johnson, N., and Chilvers, E. R., Hypoxia-induced neutrophil survival is mediated by HIF-1alpha-dependent NF-kappaB activity. *J. Exp. Med.*, **201**, pp. 105–115, 2005.

138. Wang, C., Lee, J. H., and Kim, C. H., Optimal population of FoxP3+ T cells in tumors requires an antigen priming-dependent trafficking receptor switch. *PLoS One*, **7**, p. e30793, 2012.

139. Wang, G. L., Jiang, B. H., Rue, E. A., and Semenza, G. L., Hypoxia-inducible factor 1 is a basic-helix-loop-helix-PAS heterodimer regulated by cellular O2 tension. *P. Natl. Acad. Sci., USA*, **92**, pp. 5510–5514, 1995.

140. Wang, H., Flach, H., Onizawa, M., Wei, L., McManus, M. T., and Weiss, A., Negative regulation of Hif1a expression and TH17 differentiation by the hypoxia-regulated microRNA miR-210. *Nat. Immunol.*, **15**, pp. 393–401, 2014.

141. Wang, L., Yi, T., Zhang, W., Pardoll, D. M., and Yu, H., IL-17 enhances tumor development in carcinogen-induced skin cancer. *Cancer Res.*, **70**, pp. 10112–10120, 2010.

142. Wejksza, K., Lee-Chang, C., Bodogai, M., Bonzo, J., Gonzalez, F. J., Lehrmann, E., Becker, K., and Biragyn, A., Cancer-produced metabolites of 5-lipoxygenase induce tumor-evoked regulatory B cells via peroxisome proliferator-activated receptor alpha. *J Immunol.*, **190**, pp. 2575–2584, 2013.

143. Welch, D. R., Schissel, D. J., Howrey, R. P., and Aeed, P. A., Tumor-elicited polymorphonuclear cells, in contrast to "normal" circulating poly-morphonuclear cells, stimulate invasive and metastatic potentials of rat mammary adenocarcinoma cells. *P. Natl. Acad. Sci., USA*, **86**, pp. 5859–5863, 1989.

144. Werno, C., Menrad, H., Weigert, A., Dehne, N., Goerdt, S., Schledzewski, K., Kzhyshkowska, J., and Brune, B., Knockout of HIF-1α in tumor-associated macrophages enhances M2 polarization and attenuates their pro-angiogenic responses. *Carcinogenesis*, **31**, pp. 1863–1872, 2010.

145. Wilke, C. M., Kryczek, I., Wei, S., Zhao, E., Wu, K., Wang, G., and Zou, W., Th17 cells in cancer: help or hindrance? *Carcinogenesis*, **32**, pp. 643–649, 2011.

146. Williams, M. A., and Bevan, M. J., Effector and memory CTL differentiation. *Annu Rev. Immunol.*, **25**, pp. 171–192, 2007.

147. Xu, Q., Briggs, J., Park, S., Niu, G., Kortylewski, M., Zhang, S., Gritsko, T., Turkson, J., Kay, H., Semenza, G. L., Cheng, J. Q., Jove, R., and Yu H., Targeting Stat3 blocks both HIF-1 and VEGF expression induced by multiple oncogenic growth signaling pathways. *Oncogene*, **24**, pp. 5552–5560, 2005.

148. Yang, M., Ma, C., Liu, S., Shao, Q., Gao, W., Song, B., Sun, J., Xie, Q., Zhang, Y., Feng, A., Liu, Y., Hu, W., and Qu, X., HIF-dependent induction of adenosine receptor A2b skews human dendritic cells to a Th2-stimulating phenotype under hypoxia. *Immunol. Cell. Biol.*, **88**, pp. 165–171, 2010.

149. Zea, A. H., Rodriguez, P. C., Atkins, M. B., Hernandez, C., Signoretti, S., Zabaleta, J., McDermott, D., Quiceno, D., Youmans, A., O'Neill, A., Mier, J., and Ochoa, A. C., Arginase-producing myeloid suppressor cells in renal cell carcinoma patients: a mechanism of tumor evasion. *Cancer Res.*, **65**, pp. 3044–3048, 2005.

150. Zhang, H., Qian, D. Z., Tan, Y. S., Lee, K., Gao, P., Ren, Y. R., Rey, S., Hammers, H., Chang, D., Pili, R., Dang, C. V., Liu, J. O., and Semenza, G. L., Digoxin and other cardiac glycosides inhibit HIF-1alpha synthesis and block tumor growth. *P. Natl. Acad Sci.*, *USA*, **105**, pp. 19579–19586, 2008.

151. Zhou, L., Lopes, J. E., Chong, M. M., Ivanov, II, Min, R., Victora, G. D., Shen, Y., Du, J., Rubtsov, Y. P., Rudensky, A. Y., Ziegler, S. F., and Littman, D. R., TGF-beta-induced Foxp3 inhibits T(H)17 cell differentiation by antagonizing, R.O.Rgammat function. *Nature*, **453**, pp. 236–240, 2008.

152. Zhou, S. L., Zhou, Z. J., Hu, Z. Q., Huang, X. W., Wang, Z., Chen, E. B., Fan, J., Cao, Y., Dai, Z., and Zhou, J., Tumor-associated neutrophils recruit macrophages and T-regulatory cells to promote progression of hepatocellular carcinoma and resistance to sorafenib. *Gastroenterology*, **150**, pp. 1646–1658, 2016.

153. Zhu, G., Tang, Y., Geng, N., Zheng, M., Jiang, J., Li, L., Li, K., Lei, Z., Chen, W., Fan, Y., Ma, X., Wang, X., and Liang, X., HIF-alpha/MIF and

NF-kappaB/IL-6 axes contribute to the recruitment of CD11b+Gr-1+ myeloid cells in hypoxic microenvironment of HNSCC. *Neoplasia.*, **16**, pp. 168–179, 2014.

154. Zhu, J., Yamane, H., and Paul, W. E., Differentiation of effector CD4 T cell populations (*). *Annu. Rev. Immunol.*, **28**, pp. 445–489, 2010.

# Index


**A**

aberrant DNA synthesis, 171
   replicon misfiring, 171
acetylates, 55
acetylation, 54
acidosis, 226
action, 11
adaptive immunity, 80
adaptive responses, 235
adenosine, 263, 275
adult stem cell, 102
adverse prognosis, 207
aerobic, 2, 9–10, 14–16, 32
aggressive phenotypes, 169
aHIF, 196
AIFM3, 202
amino acid metabolism, 231
AML, 103
amyotrophic lateral sclerosis (ALS), 237
angiogenesis, 50, 57, 59, 81, 84, 90, 204–205, 234, 250, 252, 254
   leaky vessels, 84
angiopoietin 2, 85

anoikis, 78–79
   ERBB2, 79
anoxia, 233
anoxic, 3, 5–8, 10, 14, 16, 32–33
anti-angiogenic factors, 85
anti-oxidant responses, 231
anti-tumor immunity, viii
apoptosis, 131–132, 134–135, 142–143, 202, 226, 252–253, 266
arginine, 254, 256, 261
arrest-defective-1 (ARD1), 54–55
aryl hydrocarbon receptor nuclear translocator (ARNT), 251, 269
ataxia telangiectasia and Rad3-related (ATR), 172–173
ataxia telangiectasia mutated ATM, 173
ATF6, 227
autophagosome, 236
autophagy, 131–132, 134, 142, 231
autophosphorylation, 229

**B**

basement membrane, 71, 73
BCL2, 203

Bcl-2-homology domain 3 (BH-3)-
   only family protein, 79
benzotriazine di-N-oxides, 22
Bevacizumab, 90
biological effect, 7, 19, 27
biological target volume (BTV), 23
biomarker, 208–209
biophysical models, 31, 33
bioreductive drugs, 12
BIX, 239
BNIP3, 79
bone marrow, 104
bone marrow niche, 115
boosting, 14
bortezomib, 57, 240
BRAF, 135
BRCA1, 174, 178, 180–181
breast cancer, 109–110
breast cancer metastasis, 193
BTV, 24

**C**
64Cu–ATSM, 25
CAD domain, 57
cadherin switch, 76–77
   cell adhesion, 76
   E-cadherin, 76–77, 79, 83
   mesenchymal marker, 76
   N-cadherin, 76–77
cancer-fighting, 276
cancer stem cell(s), 83, 101, 103
   differentiation, vii
   self-renewal, vii
   stem cell niche, vii
   stemness, vii
cancer stem cell model, 102–103
cancer therapeutics targeting, 226
cap binding eIF4E2, 108
carbonic anhydrase 9 (CA9), 235

carbon ions, 28–30
carbon ion therapy, 14
carcinoma, 254
cardiac myocyte model, 236
CASP8AP2, 202
CBP, 107
CBP/p300, 53, 56
CCL19, 82
CCR7, 82
ccRCC, 137–138, 209
CD4+, 254, 263, 265–267, 269, 271
CD8+, 254, 270–273, 275–277
CD39, 263
CD73, 263
Cdh2, 83
CDK1, 57
Cell cycle, 127, 129, 132, 134–137,
   139, 141–144, 203
cell death, vi
cell-free miRNAs, 208
cell proliferation, 81
cells, 16
Cezanne, 54
chemical chaperones, 237
chemokine, 80–81, 138, 254–255,
   257, 260, 262, 268
chemoradiation, 11
chemotaxis, 84
chemotherapy, 85, 275–276
chromosomal aberrations, viii
circulating miR-210, 208–209
clear cell renal cell carcinoma, 109,
   113
clonal evolution, viii
clonal evolution model, 102–103
clonal heterogeneity, viii
clonal selection, vi
cofactor p300, 58
colitis, 270

combination, 240

conditions, 8

connective tissue growth factor
(CTGF), 75

constitutive HIF alpha protein
expression, 109

conventional fractionation, 16

conventional radiotherapy, 8, 21

COOH-terminal activation domain
(CAD), 50

COX10, 206

C-TAD, 53

CTC(s), 78–79
hemodynamic shear forces, 78

CTGF, 90
CCN2, 75
CCN family of matricellular
proteins, 75
multimodular, 75

CTL, 271–272

cullin-2, 54

CXC chemokine family, 81

CXCL12, 82

CXCR4, 81–82

CXCR7, 82

cyclin dependent kinase 1, 55

cysteine, 256

cytokine, 80–81, 146, 253

cytotoxins, 17

**D**

DAHANCA, 20

DCs, 255, 257, 261–263

DDR, 134–135

dedifferentiation, 103, 105, 110

deletions of VHL, 111

Deltex, 270

desferrioxamine (DFX), 59

diabetes, 237

diabetic, 58

diffusion limit for oxygen, 105

dilution assay technique, 9

dimethyl–oxalylglycine, 59

dissolution of adherens junctions, 76

disulfide bond, 233

DNA cytosine methylation, 176

DNA damage(s), vi, 3–6, 11, 27–28,
31, 129, 132, 134–135, 143, 170,
173, 182, 202
aberrations, 170
DDR, 132
DNA breaks, 172
small-scale DNA mutations, 170

DNA methylation, 176
DNMT3A, 176
DNMT3B, 176

DNA mutations, viii

DNA over-replication, 172

DNA repair, 172

dose escalation, 24–26

dose-response curve, 9–10, 31

drug resistance, 103, 233

DSB induction, 27–28, 31

**E**

E2F1, 109

E2F3, 202–204

E3 ligase, 251, 270

EAE, 265

ECM, 71, 73, 79
dynamic 3D structure, 71

effectors, 240

EFNA3, 205

EFNA3 lncRNA, 205

EGF, 108

eIF2$\alpha$, 230

electron transport chain (ETC), 206

elongin B, 54

elongin C, 54
embryonic cells already, 103
embryonic human sympathetic chain
	ganglia, 113
embryonic stem cells, 104
EMT, 76–77, 83, 90, 234
	mesenchymal phenotype, 76
	non-polarized mesenchymal
		cells, 76
	polarized epithelial cells, 76
endocytosis, 229
endogenous markers, 12
endoplasmic reticulum (ER) stress,
	viii
endoribonuclease, 229
endothelial progenitor cells (EPCs),
	84
energy metabolism, vii
	fatty acid synthesis, viii
	metabolic pathways, viii
	metabolism, viii
	oxidative phosphorylation, vii
epigenetic, 174
epigenetic modification(s), vi, viii,
	170
	epigenetic regulation, 180
	DNA methylation, 170
	histone modification, 170
epigenetic regulation, 176
epigenetic therapy, 182
epithelial-to-mesenchymal transition
	(EMT), vii, 70
Eppendorf pO2 electrode, 12
ERAD, 229
ErbB4, 79
ER folding capacity, 235
ERK, 79
ER stress, 225

ER stress-induced cell death, 239
erythropoietin (EPO), 49
exogenous markers, 12
extracellular matrix (ECM), 70
extravasation, 82, 90


**F**
$^{18}$F-FAZA, 25, 30
$^{18}$F-FDG, 30
$^{18}$F-FMISO, 22, 25–26, 30–31
$^{18}$F-FMISO PET, 23
factor inhibiting HIF-1, 53
FAK, 74
fatty acid, 265, 271
F-fluoromisonidazole (F-FMISO), 13
FGFRL1, 203–204
fibroblat growth factor (FGF), 84
fibrosarcoma, 144
FIH, 55
FIH-1, 54, 57
FIH1, 107, 114
fluid stresses, 79
fluoro-deoxyglucose (FDG), 26
Foxp3, 264–268, 270
fractionated irradiation, 33
fractionated radiotherapy, 15–16
fractioned radiation, 16
fractioned radiotherapy, 19
free radicals, vi, 3–4
fully aerobic, 8
fully aerobic conditions, 7
fumarate, 111
fumarate hydroxylase (FH), 111
function by oxygen, 252


**G**
gas explosion technique, 3
GATA3, 264

geldanamycin, 58
gene amplification, 171–172
  DNA over-replication, 171
  double minutes (DMs), 171
  homogenously staining regions
    (HSRs), 171
genetic instability, 85, 170
genetic manipulation, 240
genetic mutations, vi
genotoxic stress, 132, 138
geroconversion, 139, 143
glioblastoma stem cell populations,
  114
glioma, 111, 113, 115
glucose, 147, 150–153, 155–160
glucose metabolism, 59
glucose uptake, vii
Glut1, 265, 271
glutamine, vii, 147, 150, 155–157,
  159–160
glutathione, 235
glycogen, 156, 158
glycolysis, vii, 250, 259, 265–266,
  269–271, 273
glycolytic, 152
glycosylation, 233
golgi, 231
GPD1L, 207
growth factor-induced HIF
  expression, 108
GRP78, 227
GTV, 25

**H**
H19, 194
halogenated pyrimidines, 17–18
Hayflick, Leonard, 127–128, 140
heat-shock protein 90 (HSP90), 58

helix-loop-helix-Per-ARNT-Sim, 50
hematopoietic stem cell, 102, 104
hematopoietic stem cell niche, 83,
  104, 115
heparin sulfate proteoglycans, 75
hepatic stellate cells (HSCs), 85
hepatocyte growth factor (HGF), 84
HERP, 232
heterogeneity, 1–2, 26, 33–34
heterogeneous, 232
HIF, 59–60, 86, 136–139, 143–146
    HIF-1, 49–50, 52, 54, 57–59
    HIF-1/2a, 52
    HIF-1a, 49–51, 53–59
    HIF-1b, 49–50, 55
    HIF-1$\alpha$, 74
    HIF-2, 50–51
    HIF-2/3a, 50
    HIF-2/3b, 50
    HIF-2a, 51, 55–56
    HIF-2$\alpha$, 74
    HIF-3a, 51
    HIF-a, 52, 58–60
    HIF-as, 52
    N-TAD, 51
HIF-1a, 196, 198–199, 207, 251, 253,
  256, 260, 262
HIF-1aflox, 265
HIF1alpha, 145
HIF-1$\alpha$, 73, 75–77, 79, 83–86, 233,
  258–259, 269, 271
HIF-1$\beta$, 251, 269
HIF-2a, 54, 251
HIF2A gain-of-function mutations,
  113
HIF-2$\alpha$, 75–76, 80, 86, 259
HIF-2$\alpha$ positive tumor cells, 114
HIF-mediated, 139

HIF proteasomal degradation, 106
HIF Ubiquitination, 106
high doses, 14, 33–34
high-LET radiotherapy, 26
high-linear energy transfer (LET), 14
HINCUT-1, 196
histone modification(s), 174,
    176–178
    acetylation, 175, 178
    dimethylation, 175
    epigenetic regulation, 180
    H3K4 demethylation, 181
    H3K4 demethylation and H3K9
        deacetylation, 178
    H3K4 methylation, 181
    H3K4 methylation and H3K9
        acetylation, 179
    methylation, 178
    trimethylation, 175
histone modifiers, 175
    JARID1A/RBP2, 180
    methyltransferase, 175–176
    lysine demethylases, 175
homeostasis, 226
homing, 81
homogenous, 1, 25
homologous recombination (HR),
    174
homology-dependent repair, 174
Howard-Flanders and Moore, 2
HOXA1, 200
H-RAS, 135
HRE, 85, 199
HRF, 8–9, 27–28
human breast epithelial precursor
    cells, 110
human hematopoietic stem cells, 115
HX4, 24–25

hydroxylases, 107
hydroxylation, vi, 51–54
hyperoxia, 275
    HBO chambers, 86
    hyperbaric oxygen (HBO), 83
hyperproliferation, 134–135
hypofractionated, 16
hypofractionated radiotherapy, 21,
    25, 33
hypofractionation, 26
hypoglycemia, 226
hypoxia, v, vii–viii, 49, 54, 56–57,
    70–71, 73, 76–79, 81, 83, 85–86,
    90, 136–139, 143–146, 189–190,
    200, 204, 225
    anoxic conditions, 85
    HIF, 136–138
    hypoxia gene signatures, 85
    hypoxia signatures, 86
    pathological hypoxia, 85
    physiological hypoxia, 85
    radiobiological hypoxia, 85
hypoxia-activated cytotoxins, vi
hypoxia and reoxygenation, 170
hypoxia develops, v
hypoxia-induced non-coding
    ultraconserved transcripts
    (HINCUTs), 195
hypoxia-inducible factor (HIF), vi,
    49, 190
    HIF-1a, vi
    HIF-1b, vi
    HIF-2a, vi
    HIF-3a, vi
hypoxia-inducible family of
    transcription factors (HIFs), 71
hypoxia-inducible lncRNAs, 194
hypoxia reduction factor (HRF), 7

hypoxia-reoxygenation, 171

hypoxia response element (HRE), 49, 77, 84, 251

hypoxia-selective, 21

hypoxia-selective drugs, 14

hypoxic, 51, 55, 59, 74

hypoxic cell cytotoxins, 21
    nitroaromatic compounds, 22

hypoxic cell radiosensitizers, 17–19, 21

hypoxic cytotoxins, 22

hypoxic fraction, 9, 12, 14–16, 19, 25–26

hypoxic-ischemic encephalopathy (HIE), 236

hypoxic niches, 104

hypoxic radiosensitizer, 14
    nimorazole, 14


**I**

Ifng, 270

IFN$\gamma$, 258–259, 264, 271

IGF-1/2, 75

IGF-I, 108

IL-10, 256–257, 259, 261, 268, 273

immune-mediated attack, 78

immune surveillance, vi, viii,

immunotherapeutic, 276

immunotherapies, 266, 275

inflammatory responses, 230

inheritable cancer, 102

iNOS, 256–257, 259

insulin, 108

integrin, 73, 75
    adhesion proteins, 72
    heterodimeric transmembrane proteins, 72

$\alpha v\beta 3$ integrin, 72

$\alpha v\beta 6$, 73

$\beta 1$-integrin, 73

integrins, 72

$\alpha v\beta 5$, 73

$\alpha v\beta 3$, 76

interferons, 80

interleukins, 80–81
    IL-6, 81
    IL-10, 81
    IL-11, 81
    IL-18, 81
    IL-19, 81

intravasation, 90

invasive hypoxia measurements, 12
    Oxylite fiber-optic sensor, 12
    polarographic needle electrode measurements, 12

IRE1, 227

ischemia, 236

ISCU, 206

ISR, 235


**J**

JARKD1B/PLU-1, 180

JmjC–KDMs, 139


**K**

a-ketoglutarate, 111

KF58333, 58


**L**

lactate, 151–153, 157

leaky vasculature, 80, 85

LET, 27

lethal DNA damage, 11, 27

lethal effects of radiation, 17

ligands, 208

lincRNA-p21, 194–195
lipid, 158–160
liquid biopsy, 209
lncRNA-LET, 195
lncRNAs, 193
local control, 22–23, 26
LOX, 75–76, 90
    AB0023, 75
    amine oxidase, 74
    extracellular collagen and elastin, 74
    GS-6624, 75
    idiopathic pulmonary fibrosis (IPF), 75
    LOXL, 74
    LOXL2, 74
    LOXL3, 74
    LOXL4, 74
    proteolytic cleavage, 74
    $\beta$-aminoproprionitrile, 75
LPS, 258–259, 262
LQ model, 33
LSD1, 180–182
LSD1/KDM1A, 180
lysine demethylases, 146
    JmjC–KDMs, 139
lysyl oxidase (LOX), vii, 74

**M**
M2-polarized macrophages, 80
macrometastases, 83
macrophages, 254–261
malignant progression, vii
mammosphere, 234
MAPK, 55
matrix metalloproteinases (MMPs), vii
MDM2, 132, 136, 139, 142, 144–145
MDSCs, 256, 261, 276

MEK/ERK, 76
    ERK1/2, 76
mesenchymal and cancer stem cell-like phenotype, 114
mesenchymal to epithelial transition, 81, 83
mesothelioma, 254
metabolism, 128, 132, 134–135, 137, 140, 146
metalloproteinase, 236
metastases, 73
metastasis, vii, 69–71, 76, 80, 90, 232
    grow undetected, 69
    invasive, 70
    journey to a distant organ, 70
    metastasis signature, 86
    metastatic cascade, 86, 90
    signatures of metastasis, 86
metastatic, 74
metastatic disease, 71
metastatic potential, 86
methylation, 131, 139
    lysine demethylases, 139
methylglyoxalation, 58
MG132, 240
MHC, 255, 262, 272, 275
Michaelis constant, 53
microenvironment, 230
micrometastases, 83
micrometastasis, 84
microRNA, 269
microvascular endothelial cells, 85
miR-210, 199–200, 202–203
miR-210/MNT axis, 204
miR-210 target, 200
miR-210 target genes, 201
miR-494, 199
miR-519d, 76

miRNA, 159, 196, 198
miRNP-IP, 201
miRNP-IP/CLIP, 201
mismatch repair (MMR), 173, 178
misonidazole, 19–20, 22
mitochondria, vii
mitochondrial deterioration, 132
mitochondrial metabolism, 206
mitochondrial respiration, 207
mitogenic factors, 84
mitomycin C, 22
MLH1, 173, 179, 181
MMP, 73–74, 90
    metalloproteinases, 73
    MMP-1, 74
    MMP-2, 73–74, 76
    MMP-3, 76
    MMP-9, 73–74
    MT1–MMP, 74
    Type IV collagen, 73
MNT, 204
monocarboxylate, 138
monocytes, 260–261
mtDNA damage, 134
mTOR, 252, 266, 271
mutagenesis, viii
Myc, 271
myeloid-derived suppressor cell
  (MDSC), 255
myeloma, 239

**N**
2-nitroimidazole, 19
NATs, 196
ncRNAs, 191, 209
NDUFA4, 206
near-physiological oxygen tensions,
  114

neovascularization, 250, 254, 261, 275
neuroblastoma, 110 111, 113–115
neurodegenerative, 237
neutrophils, 253–255, 258
NF$\kappa$B, 263
NF$\kappa$B signaling, 80
nitrobenzenes, 19
NO, 57
nomoxic, 58
non-coding RNA
    lncRNAs, viii
    long ncRNAs, viii
    microRNA-210, viii
    microRNAs, viii
non-coding RNAs, viii, 189, 191
non-invasive, 12–13, 30
non-invasive hypoxia measurements
    positron emission tomography
      (PET), single-photon emission
      computed tomography
      (SPECT), magnetic resonance
      imaging (MRI), and optical
      imaging, 12
normal tissue constraints, 25
normal tissues, 8, 18–19, 22–23, 29,
  31
normal tissue tolerance, 25
normoxia, 53–54
normoxic, 3, 8, 15–16, 32, 51, 55–56
normoxic cells, 22
normoxic conditions, 6–7, 19–20, 27,
  33
Notch, 266
Notch signaling, 77

**O**
2-oxoglutarate (2-OG)-dependent
  dioxygenases, 52

ODD, 52, 54, 57
OER, 8, 16, 27, 31–32
oncogene-induced senescence, 134
    OIS, 134–135, 138
oxidative phosphorylation, 140
oxidative phosphorylation is
  hypothesized, 128
oxidative phosphorylation OXPHOS
    OXPHOS, 128, 134
oxidative stress, 132, 134, 136, 138,
  144
    oxidative stress, 136
    ROS, 134, 136, 138
OXPHOS, 206
Oxygen, v, 249–253, 256, 265,
  267–269, 272–275, 277
oxygen consumption, 148, 152–154
oxygen-dependent, 2
oxygen-dependent degradation
  domain (ODD), 50
oxygen-dependent proteasomal
  degradation, 111
oxygen effect, 3, 5
oxygen enhancement ratio (OER), 7
oxygen fixation, 3–4
oxygen-independent mechanisms,
  108
oxygen partial pressure, vi

**P**
p16, 129, 131–134, 141–142
p16I, 132
p16INK4a, 142
p21, 129, 131–133, 136, 138
p38 kinases, 55
p42/44, 55
p53, 129, 132–136, 138–139
p300, 55
p300 coactivator, 57

pancreatic adenocarcinomas, 234
pancreatic cancer, 209
paraganglioma, 111, 113
Parkinson's disease, 237
PAS, 105
PAS domain, 56
pathogen infection, 230
pericytes, 84
perivascularly located glioma cells, 114
perivascular niche, 104, 111
PERK, 227
PET radiotracer, 23, 26, 30
phagocytosis, 229
PHD, 55, 58–59, 251–252
    Egg-laying Nine (EGLN), 53
    HIF-prolyl hydroxylase (HPH), 53
    PHD1/2/3, 53
    PHD-3, 59
PHD activity, 111
PHD hydroxylation site, 113
phenotype, 128–130, 132, 135–138,
  141
pheochromocytoma, 111, 113
phosphorylation, 51, 55–56
photon radiation, 26
physiological end capillary oxygen
  levels, 111
PI3K/Akt, 79
pimonidazole staining, 12
pimonizadole, 20, 84
platelet-derived growth factor
  (PDGF), 84
PLU-1, 181, 182
polyubiquitination, 54
post-translational modifications
  (PTMs), vi, vii, 51–52, 57–59, 172,
  226
    acetylation, vi
    phosphorylation, vi

S-nitrosylation, vi
SUMOylation, vi
PTMs, 172–173
Powers and Tolmach, 9
preirradiation, 15–16
pre-miRNAs, 197
pri-miRNAs, 197
proapoptotic signaling, 232
prognostic factor, 200
programmed death-ligand 1(PD-L1), 256
prolyl hydroxylase domain (PHD), 53
proteasomal degradation-independent, 109
proteasome, 251–252
protein clearance, 239
proteolytic cleavage, 231
proteomic profiling, 201
pseudohypoxia, 110
pseudo-hypoxic phenotype, 102, 111–113
PTMs, 60
Ptp1b, 202, 205
pVHL, 53–55, 57
pVHL E3 ligase complex, 56
pyruvate, 147, 150–151, 153, 155, 157, 160

**Q**
quantifying hypoxia, 12
quiescence, 136, 139
quiescense, 127

**R**
'R's (radiosensitivity, repair, redistribution, reoxygenation, and repopulation), 28
RAD52, 202

radiation
    hypoxic conditions, 2
    ionizing radiation, 6, 31
    irradiation, 2–3, 5–6, 8–9, 11, 14–23, 27, 31
    radiation damage, 3, 7, 19
    radiation delivery, 9, 25, 33
    radiation dose, 5–7, 14, 21, 23, 26
    high doses, 9
    radiation resistance, 6, 12, 17
    radiation response, 7, 20, 31
radiation field, 31
radiation-induced tumor cell killing, 22
radiation-induced tumor inflammation, 26
radiation killing, 16
radiation sensitivity, 31
radiation therapy, vi, 11, 14, 26–27
    carbon ions, 27
    linear energy transfer, vi
    X-ray irradiation, vi
radiation treatment, 10, 20, 22, 24, 30
radiation treatment plans, 25
radioprotective effect, 7, 9, 21
radioresistance, 2, 16, 22–25
radioresistant, 9, 27
radioresistant effect, 30
radiosensitive, 14
radiosensitivity, vi, 3, 6, 8–9, 16–19, 32–34
radiosensitivity parameters, 31–32
radiosensitization, 3, 19–20
radiosensitizers, vi, 17, 20, 22
radiosensitizing effect, 2–3, 20, 22
radiotherapy, 1, 13, 15–17, 20, 22
radiotracer, 24
rapamycin, 266

Rb, 128–129, 132–133, 140
RBE, 27–30
Rbx1, 54
reactive oxygen species (ROS), 231
regulatory T cells, 255, 261, 266
relative biological effectiveness
    (RBE), 26
reoxygenation, 14–17, 19, 34
repair–misrepair-fixation (RMF)
    model, 27
replication, 171
response to radiation, 16
RIDD, 230
RNA binding protein RBM4, 108
RORgt, 264–265
ROS, 134–135, 138, 256–257
Rosenzweig, 143
Roskelley, 141
Rossum, 140
rotation and movement of CTCs, 80
RSU-1069, 22

**S**
S100A4, 76
SAHF, 128–129, 131, 140
SASP, 129, 133, 135, 138, 145
    chemokines, 129
    cytokines, 129
    growth factors, 129
    proteases, 129
SBRT, 17, 21, 33–34
SDHD, 206
seed region, 197
senecence-associated b-gal, 129
senescence, 127–145
senescence-associated, 141
senescence-associated b-gal
    SA-$\beta$-gal signal, 130

senescence-associated
    heterochromatic foci
        SAHF, 128–130, 139
senescence-associated secretory
    phenotype, 129, 141
        SASP, 129, 134–135, 138
senescence-associated $\beta$-gal
    SA-$\beta$-gal, 129
sensitizer enhancement ratio (SER),
    19–21
Ser/Thr kinase, 230
shear forces, 79
    interstitial pressure, 80
shear stress, 80
side effects, 18, 23
signaling cascades, 227
signal transduction, vi
silencing, 178–179, 182
simvastatin, 59
single nucleotide polymorphisms
    (SNPs), 109
sinusoid, 104
SIRT1-7, 55
Slug, 77
small UB-like modifier (SUMO)-1, 56
Snai1, 83
S-nitrosylation, 51, 56–57
solid tumors, 69
spectroscopy, 140
sphere-forming capacity, 103
spleen colony-forming (CFU-S)
    assay, 104
STAT3, 264–265, 272
stem cell niche, 104
stereotactic ablative radiotherapy
    (SABR), 16
stereotactic body radiotherapy
    (SBRT), 16

stereotactic radiosurgery (SRS),
   21
stratify patients, 13
stress sensors, 227
stromal cell-derived factor-1 (SDF-1,
   CXCL12), 81
succinate, 111
succinyl dehydrogenase (SDH)
   subunits, 111
SUMOylation, 51, 56
surrounding normal, 17
survival curve
      clonogenic survival curve, 5,
         7–9, 19, 21
surviving fraction, 5–6, 16, 32
sympathetic nervous system
   development, 110
sympathoadrenal precursor cells,
   113
synergistic, 240

**T**
TAMs, 81
T-bet, 264, 272
TCP, 25, 33
TCPs, 34
TCR, 252, 264, 271
telomeric dysfunction, 132
      end replication problem, 133
      Okazaki fragments, 133
TERT, 139, 145
TGF-b, 268
TGFb, 264
TGF$\beta$, 254, 259, 261
Th1, 258–259, 262, 264–265, 270
Th2, 259, 262, 265
Th17, 264–266, 269, 277
thapsigargin, 237

therapeutic, 21
therapeutic target, 207
therapy resistance, vi
thermal, 275
thrombospondin-1, 85
TIE2, 85
tirapazamine, 14, 22–23, 30
tissue, 17
tissue inhibitors of metalloproteinases
   (TIMPs), 73
tissue microenvironment, 104
tissue stem cells, 102
TLR, 252, 258–259
TNF$\alpha$, 254, 259, 271
toll-like receptor, 208
transactivation domains, 50
transcriptional shift, 105
transfer RNA-Derived RNA
      Fragments (tRFs), 193
transforming growth factor beta
      (TGF-$\beta$), 75
Tregs, 264–265, 267–268, 270
triple-negative breast cancer (TNBC),
   234
tubulogenesis, 205
tumor(s), v, 1–2, 6, 9–11, 14–20,
   22–25, 27, 29–33
      Hypoxic cancer cells, 169
      hypoxic tumors, 169
      metastasis, v
      solid tumors, v, 169
tumor-associated macrophages
      (TAMs), 80
tumor-associated vessels, 105
tumor associate macrophages, 57
tumor cell death, 26, 34
      radiation-induced, 20
tumor cell immaturity, 103

tumor cells, v
  clonal, v
  clonal expansion, v
tumor-control probability (TCP), 24
tumor hypoxia, 1–2, 10–12, 17, 21,
  23–24, 26, 30, 33, 84, 209
  acute hypoxia, 1
  chronic hypoxia, 1
  hypoxia-selective drugs, 14
  hypoxic fractions, 11
  radioresistance, 11
tumorigenesis, 58, 200
tumorigenic, vii
tumorigenicity
  cancer stem cells, vii
tumor immunotherapy, viii
tumor-initiating capacity, 103
tumor microenvironment, v, viii,
  70–71, 73, 76–77, 81, 90, 191, 232
tumor necrosis factor-$\alpha$ (TNF-$\alpha$), 80
tumor progression, v, 170
tumor seeding, 80
tumor suppressor, 129, 134, 137–138,
  141–142, 145
tumor xenografts, 239
twist, 77
twist2, 83
twist-related protein 1, 76

**U**
ubiquitylation, 56
ultraconserved regions (UCRs), 195
unfolded protein response (UPR),
  viii, 225

**V**
Van Putten and Kallman, 14, 15
vascular endothelial growth factor
  (VEGF), 50, 75, 204, 254
vascular permeability, 84
VCB-Cul2 E3 ligase complex, 54
VEGF, 84–85, 90, 108, 260–262
  VEGF-A, 84
VEGF-A, 90, 234
VEGFR1, 84
vesicular transport, 229
VHL, 137–138, 144, 252, 270
von Hippel–Lindau
  pVHL ubiquitin (UB) E3 ligase
    complex, 52
von Hippel–Lindau (VHL), 52, 74,
  251

**W**
Warburg Effect, vii, 137, 151, 154
Wouters and Brown, 15

**X**
XBP1, 229
X-ray doses, 7–8

**Z**
zinc-finger E-box-binding homeobox
  1 and 2, 77
zinc-finger protein SNAIL1, 77